QUINTESSENCE
INTERNATIONAL

QUINTESSENCE
INTERNATIONAL

Editorial board articles' selection

Volume 1

Eli Eliav (ed)

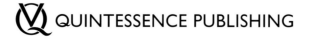

Berlin | Chicago | Tokyo
Barcelona | London | Milan | Mexico City | Paris | Prague | Seoul | Warsaw
Beijing | Istanbul | Sao Paulo | Zagreb

One book, one tree: In support of reforestation worldwide and to address the climate crisis, for every book sold Quintessence Publishing will plant a tree (https://onetreeplanted.org/).

A CIP record for this book is available from the British Library.
ISBN 978-1-78698-143-1

QUINTESSENCE PUBLISHING DEUTSCHLAND

Quintessenz Verlags-GmbH
Ifenpfad 2–4
12107 Berlin
Germany
www.quintessence-publishing.com

Quintessence Publishing Co Ltd
Grafton Road, New Malden
Surrey KT3 3AB
United Kingdom
www.quintessence-publishing.com

Editing, Layout, Production and Reproduction:
Quintessenz Verlags-GmbH, Berlin, Germany

Printed and bound in Croatia by Grafički zavod Hrvatske d.o.o.

::: PREFACE

This year marks a significant milestone, as Quintessence International is now offered exclusively as an online subscription. We are also delighted to introduce this first printed version of our annual yearbook, a compilation of selected articles from the past year.

Quintessence International caters to the global community of general dental practitioners, covering a wide array of topics and dentistry disciplines. Our team of editors, in collaboration with hundreds of reviewers from around the world, perform a remarkable job of reviewing and evaluating these submissions.

A key feature of our review process at Quintessence International is its anonymity. The double-blind process ensures that reviewers do not have access to information about the authors and are requested to assess the manuscripts solely based on their quality and content.

I have had the privilege of serving as the Editor in Chief of Quintessence International since 2008. It is both challenging and incredibly rewarding. Every month, we receive a significant number of manuscript submissions that demand careful review, assessment, and the selection of those suitable for publication.

Choosing manuscripts for publication from the multitude of outstanding submissions is a difficult task. Even more challenging was the selection of the 20 articles to be featured in the yearbook. To achieve this, we endeavored to represent the most significant work from the current year. Each of the Associate Editors selected articles from their respective disciplines and areas of interest, and we reached a collective decision on the final selection. We recognize that there are many other deserving manuscripts.

The articles in the yearbook are organized by disciplines and topics, with the aim of providing a valuable and user-friendly resource for our readers. We sincerely hope that you find it both enjoyable and informative. Looking ahead, we eagerly anticipate the manuscripts that will be submitted to Quintessence International in the coming year.

Thank you for your continued support and readership.

Eli Eliav
Editor in Chief

::: TABLE OF CONTENTS

GENERAL DENTISTRY AND RESTORATIVE DENTISTRY

Effectiveness of oral premedication of meloxicam, ketorolac, dexamethasone, and ibuprofen on the success rate of inferior alveolar nerve block in patients with symptomatic irreversible pulpitis: a prospective, double-blind, randomized controlled trial

Amr M. Elnaghy, BDS, MSc, PhD/Alaa H. Elshazli, BDS, MSc, PhD/Shaymaa E. Elsaka, BDS, MSc, PhD

Objective: The aim of this prospective, double-blind, randomized controlled trial was to compare the effect of oral premedication of meloxicam, ketorolac, dexamethasone, ibuprofen, or placebo on the success of inferior alveolar nerve blocks (IANB) of mandibular posterior teeth in patients experiencing symptomatic irreversible pulpitis. **Method and materials:** Two hundred and fifty emergency patients in moderate to severe pain diagnosed with symptomatic irreversible pulpitis of a mandibular first or second molar randomly received, in a double-blind manner, identical capsules containing either meloxicam 7.5 mg, ketorolac 10 mg, dexamethasone 0.5 mg, ibuprofen 600 mg, or placebo 60 minutes before the administration of an IANB. Profound lip numbness was assessed after 15 minutes. Access cavities were then prepared and success of IANB was defined as no or mild pain (Heft-Parker visual analog scale recordings) during access preparation and root canal instrumentation. The data were analyzed using chi-square and Kruskal-Wallis tests. **Results:** The overall success rates for the meloxicam 7.5 mg, ketorolac 10 mg, dexamethasone 0.5 mg, and ibuprofen 600 mg groups were 52%, 64%, 54%, and 58%, respectively, with no significant differences in success rates among the premedications groups ($P > .05$). However, the tested premedications revealed significant differences compared with the placebo group (32% success rate) ($P < .05$). **Conclusion:** Premedication with meloxicam, ketorolac, dexamethasone, and ibuprofen increased the efficacy of IANB in mandibular molars with symptomatic irreversible pulpitis. (Quintessence Int 2023;54:92–99; doi: 10.3290/j.qi.b3605097)

Key words: anesthesia, dexamethasone, inferior alveolar nerve block, ketorolac, meloxicam, symptomatic irreversible pulpitis

The inferior alveolar nerve block (IANB) is utilized to achieve pulpal anesthesia of mandibular teeth for endodontic treatments.[1] Pain management and achieving anesthesia are more challenging in mandibular molar teeth with symptomatic irreversible pulpitis.[2,3] It has been reported that the failure rate for IANB in patients with symptomatic irreversible pulpitis was between 43% and 83% because of inflammatory changes in the pulp.[1,4] Buccal infiltration,[5] intraosseous anesthesia,[6] and oral premedication[2] have been used to enhance the success of anesthesia for mandibular teeth.

Various pharmacologic agents such as nonsteroidal anti-inflammatory drugs (NSAIDs) and steroids have been investigated as oral premedications to improve the success of anesthesia in randomized controlled trials.[2,7,8] However, there are contradictory results about the effectiveness of oral premedications before administrating an IANB.[8] It was reported that considerable enhancements in the success rate of IANBs in mandibular molars with inflamed pulps after premedication with ibuprofen and indomethacin.[9] There was an improvement in the success rates in IANB anesthesia of mandibular molars with inflamed pulps after premedication with ibuprofen and acetaminophen while there was no considerable difference between the medicament and placebo groups.[10] On the other hand, there were no significant differences in the success rates of IANB anesthesia of mandibular molars with inflamed pulps where the patients were premedicated with analgesics.[11,12]

Meloxicam is an NSAID with preferential activity on the cyclooxygenase 2 (COX-2) system.[13] Shantiaee et al[3] reported that premedication with meloxicam and ibuprofen significantly improved the success rates of IANB anesthesia for mandibular molars with irreversible pulpitis; however, neither drug provided profound anesthesia. Dexamethasone, a glucocorticoid with an anti-inflammatory effect, increased the efficiency of IANB compared to ibuprofen.[8] Dexamethasone influences the acute inflammatory reaction by suppressing vasodilation, inhibiting the migration and phagocytosis of polymorphonuclear leucocytes, and preventing the production of prostaglandins and leukotrienes by blocking COX and lipoxygenase routes of inflammation.[1,8]

Ketorolac was developed as an intramuscular NSAID with potent prostaglandin synthesis inhibition efficacy. Ketorolac is a pyrrolo-pyrrole derivative and is as effective as morphine or meperidine for pain relief after orthopedic or disc surgery.[14-16] It was reported that the administration of ibuprofen or ketorolac has no significant effect on the success rate of IANB in patients with irreversible pulpitis.[12] On the other hand, in another clinical trial, it was shown that ketorolac revealed a higher success rate of 70% while ibuprofen gave 50%.[17]

Previous studies showed that the use of oral premedication with NSAIDs enhanced the success rate of IANB in patients with irreversible pulpitis.[18-21] However, more trials are required to compare dexamethasone and other oral premedications to validate their relative efficacy[1] in the treatment of symptomatic irreversible pulpitis. Accordingly, the purpose of this prospective, randomized, double-blind study was to compare the efficacy of oral premedication of dexamethasone, meloxicam, ketorolac, ibuprofen, or placebo on anesthetic efficacy of IANB of mandibular posterior teeth in patients with symptomatic irreversible pulpitis.

Method and materials

The clinical trial protocol and informed consent were approved by the Vision Medical College Research Ethics Committee (approval number 21-8/1). The protocol was registered at clinicaltrials.gov under the code NCT05097768. The sample size was determined using the superiority trial mode of the sealed envelope calculator (www.sealedenvelope.com) based on the data from a previous study,[8] with percentages of success in control and experimental groups 12.7% and 38.2%, respectively. The sample size was determined with a type I error of 5% and statistical power of 80%. The required sample size was 42 participants per group; however, the number was increased to 50 participants with a total sample size of 250 patients being de-

termined (allocation ratio of 1:1). A postgraduate dentistry student who was not involved in the trial screened 290 adult patients for participation in the study (Fig 1). They were emergency patients at the Faculty of Dentistry, Vision Colleges, Jeddah, Saudi Arabia, and were in good health based on their medical histories and oral questioning. The differential diagnostic criteria for symptomatic irreversible pulpitis were followed according to the American Association of Endodontists.[22] Patient exclusion criteria included those with a known allergy, sensitivity, or contraindications to an opioid or nonopioid analgesic including aspirin or NSAIDs, those with a history of the active peptic ulcer within the preceding 12 months, a history of bleeding problems or anticoagulant use within the last month, patients who were pregnant or breast-feeding, a history of known or suspected drug abuse, and those who had taken NSAIDs with 12 hours before administration of the study drugs.[12] The approved consent form was signed by all the patients.

The inclusion criteria included healthy patients experiencing pain in the first or second mandibular molar with prolonged response to cold testing (Endo-frost, Roeko), teeth with a vital pulp, and the absence of periapical radiolucency on radiographs.[2] The Modified Dental Anxiety Scale[23] was used to assess the patients' anxiety levels. The pain of the patients was classified into four types using the Heft-Parker visual analog scale (HP VAS)[12,24] as follows: no pain corresponded to 0 mm; faint, weak, or mild pain corresponded to 0 to 54 mm; moderate pain corresponded to 55 to 114 mm; and strong, intense, and maximum possible pain corresponded to more than 114 mm.

Randomization of patients was performed by using permuted block randomization (www.sealedenvelope.com) to ensure the consistency of the five groups. The patients were randomly given meloxicam 7.5 mg, ketorolac 10 mg, dexamethasone 0.5 mg, ibuprofen 600 mg, or placebo by mouth 60 minutes before administering IANB.[1] To blind the study, each of the 50 patients in each group was randomly allocated a code consisting of two letters and one number. Only the random codes identified the medications; thus, the patient and clinicians were uninformed of which medication was given to them.[25,26] The medication and placebo were blinded as follows: in opaque yellow size "000" capsules, a certified pharmacist prepared identical-appearing capsules of the medications and placebo in identical separate containers for each medication.[25] After 1 hour of oral administration of the capsules or placebo, all patients received standard IANB injections and 0.9 mL long buccal injections containing 2% lidocaine and 1:100,000 epinephrine (Xylocaine, Astra Zeneca). The solution was injected by the same clinician (first author) by using self-aspirating sy-

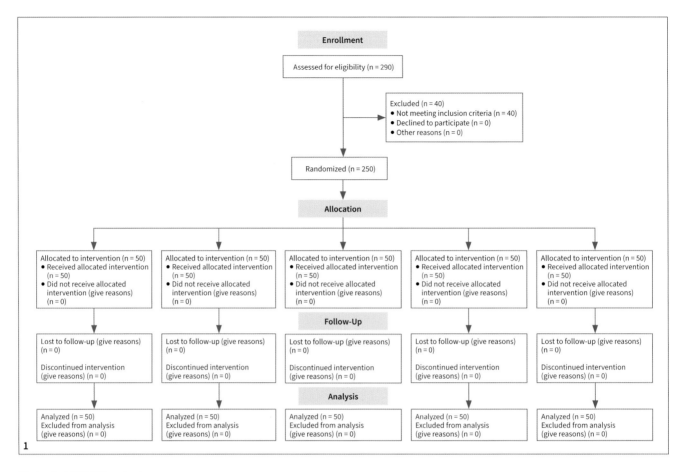

Fig 1 CONSORT flowchart.

ringes (Septodont) and 27-G long needles to inject the anesthetic solution (Septoject, Septodont).[7] Every 5 minutes for 15 minutes, each patient was asked for lip numbness after the IANB.[27] If profound lip numbness was not recorded within 15 minutes, the block was considered unsuccessful, and the patients were excluded from the study.[25,28] After the lip numbness was determined, the tooth was isolated and a second cold test was performed to verify the presence or absence of any painful reaction.[29]

Then, the endodontic access cavity was begun. If the patient felt pain during access, the treatment was stopped, and the patient used the HP VAS to rate his/her discomfort. The success of the IANB is identified by the capability to access and clean and shape the root canal space without pain (VAS score of 0) or mild pain (VAS rating ≤ 54 mm).[25,27] Rubber dam was removed if the patient had moderate or severe pain (VAS rating ≥ 55 mm).[25] Next, a buccal infiltration of a cartridge containing 4% articaine with 1:100,000 epinephrine (Septocaine, Septodont) was given

buccally to the tooth.[25] After 5 minutes, rubber dam was replaced, and endodontic access was resumed. Once access was gained, the glide path was created up to K-file ISO size 15 (Dentsply Sirona). The working length (WL) was performed up to the apical foramen as determined with a Root ZX II apex locator (J Morita). Then, the file was withdrawn, and 0.5 mm subtracted from the length. The WL was verified radiographically. Rotary file systems were utilized to prepare the root canals. The instrumentation sequence followed the manufacturer's instructions.[11] The capability to access and instrument the tooth without pain (VAS score of 0) or with mild pain (VAS rating ≤ 54 mm) was considered a success of the buccal infiltration.[25] Intraosseous anesthesia (Stabident intraosseous anesthetic system, Fairfax Dental) was given to patients who still had moderate to severe pain.[25] If that did not work, an intrapulpal injection was given, followed by endodontic debridement.[25] The extent of access preparation and/or instrumentation was recorded as within dentin, within pulp space, and instrumentation of canals.[12]

Table 1 Baseline demographics of distribution of patients among the groups

Variable		Meloxicam 7.5 mg	Ketorolac 10 mg	Dexamethasone 0.5 mg	Ibuprofen 600 mg	Placebo	P value*
Age, y (mean ± SD)		33 ± 10	32 ± 10	31 ± 10	34 ± 11	32 ± 10	.647
Sex (n)	Female	26	28	23	24	30	.622
	Male	24	22	27	26	20	
Initial pain (mean ± SD)		125 ± 18.4	118 ± 17.8	121 ± 17.3	124 ± 17.7	123 ± 19.2	.545
Modified Dental Anxiety Scale (median)		10	11	10	11	11	.201
Tooth type, (n) %	First molar	(34/50) 68%	(36/50) 72%	(32/50) 64%	(30/50) 60%	(37/50) 74%	.559
	Second molar	(16/50) 32%	(14/50) 28%	(18/50) 36%	(20/50) 40%	(13/50) 26%	

*Statistically significant at P < .05.

Statistical analysis

A chi-square test was used to compare different groups for anesthetic success, sex, and tooth type (SPSS 22.0 software, IBM). The normality of data was evaluated by the Shapiro–Wilk test. The Kruskal–Wallis test was used to analyze the Modified Dental Anxiety Scale, age, and initial pain ratings. The level of statistical significance was set at $P < .05$.

Results

The current clinical trial began in August 2021 and ended in January 2022, when the final sample size was reached. The baseline demographic data and clinical features were presented in Table 1. The flow of patients during each phase of the trial was reported according to the Consolidated Standards of Reporting Trials (Fig 1). There were no significant differences between the groups regarding age, sex, initial pain, initial Modified Dental Anxiety ratings, or tooth type ($P > .05$) (Table 1). The overall success rates for the meloxicam 7.5 mg, ketorolac 10 mg, dexamethasone 0.5 mg, and ibuprofen 600 mg groups were 52% (26/50), 64% (32/50), 54% (27/50), and 58% (29/50), respectively, with no significant differences in success rates among the premedications groups ($P > .05$) (Table 2). However, the tested premedications revealed significant differences compared with the placebo group (32% success rate; 16/50) ($P < .05$). Articaine buccal infiltration success was 38% for the meloxicam 7.5 mg, 33% for the ketorolac 10 mg, 43% for the dexamethasone 0.5 mg, 38% for the ibuprofen 600 mg, and 44% for the placebo groups. Intraosseous success rates for the meloxicam 7.5 mg, ketorolac 10 mg, dexamethasone 0.5 mg, ibuprofen 600 mg, and placebo groups

were 93%, 83%, 92%, 85%, and 89%, respectively. The pain and discomfort ratings of patients with unsuccessful anesthesia (Heft-Parker VAS score > 54) in relation to the extent of access preparation and/or instrumentation are presented in Table 3. In all groups, the patients reported initial moderate to severe pain. The IANB provided subjective lip anesthesia to all the patients involved in the data analysis. None of the patients were excluded because of a lack of lip numbness and pain during the cold test.

Discussion

The current trial compared the efficacy of preoperative oral dexamethasone, ketorolac, meloxicam, and ibuprofen drugs on the success of IANB in patients with symptomatic irreversible pulpitis. For enhancing the success of IANB in patients with symptomatic irreversible pulpitis; preoperative oral medication was administrated as it is a proper and effective method.[30] The present trial was a double-blind study, which reduces bias and allows for adequate comparison by having a homogenous distribution between groups based on sex, age, tooth type, and preoperative pain score.[30] There were no statistically significant differences in the influence of sex, age, initial pain, initial Modified Dental Anxiety ratings, and tooth type; consequently, these variables were decreased between the groups.[27] The mean initial pain ratings for the various groups ranged from 118 to 125 mm on the VAS, indicating severe pain. In the current trial, the Modified Dental Anxiety ratings averaged 10 and 11 as the study evaluated emergency patients in pain, revealing moderate anxiety.[25] Fullmer et al,[25] Simpson et al,[28] and Lindemann et al[26] reported that the anxiety rating in patients experi-

Table 2 Anesthetic success, n (%)

Anesthetic	Meloxicam 7.5 mg	Ketorolac 10 mg	Dexametha-sone 0.5 mg	Ibuprofen 600 mg	Placebo	P value
Inferior alveolar nerve block	26/50 (52%)	32/50 (64%)	27/50 (54%)	29/50 (58%)	16/50 (32%)	.02
Articaine buccal infiltration	9/24 (40%)	6/18 (30%)	10/23 (43%)	8/21 (38%)	15/34 (44%)	.97
Intraosseous anesthesia	14/15 (93%)	10/12 (83%)	12/13 (92%)	11/13 (85%)	17/19 (89%)	.89

*Statistically significant at P<.05

Table 3 Comparison of the number of unsuccessful anesthesia between different groups

Extent of access preparation and/or instrumentation	Group	Heft-Parker VAS score 54–114	Heft-Parker VAS score > 114
Within dentin	Meloxicam 7.5 mg	8 of 24	4 of 24
	Ketorolac 10 mg	6 of 18	2 of 18
	Dexamethasone 0.5 mg	9 of 23	3 of 23
	Ibuprofen 600 mg	5 of 21	3 of 21
	Placebo	16 of 34	6 of 34
Within pulpal space	Meloxicam 7.5 mg	2 of 24	5 of 24
	Ketorolac 10 mg	3 of 18	3 of 18
	Dexamethasone 0.5 mg	6 of 23	1 of 23
	Ibuprofen 600 mg	6 of 21	2 of 21
	Placebo	7 of 34	1 of 34
Instrumentation of canals	Meloxicam 7.5 mg	3 of 24	2 of 24
	Ketorolac 10 mg	3 of 18	1 of 18
	Dexamethasone 0.5 mg	3 of 23	1 of 23
	Ibuprofen 600 mg	4 of 21	1 of 21
	Placebo	3 of 34	1 of 34

encing symptomatic irreversible pulpitis averaged 10 and 11, which would indicate moderate anxiety. As the present study evaluated emergency patients in pain, the occurrence of moderate anxiety was expected.[25,26,28]

In the present study, 100% of the patients showed lip numbness. Lip numbness, at least in inflamed pulp, may not be a reliable sign of pulpal anesthesia.[7] Accordingly, a second cold pulp test was performed to evaluate whether or not there was any pain response.[29] The success rate was 32% with the IANB using a placebo. It has been reported that the success rate using a placebo ranged from 24% to 35%.[25] This finding could be due to differences in patient demographics.[25]

The breakdown of the damaged cell membrane in inflamed pulp triggers the release of arachidonic acid which acts on cy-clooxygenase or prostaglandin H synthase enzymes and produces prostaglandins.[31,32] Medications that inhibit prostaglandins tend to increase the effect of local anesthesia in patients with irreversible pulpitis.[18,32] The results revealed that the success rate of IANB was greater in patients premedicated with ketorolac (64%) and ibuprofen (58%) when compared with the other groups; however, there was no significant difference. Ketorolac and ibuprofen are NSAIDs that have been shown to provide significantly improved pain control over placebo.[2,14,15] Ketorolac, a pyrrolo-pyrrole derivative, is as effective as morphine or meperidine for pain relief.[2,14,15] Ketorolac inhibits the enzyme cyclooxygenase, thus lowering inflammation and pain.[2,33] Oral ketorolac is entirely absorbed, with a mean peak plasma concentration taking place at an average of 44 minutes after a single 10 mg dose.[34] In the current trial, oral premedication was given 1 hour before the procedure to allow ketorolac to attain an adequate plasma concentration.[2] Saha et al[22] reported the efficacy of preoperative ketorolac 10 mg in achieving IANB success in patients with irreversible pulpitis compared with the placebo group. On the other hand, Aggarwal et al[12] reported that the preoperative administration of ketorolac has no significant effect on the success rate of IANB in patients with irreversible pulpitis.

Premedication with ibuprofen, which inhibits prostaglandin production, can enhance the efficiency of IANB.[35] Ibuprofen is a nonselective drug that inhibits the cyclooxygenase enzyme that inhibits both COX1 and COX2 isoform.[3] It has been reported in previous studies that premedication with ibuprofen enhanced the success rate of IANB,[9,29] in agreement with the present study. Bidar et al,[32] Parirokh et al,[9] and Shantiaee et al[3] reported superior efficacy of premedication ibuprofen compared with placebo in achieving IANB success in mandibular molars with irreversible pulpitis. In these studies, ibuprofen was effective at lower dosages (400 mg and 600 mg) compared with the dosage of the current study (800 mg). On the other hand, Kumar et al[36] reported that there were no significant differences between placebo and ibuprofen 800 mg groups. The differences in results might be attributed to the different inclusion criteria of patients in these studies.[36]

Glucocorticoids are another class of drugs that are known to reduce the acute inflammatory response by suppressing vasodilation, the migration of polymorphonuclear leucocytes, and phagocytosis and by inhibiting the formation of arachidonic acid, consequently blocking the COX pathways and the respective synthesis of prostaglandins and leukotrienes.[8,32,37] Dexamethasone is a potent glucocorticoid with anti-inflammatory efficacy 25 times that of hydrocortisone.[12] It was reported that dexamethasone reduces or prevents postoperative endodontic pain.[38,39] In the present study, premedication with dexamethasone enhanced the anesthetic success rate of IANB to 54% compared with the placebo (32%). Shahi et al[8] reported that dexamethasone enhanced the success of IANB compared with placebo or ibuprofen; however, the study was performed in teeth with asymptomatic irreversible pulpitis. Kumar et al[36] reported that a combination of preoperative ibuprofen 800 mg and dexamethasone 0.5 mg can enhance the success rate of IANB in patients with symptomatic irreversible pulpitis.

Meloxicam is an NSAID that it is a moderately selective COX2 inhibitor and has a less disturbing influence on the gastrointestinal system compared with other NSAIDs.[3] Even though a higher probability of myocardial infarction and stroke correlated with the use of selective COX2 inhibitors, such as rofecoxib and celecoxib, has been reported, meloxicam is safer for the cardiovascular system.[3,40,41] In the present study, premedication with meloxicam enhanced the anesthetic success rate of IANB to 52% compared with the placebo (32%). Shantiaee et al[3] showed that premedication with meloxicam significantly enhanced the success rates of IANB for teeth with irreversible pulpitis.

Most unsuccessful patients had pain during dentin penetration, preventing pulpal chamber penetration, and they were given intraosseous injections for pain control.[12,25] The IANB was shown to have a 32% to 71% incidence of moderate to severe pain upon access to dentin in patients with symptomatic irreversible pulpitis.[12,25]

The IANB was not the only anesthetic method that did not seem to benefit from premedication administration. Articaine buccal infiltration success ranged between 33% and 44%. Simpson et al[28] showed the range of articaine infiltration success rate of 38% for the acetaminophen/ibuprofen group. Matthews et al,[42] Oleson et al,[11] Simpson et al,[28] and the current study showed that only modest success rates can be anticipated when a supplemental buccal infiltration of articaine is added to the IANB in patients with symptomatic irreversible pulpitis. The intraosseous success rates were similar to the previously mentioned success rates of 83% to 93%.[11,28,42] Even though intraosseous anesthesia had the highest success rate of the three techniques, it was not entirely successful; some patients still needed intrapulpal injections.[25] This finding is in agreement with Fullmer et al.[25]

The findings of the current trial may not apply to the elderly or children as the patients' average ages were 31 to 35 years.[25] Future clinical trials should take into consideration broader age groups and different dosages or combinations of drugs to explain the capability of these premedications in the anesthetic success of IANB in cases of mandibular posterior teeth in patients with symptomatic irreversible pulpitis.

Conclusion

Within the limitations of the present study, it could be concluded that premedication with meloxicam, ketorolac, dexamethasone, and ibuprofen increased the success rate of IANB in mandibular molars with symptomatic irreversible pulpitis.

Disclosure

The authors deny any conflict of interests related to this study.

References

1.   Pulikkotil SJ, Nagendrababu V, Veettil SK, Jinatongthai P, Setzer FC. Effect of oral premedication on the anaesthetic efficacy of inferior alveolar nerve block in patients with irreversible pulpitis: A systematic review and network meta-analysis of randomized controlled trials. Int Endod J 2018;51:989–1004.

2.   Yadav M, Grewal MS, Grewal S, Deshwal P. Comparison of preoperative oral ketorolac on anesthetic efficacy of inferior alveolar nerve block and buccal and lingual infiltration with articaine and lidocaine in patients with irreversible pulpitis: A prospective, randomized, controlled, double-blind study. J Endod 2015;41:1773–1777.

3.   Shantiaee Y, Javaheri S, Movahhedian A, Eslami S, Dianat O. Efficacy of preoperative ibuprofen and meloxicam on the success rate of inferior alveolar nerve block for teeth with irreversible pulpitis. Int Dent J 2017;67:85–90.

4.   Fowler S, Drum M, Reader A, Beck M. Anesthetic success of an inferior alveolar nerve block and supplemental articaine buccal infiltration for molars and premolars in patients with symptomatic irreversible pulpitis. J Endod 2016;42:390–392.

5.   Aggarwal V, Jain A, Kabi D. Anesthetic efficacy of supplemental buccal and lingual infiltrations of articaine and lidocaine after an inferior alveolar nerve block in patients with irreversible pulpitis. J Endod 2009;35:925–929.

6.   Nusstein J, Kennedy S, Reader A, Beck M, Weaver J. Anesthetic efficacy of the supplemental X-tip intraosseous injection in patients with irreversible pulpitis. J Endod 2003;29: 724–728.

7.   Prasanna N, Subbarao CV, Gutmann JL. The efficacy of pre-operative oral medication of lornoxicam and diclofenac potassium on the success of inferior alveolar nerve block in patients with irreversible pulpitis: a double-blind, randomised controlled clinical trial. Int Endod J 2011;44:330–336.

8.   Shahi S, Mokhtari H, Rahimi S, et al. Effect of premedication with ibuprofen and dexamethasone on success rate of inferior alveolar nerve block for teeth with asymptomatic irreversible pulpitis: a randomized clinical trial. J Endod 2013;39:160–162.

9.   Parirokh M, Ashouri R, Rekabi AR, et al. The effect of premedication with ibuprofen and indomethacin on the success of inferior alveolar nerve block for teeth with irreversible pulpitis. J Endod 2010;36:1450–1454.

10.   Ianiro SR, Jeansonne BG, McNeal SF, Eleazer PD. The effect of preoperative acetaminophen or a combination of acetaminophen and Ibuprofen on the success of inferior alveolar nerve block for teeth with irreversible pulpitis. J Endod 2007;33:11–14.

11.   Oleson M, Drum M, Reader A, Nusstein J, Beck M. Effect of preoperative ibuprofen on the success of the inferior alveolar nerve block in patients with irreversible pulpitis. J Endod 2010;36:379–382.

12.   Aggarwal V, Singla M, Kabi D. Comparative evaluation of effect of preoperative oral medication of ibuprofen and ketorolac on anesthetic efficacy of inferior alveolar nerve block with lidocaine in patients with irreversible pulpitis: a prospective, double-blind, randomized clinical trial. J Endod 2010;36:375–378.

13.   Thompson JP, Sharpe P, Kiani S, Owen-Smith O. Effect of meloxicam on postoperative pain after abdominal hysterectomy. Br J Anaesth 2000;84:151–154.

14.   McQuay HJ, Poppleton P, Carroll D, Summerfield RJ, Bullingham RE, Moore RA. Ketorolac and acetaminophen for orthopedic postoperative pain. Clin Pharmacol Ther 1986;39:89–93.

15.   Fletcher D, Negre I, Barbin C, et al. Postoperative analgesia with i.v. propacetamol and ketoprofen combination after disc surgery. Can J Anaesth 1997;44:479–485.

16.   Aggarwal V, Singla M, Rizvi A, Miglani S. Comparative evaluation of local infiltration of articaine, articaine plus ketorolac, and dexamethasone on anesthetic efficacy of inferior alveolar nerve block with lidocaine in patients with irreversible pulpitis. J Endod 2011;37:445–449.

17.   Jena A, Shashirekha G. Effect of preoperative medications on the efficacy of inferior alveolar nerve block in patients with irreversible pulpitis: A placebo-controlled clinical study. J Conserv Dent 2013;16:171–174.

18.   Lapidus D, Goldberg J, Hobbs EH, Ram S, Clark GT, Enciso R. Effect of premedication to provide analgesia as a supplement to inferior alveolar nerve block in patients with irreversible pulpitis. J Am Dent Assoc 2016;147:427–437.

19.   Li C, Yang X, Ma X, Li L, Shi Z. Preoperative oral nonsteroidal anti-inflammatory drugs for the success of the inferior alveolar nerve block in irreversible pulpitis treatment: a systematic review and meta-analysis based on randomized controlled trials. Quintessence Int 2012;43:209–219.

20.   Corbella S, Taschieri S, Mannocci F, Rosen E, Tsesis I, Del Fabbro M. Inferior alveolar nerve block for the treatment of teeth presenting with irreversible pulpitis: A systematic review of the literature and meta-analysis. Quintessence Int 2017;48:69–82.

21.   Shirvani A, Shamszadeh S, Eghbal MJ, Marvasti LA, Asgary S. Effect of preoperative oral analgesics on pulpal anesthesia in patients with irreversible pulpitis: a systematic review and meta-analysis. Clin Oral Investig 2017;21:43–52.

22.   Saha SG, Jain S, Dubey S, Kala S, Misuriya A, Kataria D. Effect of oral premedication on the efficacy of inferior alveolar nerve block in patients with symptomatic irreversible pulpitis: a prospective, double-blind, randomized controlled clinical trial. J Clin Diagn Res 2016;10:ZC25–ZC29.

23.   Humphris GM, Morrison T, Lindsay SJ. The Modified Dental Anxiety Scale: validation and United Kingdom norms. Community Dent Health 1995;12:143–150.

24.   Heft MW, Parker SR. An experimental basis for revising the graphic rating scale for pain. Pain 1984;19:153–161.

25.   Fullmer S, Drum M, Reader A, Nusstein J, Beck M. Effect of preoperative acetaminophen/hydrocodone on the efficacy of the inferior alveolar nerve block in patients with symptomatic irreversible pulpitis: a prospective, randomized, double-blind, placebo-controlled study. J Endod 2014;40:1–5.

26.   Lindemann M, Reader A, Nusstein J, Drum M, Beck M. Effect of sublingual triazolam on the success of inferior alveolar nerve block in patients with irreversible pulpitis. J Endod 2008;34:1167–1170.

27.   Stanley W, Drum M, Nusstein J, Reader A, Beck M. Effect of nitrous oxide on the efficacy of the inferior alveolar nerve block in patients with symptomatic irreversible pulpitis. J Endod 2012;38:565–569.

28.   Simpson M, Drum M, Nusstein J, Reader A, Beck M. Effect of combination of preoperative ibuprofen/acetaminophen on the success of the inferior alveolar nerve block in patients with symptomatic irreversible pulpitis. J Endod 2011;37:593–597.

29.   Noguera-Gonzalez D, Cerda-Cristerna BI, Chavarria-Bolanos D, Flores-Reyes H, Pozos-Guillen A. Efficacy of preoperative ibuprofen on the success of inferior alveolar nerve block in patients with symptomatic irreversible pulpitis: a randomized clinical trial. Int Endod J 2013;46:1056–1062.

30.   Suresh N, Nagendrababu V, Koteeswaran V, et al. Effect of preoperative oral administration of steroids in comparison to an anti-inflammatory drug on postoperative pain following single-visit root canal treatment: a double-blind, randomized clinical trial. Int Endod J 2021;54:198–209.

31.   Pilbeam CC, Fall PM, Alander CB, Raisz LG. Differential effects of nonsteroidal anti-inflammatory drugs on constitutive and inducible prostaglandin G/H synthase in cultured bone cells. J Bone Miner Res 1997;12:1198–1203.

32.   Bidar M, Mortazavi S, Forghani M, Akhlaghi S. Comparison of effect of oral premedication with ibuprofen or dexamethasone on anesthetic efficacy of inferior alveolar nerve block in patients with irreversible pulpitis: a prospective, randomized, controlled, double-blind study. Bull Tokyo Dent Coll 2017;58:231–236.

33.   Mishra H, Khan FA. A double-blind, placebo-controlled randomized comparison of pre and postoperative administration of ketorolac and tramadol for dental extraction pain. J Anaesthesiol Clin Pharmacol 2012; 28:221–225.

34.   Johansson S, Josefsson G, Malstam J, Lindstrand A, Stenstroem A. Analgesic efficacy and safety comparison of ketorolac tromethamine and Doleron for the alleviation of orthopaedic post-operative pain. J Int Med Res 1989;17:324–332.

35.   Mahajan P, Singh G, Kaur R, Monga P, Bhandari S. A comparative clinical study to evaluate the effect of premedication with ibuprofen, tramadol and combination of ibuprofen and acetaminophen on success of inferior alveolar nerve block in patients with asymptomatic irreversible pulpitis. Bangladesh J Med Sci 2017;16:370–374.

36.   Kumar M, Singla R, Gill GS, Kalra T, Jain N. Evaluating combined effect of oral premedication with ibuprofen and dexamethasone on success of inferior alveolar nerve block in mandibular molars with symptomatic irreversible pulpitis: a prospective, double-blind, randomized clinical trial. J Endod 2021;47:705–710.

37.   Remmers T, Glickman G, Spears R, He J. The efficacy of intraFlow intraosseous injection as a primary anesthesia technique. J Endod 2008;34:280–283.

38.   Mehrvarzfar P, Esnashari E, Salmanzadeh R, Fazlyab M, Fazlyab M. Effect of dexamethasone intraligamentary injection on post-endodontic pain in patients with symptomatic irreversible pulpitis: a randomized controlled clinical trial. Iran Endod J 2016; 11: 261–266.

39.   Pochapski MT, Santos FA, de Andrade ED, Sydney GB. Effect of pretreatment dexamethasone on postendodontic pain. Oral Surg Oral Med Oral Pathol Oral Radiol Endod 2009;108:790–795.

40.   Zarif Najafi H, Oshagh M, Salehi P, Babanouri N, Torkan S. Comparison of the effects of preemptive acetaminophen, ibuprofen, and meloxicam on pain after separator placement: a randomized clinical trial. Prog Orthod 2015;16:34.

41.   Asghar W, Jamali F. The effect of COX-2-selective meloxicam on the myocardial, vascular and renal risks: a systematic review. Inflammopharmacology 2015;23:1–16.

42.   Matthews R, Drum M, Reader A, Nusstein J, Beck M. Articaine for supplemental buccal mandibular infiltration anesthesia in patients with irreversible pulpitis when the inferior alveolar nerve block fails. J Endod 2009;35:343–346.

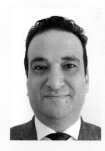

Amr M. Elnaghy

Amr M. Elnaghy   Professor, Department of Endodontics, Faculty of Dentistry, Mansoura University, Mansoura, Egypt

Shaymaa E. Elsaka   Professor, Department of Dental Biomaterials, Faculty of Dentistry, Mansoura University, Mansoura, Egypt; and Professor, Department of Restorative Dental Sciences, Vision Medical College, Jeddah, Saudi Arabia

Alaa H. Elshazli   Assistant Professor, Department of Endodontics, Faculty of Dentistry, Mansoura University, Mansoura, Egypt

Correspondence: Professor, Dr Amr M. Elnaghy, Department of Endodontics, Faculty of Dentistry, Mansoura University, Mansoura PC 35516, Egypt. Email: aelnaghy@mans.edu.eg

First submission: 26 Apr 2022
Acceptance: 24 Sep 2022
Online publication: 24 Nov 2022

Effectiveness of oral hygiene educational interventional programs on participants with Parkinson disease: a randomized controlled study

Stella Spurthi, MDS/Srirangarajan Sridharan, MDS/Rajesh Hosadurga, PhD/Ravi J. Rao, MDS/Srikumar Prabhu, MDS/
Pramod Kumar Pal, DM, DNB/Nitish Kamble, DM/Kempaiah Rakesh, DM/Amit Kumar, MDS

Objective: The objective was to evaluate oral health-related knowledge, and to compare the effectiveness of three different oral health education interventions (OHEI) on plaque removal in a cohort with Parkinson disease. **Method and materials:** The three-arm, parallel-group, randomized controlled trial included 63 Parkinson disease stage 1 and 2 patients aged ≥40 years and scores ≥26 in both Montreal Cognitive Assessment test and Mini-Mental State Exam. These patients were allocated to three OHEI groups: lectures, presentation, and demonstration. The validated questionnaire assessed knowledge level at baseline (0), 1, 2, and 3 months. Oral hygiene at 0 and 3 months was assessed by the Plaque Index and the Patient Hygiene Performance Index (PHPI). Unstimulated whole saliva was collected to assess the salivary flow rate. **Results:** Pairwise comparison using ANOVA showed a significant decrease in mean percentage knowledge 0, 1, 2, and 3 months in all three groups ($P<.001$). After Tukey post-hoc analysis the presentation group had significantly higher knowledge ($P=.030$). ANOVA showed that the percentage of knowledge decreased as time passed ($P=.001$). Comparison of means of Plaque Index and PHPI scores by MANOVA followed by Tukey post-hoc analysis showed significant decrease in Plaque Index scores from 0 to 3 months ($P=.001$). No significant change in the salivary flow rate was noted. **Conclusion:** Pictorial representation of OHEI is a better mode of intervention compared to lectures and demonstrations in Parkinson disease stage 1 and 2 patients. Despite the decline in knowledge with time, Plaque Index scores reduced significantly, implying that this form OHEI offers positive benefits. (*Quintessence Int 2023;54:428–437; doi: 10.3290/j.qi.b3840763*)

Key words: cohort, intervention, knowledge, oral hygiene, Parkinson disease, salivary rate

Parkinson disease (PD), the second most common neurodegenerative disease after Alzheimer disease, is a complex neurologic disorder characterized by the classic motor features of parkinsonism associated with Lewy bodies and loss of dopaminergic neurons in the substantia nigra.[1] The current belief is that the symptomatology of PD is clinically heterogenous with significant nonmotor features.[1] The motor symptoms of PD include bradykinesia, resting tremor, stiffness, postural instability, and difficulty in walking.[1] The cause of PD remains unknown and is thought to be resulting from a complex interplay of genetic and environmental factors affecting numerous cellular processes.[1] Nonmotor symptoms experienced by the elderly suffering from PD include sleep disorders, pain, cognitive symptoms, neuropsychiatric dysfunctions, and gastrointestinal symptoms.[2] A strong diurnal oscillation is seen in both motor and nonmotor symptoms, which may be related to dopamine levels.[3] Poor sleepers with PD seem to have more problems like low mood, apathy, impaired cognition, cognitive decline, and amnesia.[4] The global prevalence increases with age, and it is about 1% in those above 60 years.[5] Prevalence is increasing rapidly in many Asian countries at an alarming level, and it is 1.5 times more common in males than females.[6] Males have significantly greater executive and processing speed impairments.[6]

A multitude of oral health problems like dental caries, periodontitis, sialorrhea, xerostomia, impairment of taste, chewing alterations, jaw opening, bruxism, dysphagia, burning mouth syndrome, orofacial pain, and denture retention problems are frequently seen.[7] Drooling is another distressing and debilitating complication leading to social isolation, depression, skin infection, and aspiration pneumonia.[8] Oral dysbiosis was noted in the early and midstage phases of PD. The relationship between oral dysbiosis, inflammation, and pathogenesis might be interrelated and requires further study.[9]

PD affects the automatic movements of the hands, posing difficulties in maintaining good oral health.[10] Older people with PD face several challenges in maintaining good oral health. Hence, emphasis should be laid on the need to cultivate good oral hygiene practices.[11] Educational programs appear to improve perceived health and wellbeing. These education programs have proven to be a useful adjunct to medical therapy of PD not only by reducing cost but also by improving intermediate term outcomes.[12,13]

Deterioration in motor skills (tremors, instability, and bradykinesia) inhibits the ability to hold a toothbrush and move it properly while keeping the mouth open.[14] Educational intervention consisting of individual instruction in oral hygiene and exercises improved oral hygiene, masticatory function, and objective measurements of jaw mobility.[14] Most of these studies have been conducted in developed countries. To the best of the present authors' knowledge, in underdeveloped and developing countries there is a dearth of studies that assess the effectiveness of oral health education interventions (OHEI) in PD. Therefore, the objectives of this study were to evaluate oral health-related knowledge, compare the effectiveness of three different OHEI, and estimate the salivary flow rate in a cohort with PD.

Method and materials

This three-arm parallel design randomized controlled trial study with 1:1 allocation of patients was conducted after receiving ethical approval from the Institutional Review Board of the Bangalore Institute of Dental Sciences and Post Graduate Research Center. All procedures were conducted in accordance with the declaration of Helsinki of 1975 as revised in 2013. The study was conducted between September 2019 and October 2021 at the Bangalore Institute of Dental Sciences and Post Graduate Research Center. It has been reported in accordance with Consolidated Standards of Reporting Randomized Trials (CONSORT) guidelines The inclusion criteria were participants aged 40 years and above with a minimum of 20 permanent teeth and a minimum cognitive

ability score of 26 as per the Montreal Cognitive Assessment (MoCA) test and Mini-Mental State Exam (MMSE), clinical severity Stage1 and 2 as per the Unified Parkinson Disease Rating Scale (UPDRS) III and Hoehn and Yahr (HY) scale; diagnosed with PD using UK Parkinson Disease Society Brain Bank clinical diagnostic criteria (UKPDS Brain Bank Criteria). The participants who had a persisting or recurrent malignant disease, radiation or chemotherapy for head and neck regions, Alzheimer disease, history of recent usage of antimicrobials, diabetes mellitus, Sjogren syndrome or other medical causes for xerostomia, any other systemic conditions and generalized mobility of teeth were excluded.

Out of 100 eligible patients who reported to the outpatient department of Neurology, National Institute of Mental Health and Neurosciences (NIMHANS), 63 participants were recruited for the study after obtaining informed consent. The estimated sample size with a power of 80% was 20 participants per group. The neurology specialists (PP, RK, and NK) assessed the cognitive ability of the participants using the MoCA test and MMSE. The clinical assessment of participants for motor function using UPDRS III and HY staging and monitoring of the participants were carried out throughout the study period (Fig 1).

Calibration of the examiner

Training and calibration were done prior to the initiation of the study, and intra-examiner reliability for oral health assessment achieved was greater than 90%.

Clinical examination

Self-reported sociodemographic data were collected including age, sex, educational level, socioeconomic status (SES), history of smoking and alcohol consumption, drug history, and oral hygiene practice. A single examiner (SG) examined and recorded all the clinical measurements using a mouth mirror, dental explorer, and periodontal probe. Plaque Index (PI)[15] and Patient Hygiene Performance Index (PHPI)[16] were recorded at baseline and 3 months.

Estimation of salivary flow

Unstimulated whole saliva (UWS) was collected by the examiner (SG) as per the Navazesh[17] protocol. UWS flow rate with a threshold of ≤ 0.1 mL/minute is one of the ACR/EULAR (American College of Rheumatology/European League Against Rheumatism) 2016 criteria for dryness of the mouth or primary Sjogren syndrome.[18] Participants were instructed to rinse their oral cavity thoroughly prior to the collection of saliva. They

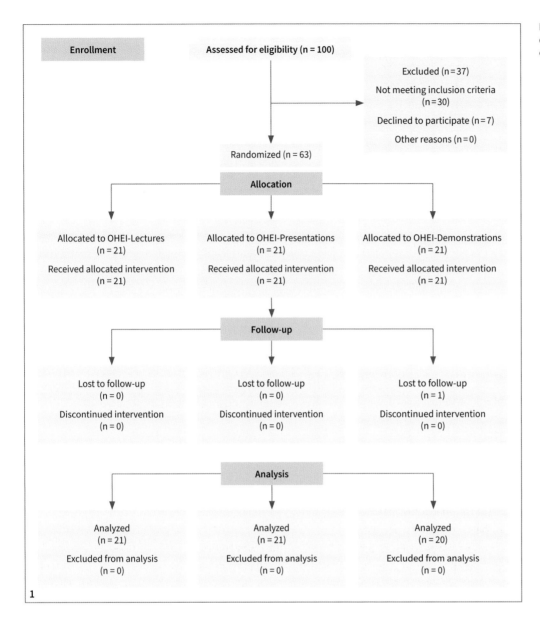

Fig 1 CONSORT flow diagram. Assessed for eligibility (n = 100).

were asked to sit comfortably with eyes open (to minimize oro-facial movements), with their head bent down and mouth open to allow the saliva to drip passively from the lower lip into a pre-weighed tube for 5 minutes. The quantity of saliva collected was measured by using the precision balance weighing method. The salivary flow rate was calculated as the difference in weight of the tube divided by time (mL per minute).

Grouping of patients

As the recruited PD patients had similar grading for cognitive and mental ability, they were randomly allocated using computer generated random numbers into three groups:

- Group 1 (n = 21) received instructions in the form of lectures
- Group 2 (n = 21) received instructions in the form of presentations
- Group 3 (n = 21) received instructions in the form of demonstrations.

Questionnaire development for assessment of knowledge

Most of the participants had received only primary education (elementary education), spoke diverse dialects, had difficulty in speaking, and to the best of the authors' knowledge no standard questionnaires suited the study participants. Hence, a closed-

Table 1 Participants' characteristics among the three groups

Characteristic		Group 1 (n = 21)	Group 2 (n = 21)	Group 3 (n = 21)	χ² value (or F where indicated)	P value
Age (y), mean ± SD		56.33 ± 6.98	54.95 ± 8.13	53.35 ± 10.36	F = 0.62	.540
Sex, n (%)	Male	17 (81.0)	12 (57.1)	14 (70.0)	2.806	.240
	Female	4 (19.0)	9 (42.9)	6 (30.0)		
Duration of illness, n (%)	<6 y	16 (76.2)	18 (85.7)	16 (80.0)	17.146	.376
	≥6 y	5 (23.8)	3 (14.3)	4 (20.0)		
Education, n (%)	Postgraduate	1 (4.8)	1 (4.8)	0 (0.0)	10.738	.217
	Graduate	3 (14.3)	3 (14.3)	3 (15.0)		
	Secondary	6 (28.6)	9 (42.9)	4 (20.0)		
	Primary	10 (47.6)	6 (28.6)	6 (30.0)		
	Illiterate	1 (4.8)	2 (9.5)	7 (35.0)		
Socioeconomic status, n (%)	High	9 (42.9)	8 (38.1)	3 (15.0)	5.300	.230
	Medium	4 (19.0)	9 (42.9)	2 (10.0)		
	Low	8 (38.1)	4 (19.0)	15 (75.0)		
Smoking, n (%)	No	17 (81.0)	21 (100.0)	19 (95.0)	5.185	.213
	Former	1 (4.8)	0 (0.0)	0 (0.0)		
	Current	3 (14.3)	0 (0.0)	1 (5.0)		
Alcohol intake, n (%)	No	18 (85.7)	21 (100.0)	19 (95.0)	4.158	.385
	Former	1 (4.8)	0 (0.0)	0 (0.0)		
	Current	2 (9.5)	0 (0.0)	1 (5.0)		

*Statistical significance set at $P < .05$.

ended multiple-choice questionnaire was prepared from the evidence in the literature. The questionnaire consisted of 18 questions based on basic knowledge about oral hygiene. Each right answer was scored one (1), with zero (0) for a wrong answer. The face and content validation were done by the specialist periodontists SR, RR, and SK. The linguistic validation was done using the back-translation method. A pilot test survey was done on the intended population. The data were analyzed using principal component analysis and the internal consistency of questions was checked and the survey was revised based on the information.

OHEI content preparation

The examiner (AK) prepared all the contents for OHEI, including questionnaires and lectures, presentations, and demonstrations. The content included the common causes of dental and oral disease, type of brush, brushing techniques, use of interdental aids, use of fluoridated dentifrices, mouth rinses, appropriate diet, and oral diseases–systemic diseases link. It was ensured that the content was uniform across the different form of oral hygiene education methods.

Questionnaire administration

The pilot study was done on five volunteers who matched the inclusion criteria (PD stage 1 and 2 patients) but were not included in the main study. Test–retest reliability was done with a gap of 2 weeks. All the participants were made to answer the questions under the supervision of one examiner (SG). The baseline knowledge was assessed, and the mean percentage was calculated.

Oral hygiene education session

Oral hygiene education to the respective group of participants was provided by the examiner (SG). Each session lasted for 20 minutes for an individual, delivered only at the baseline. At the end of the session, a new standard soft toothbrush and standard fluoridated dentifrice were provided for each participant by a dental hygienist (DN), who assessed the compliance of brushing by physical examination of the toothbrush and dentifrices of all the participants at months 1, 2, and 3, and was blinded to the participant's group allocation. If the toothbrush

Table 2 Comparison of mean percentage of knowledge between the groups at different time intervals

Time	Group	n	Mean (%)	SD	F	P value
Baseline	Group 1	21	54.76	10.66	2.82	.067
	Group 2	21	60.71	13.54		
	Group 3	20	62.25	6.58		
1 month	Group 1	21	56.43	12.06	1.05	.353
	Group 2	21	60.71	13.54		
	Group 3	20	61.00	7.36		
2 months	Group 1	21	45.71	11.43	3.7	.030*
	Group 2	21	54.52	14.31		
	Group 3	20	47.00	6.57		
3 months	Group 1	21	36.90	11.99	2.8	.069
	Group 2	21	44.29	12.38		
	Group 3	20	37.25	9.39		

*One way ANOVA; Statistical significance set at $P<.05$.

Table 3 Tukey post-hoc analysis of the mean percentage of knowledge between groups at 2 months

Group (I)	Group (J)	Mean difference (I − J)	SE	Sig.	95% CI Lower bound	Upper bound
Group 1	Group 2	−8.81	3.49	.037*	−17.19	−0.43
	Group 3	−1.29	3.53	.930	−9.77	7.20
Group 2	Group 3	7.52	3.53	.092	−0.96	16.01

*Statistical significance set at $P<.05$.
CI, confidence interval; SE, standard error.

bristles flared or the dentifrice tube was empty, they were replaced with a new toothbrush and dentifrice of the same brand.

Recall visits

The same questionnaire was re-administered at months 1, 2, and 3 to test the change in scores. The salivary flow rate was estimated and clinical indices PI[15] and PHPI[16] were recorded at the end of 3 months.

Data analysis

The data recorded from individual participants were used for analysis. All the recorded parameters were statistically analyzed using SPSS version 20 (IBM). Normality of the data was checked by Shapiro-Wilk test. The data are presented as mean ± standard deviation (SD). All the demographic data including sex, SES, duration of illness, education, and habits were analyzed using the chi-square test. One way ANOVA was performed to compare age, and the percentage of knowledge between all the groups at different time intervals and compare the means of all clinical parameters between groups at baseline and 3 months. Bonferroni post-hoc analysis was used for comparing the percentage of good knowledge among groups. PI and PHPI between the three groups at baseline and 3 months were compared using Tukey post-hoc analysis. Multivariate test (MANOVA) was done for hypothesis testing. Pearson correlation analysis was performed to measure the linear relationship between the knowledge and PI scores. Statistical significance was set at .05 ($P<.05$) for all the tests, two-tailed.

Table 4 Multivariate tests to compare at different time intervals (baseline, 1 month, 2 months, and 3 months) and between the groups

Group	Wilks λ value	F	Hypothesis df	Partial η²	P value
Group 1	0.153	33.29	3	0.847	.001*
Group 2	0.221	33.5	2	0.779	.001*
Group 3	0.097	52.94	3	0.903	.001*

Statistical significance set at $P<.05$ (MANOVA).
df, degrees of freedom; SE, standard error.

Results

One hundred eligible patients who reported to the outpatient department of Neurology, NIMHANS, with PD were screened and 63 participants consented to participate; there was one drop out during the study. The mean ages of participants were 56.33 ± 6.98, 54.95 ± 8.13, and 53.35 ± 10.36 years, respectively, in Groups 1, 2, and 3. A preponderance of male sex was seen in the study. The majority of the participants were diagnosed with PD less than 6 years and had only primary education. Few of the included participants consumed alcohol and smoked cigarettes. All the groups had participants from high-, middle-, and low-income groups (Table 1). No statistical difference was observed between the groups for the baseline characteristics ($P>.05$).

On comparison, the mean percentage of knowledge among groups showed significant decrease from baseline to 1 month, 2 months, and 3 months in all three groups ($P<.001$). A statistically significant difference between the groups was observed only at 2 months for mean percentage of knowledge ($P=.030$). Group 2 had a significantly higher mean percentage knowledge (mean difference 8.81; $P=.037$) (Tables 2 and 3). The results of the MANOVA showed a significant time effect among Group 1 (Wilks Lambda (λ) = 0.153, F (3) = 33.29, $P=.001$, $\eta^2=0.847$), Group 2 (Wilks $\lambda=0.221$, F (2) = 33.5, $P=.001$, $\eta^2=0.779$), and Group 3 (Wilks $\lambda=0.097$, F (3) = 52.94, $P=.001$, $\eta^2=0.903$). Thus, there was significant evidence to reject the null hypothesis (Table 4). Intergroup comparison of clinical parameters between the groups at baseline and after 3 months showed a significant difference of PI scores between Group 1, Group 2, and Group 3 at 3 months (F = 11.54; $P=.001$), but salivary flow rate and PHPI scores showed no significant difference (Table 5). Multiple comparisons using Tukey post-hoc analysis showed that mean PI scores remained significantly lower in Group 2 (mean difference = −0.24; $P=.027$) as compared to Group 1 and Group 3 than other groups (Group 1, mean difference = 0.3, $P=.027$; and Group 3 mean dif-

ference = −0.54; $P=.001$) (Table 6). Pearson correlation was used to assess if there was correlation between knowledge, PI, and PHPI scores at 3 months. There was no significant correlation between knowledge and PI scores in all the three groups (Fig 2). There were no adverse events reported.

Discussion

PD participants face multiple oral health-related problems along with motor and nonmotor symptoms. OHEI can be a useful adjunct along with standard dental therapy. Very few studies have addressed this issue. For effective prevention of oral health-related problems in older people with PD, the goal should be to help them perform effective daily plaque removal on a long-term basis. To the best of the present authors' knowledge this is the first study that has evaluated the effect of OHEI among a cohort of PD in an Asian population.

The participants in the study were mostly men in the age range of 53 to 56 years, which was similar to the age range and higher male predilection reported in other studies.[5,6,14] The oral hygiene was poor at baseline. This could be due to problems associated with mastication, taste impairment, xerostomia, and increased plaque, poor dexterity, increased caries lesions, and teeth mobility due to periodontal disease, increased root stumps, and reduced oral hygiene care. The duration and severity of the oral problems increase with poor oral health and hygiene care problems. Similar reasons have been reported.[18]

Mean percentage knowledge showed significant decrease from baseline to the third month in all the three groups. Mild cognitive impairment along with poor educational background, language difficulties, lack of standardized questionnaires in the local language, diverse dialects, and recall bias are an inherent problem of questionnaire studies, and not using motivational interviews addressing the five levels of Leventhal's theory might have contributed to the decline in knowledge.[19,20]

Table 5 Comparison of means of salivary flow rate, PI, and PHPI between the groups at baseline and after 3 months

Time	Group	N	Mean	SD	F	P value
Baseline	Group 1	21	0.88	0.33	1.900	.159
	Group 2	21	1.02	0.37		
	Group 3	20	1.11	0.43		
3 months	Group 1	21	1.00	0.39	1.697	.192
	Group 2	21	1.16	0.40		
	Group 3	20	1.23	0.44		
	Group 2	21	3.00	1.01		
	Group 3	20	3.02	1.16		
Baseline	Group 1	21	0.89	0.46	2.614	.082
	Group 2	21	1.03	0.38		
	Group 3	20	1.18	0.40		
3 months	Group 1	21	0.78	0.43	11.54	.001*
	Group 2	21	0.49	0.19		
	Group 3	20	1.02	0.42		
3 months	Group 1	21	1.76	0.47	3.119	.052
	Group 2	21	1.53	0.52		
	Group 3	20	1.94	0.57		

One-way ANOVA; *Statistical significance set at $P < .05$.

Table 6 Tukey post-hoc analysis for multiple comparison of means of PI between the groups at 3 months

	Groups (I)	Groups (J)	Mean difference (I-J)	SE	P value	95% CI	Groups (I)
PI 3 months	Group 1	Group 2	0.30	0.11	.027*	0.03	0.56
		Group 3	−0.24	0.11	.086	−0.51	0.03
	Group 2	Group 3	−0.54	0.11	.001*	−0.81	−0.27

*Statistical significance set at $P < .05$.
CI, confidence interval; SE, standard error.

In addition, motor fluctuations have been reported in PD ("ON" and "OFF" phases) in participants with PD alone or those who are on medication for PD.[21] These motor fluctuations can worsen the health-related quality of life (HQORL) of PD participants which in turn can lead to anxiety,[22] depression,[23] cognitive impairments,[24] sleep disturbance,[25] and psychosis.[26] These factors can affect the knowledge and oral care. It has been noted that the educational sessions can be an effective adjunct to the standard medicinal therapy to PD. The PROPATH health promotion program for medical treatment of PD reported a similar observation.[27] A study in Japan that focused on oral health education in a cohort of mental illness patients along with PD medication concluded that the oral health education showed positive effects.[28]

Instructions given in the pictorial form of presentation appeared to improve the ability to retain and recall oral hygiene information in the present study cohort. It has been reported that older people with PD have sentence comprehension difficulties.[29] This could be one of the reasons why the written instructions group did not perform better. The knowledge of the demonstration group did not meet the expectations in the present cohort despite demonstration being an effective visual and interactive intervention. The efficacy of video demonstration

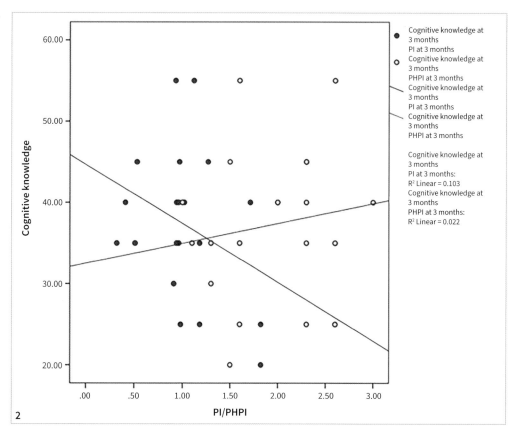

Fig 2 Correlation of cognitive knowledge with PI and PHPI at 3 months.

methods was proved in a randomized controlled trial on the oral hygiene status of children with hearing loss.[30] Attention deficits like vigilance and fluctuating attention along with a broad range of attentional phenomena are compromised in PD,[31] as well as motor fluctuations ("ON" and "OFF" phases), and this may be why demonstration was not significantly effective.[32]

Although the knowledge level declined, the PI scores decreased significantly in the present cohort. Similar results were reported in the study assessing the impact of OHEI in children with hearing loss.[30] There was no correlation between PI scores and knowledge levels in the present cohort. However, a negative correlation has been noted between oral hygiene practices and mean age, degree of dependency, and degree of institution among older people.[33] Cognitive impairment, motor and non-motor symptoms, and differences in population and study design could be the most probable reasons for lack of correlation in the present study.

Changes in salivary flow rates and difficulty in swallowing have been shown to affect the oral self-cleansing mechanisms in PD.[34] The parasympatholytic or anti-muscarinic effects of the drugs administered during PD treatment may play a role in decreased qualitative and quantitative changes in saliva.[35] The

saliva secreted by submandibular glands differs from the parotid glands in that it is more viscous and mucin-rich.[36] This was the rationale for the preference of UWS saliva over the stimulated, watery saliva produced by parotid glands. The UWS flow rate in the present cohort did not show any significant change as the study interval was short and the drug regimen also remained unchanged. The COVID-19 pandemic wave and changing guidelines could have affected the cohort and their caregivers during the study. The most recent recommendation is that tooth brushing must be done regularly and with alternate hands.[37] The present participants did not follow this recommendation.

Despite these limitations, the results of the present study do provide evidence for the need for OHEI at regular intervals to improve poor oral hygiene related problems that are mostly preventable. When interpreted with caution the results can contribute meaningful data for the effectiveness of OHEI in patients with PD. More studies are required to validate the result of the study. In the future, studies should include health-related quality of life, motor fluctuations, and tooth brushing with alternate hands to generate the evidence to prove the effectiveness of OHEI in patients with PD.

Conclusion

Pictorial presentation of OHEI appears to be a better mode of intervention when compared to lectures and demonstration in the present cohort of patients with PD. Although there was a decline in knowledge level at 3 months, plaque scores reduced significantly implying that OHEI offer tangible positive benefits.

Acknowledgment

The authors thank Dr Deepa Bullappa, Department of Biostatistics, Bangalore Institute of Dental Sciences and Post graduate Research Center, Bangalore, for the statistical evaluation.

Disclosure

The authors declare that no external funds or grants were used for this study and the study was self-funded. The authors have no conflicts of interest to declare.

References

1. Kalia LV, Lang AE, Shulman G. Parkinson's disease. Lancet 2015;386(9996):896–912.

2. Mu J, Chaudhuri KR, Bielza C, de Pedro Cuesta J, Larrañaga P, Martinez-Martin P. Parkinson's disease subtypes identified from cluster analysis of motor and non-motor symptoms. Front Aging Neurosci 2017;9: 301–306.

3. Videnovic A, Golombek D. Circadian dysregulation in Parkinson's disease. Neurobiol Sleep Circadian Rhythms 2017;2:53–58.

4. Tysnes OB, Storstein A. Epidemiology of Parkinson's disease. J Neural Transm (Vienna) 2017;124:901–905.

5. Mahmood A, Shah AA, Umair M, Wu Y, Khan A. Recalling the pathology of Parkinson's disease; lacking exact figure of prevalence and genetic evidence in Asia with an alarming outcome: A time to step-up. Clin Genet 2021; 100:659–677.

6. Reekes TH, Higginson CI, Ledbetter CR, et al. Sex specific cognitive differences in Parkinson disease. NPJ Parkinsons Dis 2020;6:7.

7. Barbe AG, Bock N, Derman SHM, Felsch M, Timmermann L, Noack MJ. Self-assessment of oral health, dental health care and oral health-related quality of life among Parkinson's disease patients. Gerodontology 2017;34: 135–143.

8. Isaacson J, Patel S, Torres-Yaghi Y, Pagán F. Sialorrhea in Parkinson's disease. Toxins (Basel) 2020;12:691.

9. Fleury V, Zekeridou A, Lazarevic V, et al. Oral dysbiosis and inflammation in Parkinson's disease. J Parkinsons Dis 2021;11:619–631.

10. Jeong E, Park JB, Park YG. Evaluation of the association between periodontitis and risk of Parkinson's disease: a nationwide retrospective cohort study. Sci Rep 2021;11:16594.

11. Auffret M, Meuric V, Boyer E, Bonnaure-Mallet M, Vérin M. Oral health disorders in Parkinson's disease: more than meets the eye. J Parkinsons Dis 2021;11:1507–1535.

12. Ueno T, Kon T, Haga R, Nishijima H, Arai A, Tomiyama M. Assessing the relationship between non-motor symptoms and health-related quality of life in Parkinson's disease: a retrospective observational cohort study. Neurol Sci 2020;41:2867–2873.

13. Cersósimo MG, Perandones C, Micheli FE, et al. Alpha-synuclein immunoreactivity in minor salivary gland biopsies of Parkinson's disease patients. Mov Disord 2011;26:188–190.

14. Baram S, Karlsborg M, Øzhayat EB, Bakke M. Effect of orofacial physiotherapeutic and hygiene interventions on oral health-related quality of life in patients with Parkinson's disease: A randomised controlled trial. J Oral Rehabil 2021;48:1035–1043.

15. Turesky S, Gilmore ND, Glickman I. Reduced plaque formation by the chloromethyl analogue of victamine C. J Periodontol 1970; 41:41–43.

16. Podshadley AG. A method for evaluating oral hygiene performance. Public Health Rep 1968;83:259–264.

17. Navazesh M. Methods for collecting saliva. Ann N Y Acad Sci 1993;69:72–77.

18. van Stiphout MAE, Marinus J, van Hilten JJ, Lobbezoo F, de Baat C. Oral health of Parkinson's disease patients: a case-control study. Parkinsons Dis 2018;18:9315285.

19. Godard A, Dufour T, Jeanne S. Application of self-regulation theory and motivational interview for improving oral hygiene: a randomized controlled trial. J Clin Periodontol 2011;38:1099–1105.

20. Rosenthal E, Brennan L, Xie S, et al. Association between cognition and function in patients with Parkinson disease with and without dementia. Mov Disord 2010;25: 1170–1176.

21. Dirks SJ, Paunovich ED, Terezhalmy GT, Chiodo LK. The patient with Parkinson's disease. Quintessence Int 2003;34(5):379-93.

22. Egan SJ, Laidlaw K, Starkstein S. Cognitive behaviour therapy for depression and anxiety in Parkinson's disease. J Parkinsons Dis 2015;5:443–451.

23. Wei YJ, Palumbo FB, Simoni-Wastila L, et al. Antiparkinson drug use and adherence in medicare part D beneficiaries with Parkinson's disease. Clin Ther 2013;35:1513–1525.

24. O'Callaghan C, Lewis SJG. Cognition in Parkinson's disease. Int Rev Neurobiol 2017;133:557–583.

25. Albers JA, Chand P, Anch AM. Multifactorial sleep disturbance in Parkinson's disease. Sleep Med 2017;35:41–48.

26. Fredericks D, Norton JC, Atchison C, Schoenhaus R, Pill MW. Parkinson's disease and Parkinson's disease psychosis: a perspective on the challenges, treatments, and economic burden. Am J Manag Care 2017; 23:S83–S92.

27. Montgomery EB Jr, Lieberman A, Singh G, Fries JF. Patient education and health promotion can be effective in Parkinson's disease: a randomized controlled trial. PROPATH Advisory Board. Am J Med 1994; 97:429–435.

28. Yoshii H, Kitamura N, Akazawa K, Saito H. Effects of an educational intervention on oral hygiene and self-care among people with mental illness in Japan: a longitudinal study. BMC Oral Health 2017;17:81.

29. Grossman M, Carvell S, Stern BM, Gollomp S, Hurtig IH. Sentence comprehension in Parkinson's disease: The role of attention and memory. Brain Lang 1992;42:347–384.

30. Moin M, Saadat S, Rafique S, et al. Impact of oral health educational interventions on oral hygiene status of children with hearing loss: a randomized controlled trial. Biomed Res Int 2021;2021:5185613.

31. Bronnick K, Ehrt U, Emre M, et al. Attentional deficits affect activities of daily living in dementia-associated with Parkinson's disease. J Neurol Neurosurg Psychiatry 2006; 77:1136–1142.

32. Thach A, Jones E, Pappert E, Pike J, Wright J, Gillespie A. Real-world assessment of the impact of "OFF" episodes on health-related quality of life among patients with Parkinson's disease in the United States. BMC Neurol 2021;21:46.

33. Vanobbergen JN, De Visschere LM. Factors contributing to the variation in oral hygiene practices and facilities in long-term care institutions for the elderly. Community Dent Health 2005;22:260–265.

34. Furuta M, Yamashita Y. Oral health and swallowing problems. Curr Phys Med Rehabil Rep 2013;1:216-222.

35. Tumilasci OR, Cersósimo MG, Belforte JE, Micheli FE, Benarroch EE, Pazo JH. Quantitative study of salivary secretion in Parkinson's disease. Mov Disord 2006;21: 660–667.

36. Pedersen A, Sørensen CE, Proctor GB, Carpenter GH. Salivary functions in mastication, taste, and textural perception, swallowing and initial digestion. Oral Dis 2018;24:1399–1416.

37. Martimbianco ALC, Prosdocimi FC, Anauate-Netto C, Dos Santos EM, Mendes GD, Fragoso YD. Evidence-based recommendations for the oral health of patients with Parkinson's disease. Neurol Ther 2021; 10:391–400.

Stella Spurthi

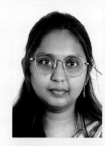

Stella Spurthi   Post graduate student, Department of Periodontics, Bangalore Institute of Dental Sciences and Postgraduate research center, Bengaluru, India

Srirangarajan Sridharan   Professor and Head, Department of Periodontics, Bangalore Institute of Dental Sciences and Postgraduate research center, Bengaluru, India

Rajesh Hosadurga   Professor, Department of Periodontics and Oral Implantology, Faculty of Dentistry, Manipal University College Malaysia (MUCM), Melaka, Malaysia

Ravi. J. Rao   Reader, Department of Periodontics, Bangalore Institute of Dental Sciences and Postgraduate research center, Bengaluru, India

Srikumar Prabhu   Reader, Department of Periodontics, Bangalore Institute of Dental Sciences and Postgraduate research center, Bengaluru, India

Pramod Kumar Pal   Professor and Head, Department of Neurology NIMHANS, Bangalore, India

Nitish Kamble   Professor, Department of Neurology NIMHANS, Bangalore, India

Kempaiah Rakesh   Associate Professor, Department of Neurology NIMHANS, Bangalore, India

Amit Kumar   Reader, National Resource Centre for Oral Health and Tobacco Cessation, Maulana Azad Institute of Dental Sciences, Delhi, India

Correspondence: Dr Srirangarajan, 5/3, Hosur road; Bangalore Institute of Dental Sciences and Postgraduate Research Center, Bangalore 560027, India. Email: docranga@yahoo.com

First submission: 2 Nov 2022
Acceptance: 22 Jan 2023
Online publication: 27 Jan 2023

Complete oral rehabilitation with direct and indirect composite resins: a minimally invasive approach on severely compromised teeth

Vinícius F. Lippert, DDS, MS/Jonas P. Andrade, DDS, MS, PhD/Ana M. Spohr, DDS, MS, PhD/ Marcel F. Kunrath, DDS, MS, PhD

The rehabilitation of severely worn teeth is a complex challenge for dental practitioners. There are many different types of dental materials and restorative techniques, and there is not a single way to achieve the desired result. This clinical report demonstrates a complete oral rehabilitation with composite resins when using an indirect application and direct techniques, with the support of the Lucia Jig technique, the Willis technique, and diagnostic waxing for the vertical dimension correction. The wide clinical improvement was achieved with the recovery of the function, the esthetics, and the increase of vertical dimension of occlusion through the planned treatment. The proposed treatment maintained the natural teeth, without the intense wear by the application of the composite resins instead of ceramics, together with excellent conditions for the patient to control the posttreatment and extend the durability, with the correct follow-up of appointments. Young patients with extensive dental wear and the loss of vertical dimension should not be directly submitted to ceramic treatments, with preparations for full crowns. Oral rehabilitation using composite resins, either directly or indirectly, allows for the recovery of the function and esthetics, without the intense predictable dental wear, and reduced financial investment.
(Quintessence Int 2022;53:824–831; doi: 10.3290/j.qi.b3315033)

Key words: direct resin, esthetic, indirect resin, occlusion, oral rehabilitation

The gradual loss of tooth enamel is a biologic condition that results from the aging process. However, the premature wear of this tissue is due to a combination of factors, such as friction (abrasion), occlusal stress (abfraction), and biocorrosion (erosion), with the last mentioned being the most predominant factor in this process.[1,2] The action of acidic drinks, gastroesophageal reflux, bulimia, medications, drugs, and reduced salivary flow all contribute to the progression of these injuries.[3]

The treatment for dental erosion depends on the amount of dental structure loss and this must address the main factors promptly, to prevent a progression of this disease.[3,4] The European Consensus Statement[5] suggests that the restorative procedures should be postponed whenever possible. However, when these procedures are performed, they must be minimally invasive for reducing the pain and restoring the function and esthetics, through mutual agreement with the patient. The treatment of severe tooth wear is not a simple approach. The planning must be conducted carefully, including the impression of the arches, photographs, and the assembly of the models in a semi-adjustable articulator and diagnostic waxing. This procedure can be performed in an analog or virtual way, to return a natural esthetic, and a stable and balanced occlusion.[6]

The restorative materials that are mainly used in the rehabilitation of patients with eroded teeth are metal-ceramic crowns, zirconia crowns, and glass ceramics, such as lithium disilicate ceramics, as well as composite resins that are made by both direct and indirect methods.[7-10] Direct composite resins are the most economical option when resorted to in situations of mandibular dental wear.[4,5] Currently, the indirect composite resins that are produced by the CAD/CAM process have been an option that has been well used for posterior teeth.[11] The literature shows countless types of treatments, and there is no consensus on which restorative technique is the best, exemplifying different advantages and disadvantages.

Figs 1a to 1d *(a)* Initial smile. *(b)* Intraoral initial view. *(c)* Intraoral occlusal maxillary view. *(d)* Intraoral occlusal mandibular view.

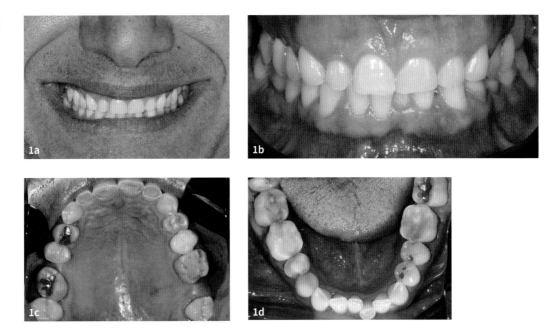

Nowadays, it is more common that patients, especially the young, look for conservative treatments, to avoid dental wear.[12] In addition, a therapeutic approach with composite resins provides better intraoral finishing and polishing, thus avoiding antagonistic tooth wear when compared to ceramics.[13-15] Some in vitro studies have shown that the fracture resistance of occlusal veneers in composite resin is greater than occlusal veneers in glass ceramics, due to the fact that they have a lower elastic modulus and a better absorbs the tensions, which is beneficial for the stomatognathic system.[16-20]

The purpose of this clinical report was to present an ultra-conservative clinical case of full-mouth rehabilitation that was made from composite resins, in a patient with extensive dental wear, using indirect (laboratory technique) and direct (stratified technique) methods.

Case presentation

A 45-year-old man who complained about frequent fractures on composite resin restorations and dental structures sought dental treatment at a private clinic. Anamnesis, clinical and radiographic examinations, photographs, and diagnostic casts were performed. These procedures revealed that the patient presented a loss of the vertical dimension of occlusion (VDO), which was associated with parafunction events and erosion (Fig 1). Due to the great dental wear and dentin exposure, a full-mouth rehabilitation treatment was proposed, with a restoration of the VDO, by applying composite resins, to recover the function and esthetics, without aggressive additional wear on the teeth. Additionally, the patient was advised to control the intake of liquids and acid foods, combined with a medical follow-up.

Initially, adequate oral health was ensured, with prophylaxis and a replacement of all patient's aged restorations. The cavities were all sealed with Flowable Dental Composite Resin A2 (Natural Flow, DFL). Subsequently, for the extraoral planning, impressions of the maxillary and mandibular dental arches were made with polyvinyl siloxane (PVS) (Variotime, Kulzer), using the two-step technique, to obtain the casts for diagnostic waxing. The casts were mounted on an articulator (Bio-Art A7 Fix) for carrying out the transfer of the skull-maxilla relationship with the facial arch (Elite Facial Arch, Bio-Art). The VDO was reestablished by the Lucia Jig technique,[21] with the posterior bilateral bite registration when using self-curing acrylic (GC Pattern Resin). The parameters that were applied were the metric method of Willis[22] when using a compass, while the determination of the VDO was performed by subtracting 3 mm (freeway space) from the vertical dimension at rest, together with the Turner and Fox esthetic method when concerning the thirds of the face.[23] In addition, an unconditioned resin veneer increment over the patient's maxillary central incisor was performed, and this was sent to the laboratory as a length reference for the diagnostic waxing. The difference that was provided after the protocols for the VDO increase when using the articulator was 3 mm from the initial measurement.

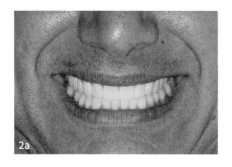
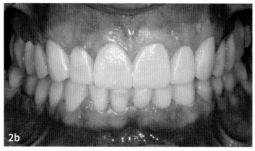

Figs 2a to 2d Immediate dental reconstruction with mock-up and bisacrylic resin. *(a)* Frontal smile. *(b)* Intraoral view. *(c)* Lateral view, right. *(d)* Lateral view, left.

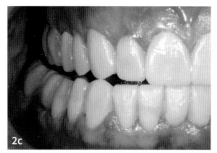
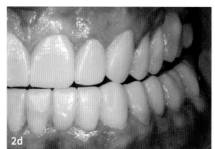

The diagnostic waxing was made by a dental technician, with the aim of performing full-mouth rehabilitation, by applying the direct and indirect composite resins, whilst recovering the dental health, the anatomy, the esthetics, and the VDO. Two PVS (Variotime) guides on the waxing were made for the mock-up by using A1 colored bisacrylic resin (Structur 2, Voco). With the reproduction of the wax-up in the mouth with bisacrylic resin, the evaluation of the esthetic aspects and the phonetic tests were performed to check the increase in the VDO. Furthermore, the contact points and the guides were both evaluated (Fig 2).

Regarding the previous esthetic procedures for the main treatment, a periodontal surgery of the maxillary anterior teeth (canine to canine) was performed, with an electric scalpel (B 100 Plus, Rhosse) but only over the soft tissue (0.5 mm in the maxillary left central incisor and 0.5 mm in the maxillary right lateral incisor), aiming at the gingival recontour by equalizing the gingival zenith. The CT scan was performed with soft tissue retraction, to precisely identify the distances between the bone crest and the gingival margin, the bone crest and the cementoenamel junction, and the gingival margin and the cementoenamel junction. From this evaluation, it was verified what would be necessary to esthetically improve the situation when using the diagnostic wax-up, and this identified the need for only the removal of the soft tissue. A duplication of the diagnostic wax-up was performed and a

surgical guide was made with an acetate plate to perform the procedure. After 30 days, a dental night guard bleaching technique was carried out for 4 weeks when using a 10% carbamide peroxide gel (Whiteness Perfect 10%, FGM Dental Group), for daily use with a 24-hour interval between each application. The patient was recommended to use a toothpaste with properties for sensitivity protection during the whitening, and there was no report of any discomfort. After the bleaching, the color of the teeth was recorded with the Vita Classical Shade Guide, for selection of the composite resin to be used in the rehabilitation procedure. An additional color investigation was carried out, by using small resin spheres to compare with the tooth substrate.

Indirect composite resins and adhesive procedure

To carry out the indirect composite resin restorations and to increase the VDO, the retentions were removed, and the acute angles of posterior teeth (15, 16, 27, 34 to 37, and 44 to 47, according to FDI notation) were rounded by finishing and polishing disks (Sof-Lex, 3M Espe), followed by impressions of the dental arches with PVS. Indirect composite resins (Ceramage, Shofu Dental) were produced in the laboratory, by using transparent guides, according to the diagnostic waxing that was previously approved, with the objective of providing better mechanical properties.[24] Initially, the indirect composite resins

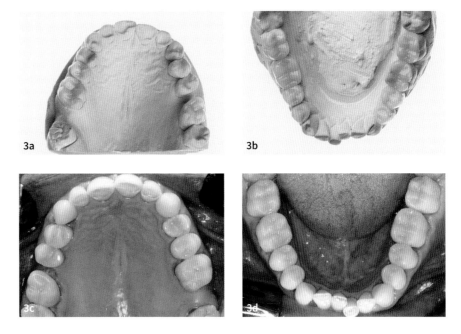

Figs 3a to 3d *(a and b)* The indirect resins at the planning stage, and *(c and d)* the indirect resins after the adhesion to the patient's teeth.

were tested without rubber dam isolation, to verify the adaptation of the margins. In sequence, under isolation with rubber dam (Madeitex, Brazil) the luting procedures were performed, and a further test was carried out to carefully observe the adaptation and contact points. The internal surface of each composite resin was blasted with 50 μm aluminum oxide, followed by an application of silane (Prosil, FGM Dental Group) for 2 minutes, with a Single Bond Universal Adhesive system (3M Espe), and a subsequent light jet of air (like a jet wash for the teeth), without photoactivation. On the dental substrate, selective etching (Ultra-Etch, Ultradent) was performed on the enamel for 30 seconds, with a subsequent washing and drying, and the Single Bond Universal Adhesive system was applied, with a subsequent light jet of air, without photoactivation. For the cementation, dual-cure resin cement (RelyX Ultimate, 3M) was used, which was positioned on the internal surface of the indirect composite resin, and then adapted for the dental substrate. The removal of the excess cement was conducted with a microbrush and dental floss, followed by photopolymerization for 60 seconds on each face, with a VALO poly-wave device (Ultradent) in a standard mode (1,000 mW/cm^2). An additional polymerization per face was carried out after applying a water-soluble gel (Power Block, BM4), thus inhibiting the contact of the resin cement with oxygen from the external environment. After removing the absolute isolation, and with the Lucia Jig in position, the occlusal adjustments were made, with the

subsequent finishing and final polishing of all the teeth (Fig 3). The EVE Diacomp Twist system (pink and gray rubber) and a felt disk with universal polishing paste (Diamond Excel, FGM Dental Group) were used for the finishing and polishing procedures. On the same day, provisional direct composite resins were performed on the teeth 13, 23, 33, and 43, to give contact with the anterior sector and the canine guides.

Direct composite resins

At the next appointment, direct restorations using the stratified technique were performed on the maxillary and mandibular anterior teeth. However, due to the inadequate position of the mandibular left central incisor (tooth 31) and the option of not performing the orthodontic treatment as first indicated, the buccal surface preparation was performed by correcting the positioning of this specific tooth. To execute these direct restorations, silicone palatal guides were made on the models of the diagnostic waxing. These helped in making the first palatal and lingual layer of all the elements. The composite resins that were used were the A1E palatal layer (Empress Direct, Ivoclar), the A2D dentin layer (Estelite Omega, Tokuyama), the Trans incisal effect (Estelite Omega), and the EB1 final layer (Estelite Omega), respectively. For the finishing process, a surgical scalpel blade no. 12, FF diamond tips (KG Sorensen), a 3M Sof-Lex disk, and multi-laminated dental burs (Jota) were used to remove the ex-

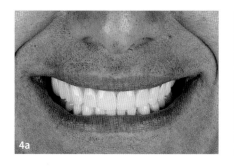
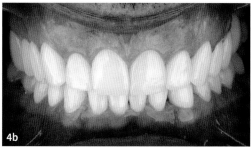
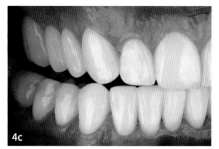
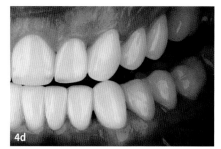

Figs 4a to 4d The final aspect of the complete rehabilitation when using the direct and indirect resins. *(a)* Frontal smile. *(b)* Intraoral view. *(c)* Lateral view, right. *(d)* Lateral view, left.

cesses and delimit the texture. Diamond spiral rubbers from Eve Diacomp Twist (pink and gray), felts, and a universal polishing paste (Diamond Excel) were used for the polishing process. Furthermore, the posterior teeth (14, 24, and 25), in which the indirect restorations were not performed, received direct restorations, reestablishing the missing occlusal contacts. The reason for applying the direct restorations on these specific teeth was diagnosed due to the small thickness of the resin that was needed for the restorations, which made it difficult to manufacture the indirect restorations in the laboratory.

All the mandibular movements and guides were checked, and an immediate protective 1-mm temporary acetate plate was made for the patient to use at night. Posteriorly, the patient returned for a final finishing and polishing appointment (Fig 4), to identify any excess that was still present. Following this procedure, a night guard was manufactured for adjusting all the occlusal contacts, with the indication of night use.

The final case registration showed an esthetic improvement and a functional rehabilitation due to the recovery of the VDO in a well-stabilized position, and the reconstruction of the teeth's natural size. Thereafter, the patient returned for a 1-year follow-up, and no damage was observed as a result of the rehabilitation. The patient agreed with the constant use of the night guard, with the intention of protecting his rehabilitation. New photographs were taken, without any repolishing, to identify any possible wear or pigmentation (Fig 5).

Discussion

The premature loss of the VDO and the severe tooth wear were not related to only one reason. There occurred a combination of factors, such as attrition (bruxism), abrasion, and erosion, which all led to this deleterious result.[2,3,26]

The wear of the posterior cusps provided an overload on the anterior teeth and the incisal wear of the anterior teeth generated an occlusal overload on the posterior teeth. In other words, the occlusal balance was directly related to a mutually protected occlusion at the maximum habitual intercuspation (formerly named centric occlusion), in a combination with the laterality and protrusion guides. The loss of the guides can cause early wear of the molar and premolar cusps, as well as the non-carious cervical lesions, known as abfraction.[25,27,28]

It has become increasingly prevalent to find severe dental wear in young patients. This is probably due to bruxism and diet changes with acidic foods, due to their current chosen lifestyle. The fact is that premature dental wear is now a reality, and how dentistry professionals should treat these patients is a challenge to be faced.[8,26]

First, it is essential to identify and treat the main etiologic factors of dental wear for the long-term success of any restorative treatment. Second, the choice of the most suitable material available in the market is important. This is controversial and can generate doubt for the dental surgeon because there is

Figs 5a to 5d   Patient follow-up (1 year). *(a)* Frontal smile. *(b)* Intraoral view. *(c)* Intraoral maxillary view. *(d)* Intraoral mandibular view.

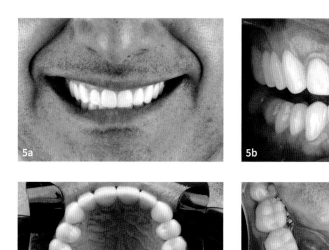

no consensus in the literature concerning the best restorative material for severely worn teeth.

The use of composite resins in patients with eroded teeth is one of the current options and this strategy is well-accepted today because it allows for minimally invasive techniques and provides adequate intraoral finishing and polishing.[4,5] It likewise prevents antagonistic teeth wear.[13,21]

The composite resin brand for the posterior teeth that was selected in this case study was Ceramage (Shofu Dental), which is a micro-hybrid composite resin for laboratory use. This composite, as well as the nano-hybrids, is indicated for the posterior teeth because it presents better mechanical properties (hardness, abrasive resistance, and flexural resistance) when compared to the microfilled composite resins, which have better polishing properties and surface gloss.[14,21] In the anterior sector, two different commercial brands were used in this case report. Empress Direct resin (nano-hybrid resin) was used in the palatal layer to provide better mechanical resistance in the excursion movements. The other commercial brand that was used was the Estelite Omega resin, and this presented better rheologic, finishing, and polishing properties. The best smoothness and surface gloss properties of the Estelite Omega resin were mainly related to the spherical and regular inorganic filler particle sizes.[29-31]

After the end of any rehabilitation, the dental practitioner must be aware of the patient's occlusion in the centric and eccentric movements. Occlusal overloads can generate failures, such as chipping and fracture.[32,33] Another relevant factor is recalling the patients periodically to adjust and repolish the composite resin restorations, while checking the occlusal contacts and for possible early wear.

The limitations of the treatment presented in this clinical report are linked to the engagement of the patient in the care of his rehabilitation, with periodic appointments, as well as the daily care at home. It is extremely important that the patient changes deleterious habits to increase the restorations' longevity, as well using a night mouth guard.   ▦

Conclusion

Within the limitations of the current clinical case, it was concluded that a full-mouth rehabilitation by using composite resins was one of the attainable options for the dental treatment because it required less dental wear. It was economical and less abrasive to the antagonistic teeth than ceramics, thus mainly benefitting the younger patients, who still need to maintain their natural teeth intact for a long time. The treatment technique requires training and attention at all stages of the execution. In addition, it is necessary to follow-up with the patients by scheduling periodic maintenance appointments (polishing, checking the occlusal contacts, and ascertaining the excursion movements), to increase the longevity of this dental rehabilitation.

Acknowledgment

The author MFK thanks the Osteology Foundation, Switzerland, for financial support. during his research period at the Department of Biomaterials, The Sahlgrenska Academy at University of Gothenburg, Gothenburg, Sweden.

Disclosure

The authors do not have any financial interest in the companies whose materials are included in this article.

References

1.   Bartlett D, Phillips K, Smith B. A difference in perspective: the North American and European interpretations of tooth wear. Int J Prosthodont 1999;12:401–408.

2.   West NX, Joiner A. Enamel mineral loss. J Dent 2014;42:2–11.

3.   Peumans M, Politano G, Van Meerbeek B. Treatment of noncarious cervical lesions: when, why, and how. Int J Esthet Dent 2020; 15:16–42.

4.   Carvalho TS, Colon P, Ganss C, et al. Consensus report of the European Federation of Conservative Dentistry: erosive tooth wear—diagnosis and management. Clin Oral Investig 2015;19:1557–1561.

5.   Loomans B, Opdam N, Attin T, et al. Severe tooth wear: European Consensus Statement on Management Guidelines. J Adhes Dent 2017;19:111–119.

6.   Vailati F, Belser UC. Full-mouth adhesive rehabilitation of a severely eroded dentition: the three step technique. Part 1. Eur J Dent 2008;3:30–44.

7.   Kavoura V, Kourtis SG, Zoidis P, Andritsakis DP, Doukoudakis A. Full-mouth rehabilitation of a patient with bulimia nervosa. A case report. Quintessence Int 2005;36: 501–510.

8.   Rinke S, Fischer C. Range of indications for translucent zirconia modifications: clinical and technical aspects. Quintessence Int 2013;44:557–566.

9.   Mesko ME, Sarkis-Onofre R, Cenci MS, et al. Rehabilitation of severely worn teeth: A systematic review. J Dent 2016;48:9–15.

10.   Edelhoff D, Ahlers MO. Occlusal onlays as a modern treatment concept for the reconstruction of severely worn occlusal surfaces. Quintessence Int 2018;49:521–533.

11.   Mainjot AK, Dupont NM, Oudkerk JC, et al. From artisanal to CAD-CAM blocks: state of the art of indirect composites. J Dent Res 2016;95:487–495.

12.   Resende TH, Reis KR, Schlichting LH, et al. Ultrathin CAD-CAM ceramic occlusal veneers and anterior bilaminar veneers for the treatment of moderate dental bio-corrosion: a 1.5-year follow-up. Oper Dent 2018;43:337–346.

13.   Wiegand A, Credé A, Tschammler C, Attin T, Tauböck TT. Enamel wear by antagonistic restorative materials under erosive conditions. Clin Oral Investig 2017;21: 2689–2693.

14.   Zhao X, Pan J, Zhang S, Malmstrom HS, Ren YF. Effectiveness of resin-based materials against erosive and abrasive enamel wear. Clin Oral Investig 2017;21:463–468.

15.   Yadav R, Kumar M. Dental restorative composite materials: A review. J Oral Biosci 2019;61:78–83.

16.   Magne P, Schlichting LH, Maia HP, et al. In vitro fatigue resistance of CAD/CAM composite resin and ceramic posterior occlusal veneers. J Prosthet Dent 2010;104:149–157.

17.   Schlichting LH, Maia HP, Baratieri LN. Novel-design ultra-thin CAD/CAM composite resin and ceramic occlusal veneers for the treatment of severe dental erosion. J Prosthet Dent 2010;105:217–226.

18.   Johnson AC, Versluis A, Tantbirojn D, et al. Fracture strength of CAD/CAM composite and composite-ceramic occlusal veneers. J Prosthodont Res 2014;58: 107–114.

19.   Egbert JS, Johnson AC, Tantbirojn D, et al. Fracture strength of ultrathin occlusal veneer restorations made from CAD/CAM composite or hybrid ceramic materials. Oral Sci Int 2015;12:53–58.

20.   Schlichting LH, Resende TH, Reis KR, et al. Simplified treatment of severe dental erosion with ultrathin CAD-CAM composite occlusal veneers and anterior bilaminar veneers. J Prosthet Dent 2016;116:474–482.

21.   Lucia VO. Centric relation: theory and practice. J Prosthet Dent 1960;10:849–856.

22.   Willis FM. Esthetic of full denture construction. J Am Dent Assoc 1930;17:633–642.

23.   Geerts GAVM, Stuhlinger ME, Nel DG. A comparison of the accuracy of two methods used by pre-doctoral students to measure vertical dimension. J Prosthet Dent 2004;91: 59–66.

24.   Yadav RD, Raisingani D, Jindal D, Mathur R. A comparative analysis of different finishing and polishing devices on nano-filled, microfilled, and hybrid composite: a scanning electron microscopy and profilometric study. Int J Clin Pediatr Dent 2016;9: 201–208.

25.   Sreekumar AV, Rupesh PL, Pradeep N. Nature of occlusion during eccentric mandibular movements in young adults. J Contemp Dent Pract 2012;13:612–617.

26.   Wetselaar P, Lobbezoo F. The tooth wear evaluation system: a modular clinical guideline for the diagnosis and management planning of worn dentitions. J Oral Rehabil 2016;43:69–80.

27.   Katona TR, Eckert GJ. The mechanics of dental occlusion and disclusion. Clin Biomech 2017;50:84–91.

28.   Kumar M, Verma R, Bansal M, et al. To evaluate the severity, distribution of occlusal tooth wear and its correlation with bite force in young North Indian adults. Open Dent J 2018;12:735–741.

29.   Ilie N, Hickel R. Investigations on the mechanical behavior of dental composites. Clin Oral Investig 2009;13:427–438.

30.   Ilie N, Rencz A, Hickel R. Investigations towards nano-hybrid resin-based composites. Clin Oral Investig 2013;17:185–193.

31.   Can Say E, Yurdagüven H, Yaman BC, et al. Surface roughness and morphology of resin composites polished with two-step polishing systems. Dent Mater J 2014;33: 332–342.

32.   Belli R, Geinzer E, Muschweck A, Petschelt A, Lohbauer U. Mechanical fatigue degradation of ceramics versus resin composites for dental restorations. Dent Mater 2014;30:424–432.

33.   Demarco FF, Collares K, Coelho K, et al. Anterior composite restorations: A systematic review on long-term survival and reasons for failure. Dent Mater 2015;31: 1214–1224.

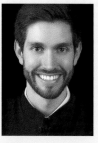

Vinícius F. Lippert

Jonas P. Andrade   Associate Clinical Researcher, Department of Restorative Dentistry, School of Health and Life Sciences, Pontifical Catholic University of Rio Grande do Sul (PUCRS), Porto Alegre, RS, Brazil

Ana M. Spohr   Full Professor, Department of Restorative Dentistry, School of Health and Life Sciences, Pontifical Catholic University of Rio Grande do Sul (PUCRS), Porto Alegre, RS, Brazil

Marcel F. Kunrath   Associate Researcher, Post-Graduate Program of Dentistry, School of Health and Life Sciences, Pontifical Catholic University of Rio Grande do Sul (PUCRS), Porto Alegre, RS, Brazil; and Postdoctoral Researcher, Department of Biomaterials, Institute of Clinical Sciences, The Sahlgrenska Academy at University of Gothenburg, Gothenburg, Sweden

Vinícius F. Lippert   Associate Professor, Department of Restorative Dentistry, School of Health and Life Sciences, Pontifical Catholic University of Rio Grande do Sul (PUCRS), Porto Alegre, RS, Brazil

Correspondence: Vinícius Funghetto Lippert, Department of Restorative Dentistry, School of Health and Life Sciences, Pontifical Catholic University of Rio Grande do Sul (PUCRS), Avenida Ipiranga, 6681 Porto Alegre, Rio Grande do Sul, 90619-900, Brazil.
Email: vinicius.lippert@pucrs.br

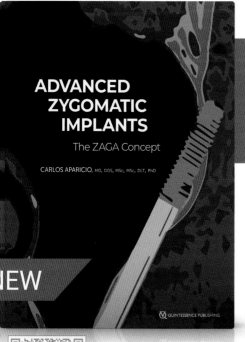

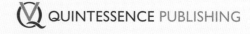

Autotransplantation of an immature mandibular third molar to a recipient site with periradicular lesion: a case report

Ahmad Mekari, DDS, MSc/Abdulkareem Almarrawi, DDS, MSc, PhD/Christian H. Splieth, Prof Dr

Tooth autotransplantation is becoming a predictable method to replace a missing tooth, especially in young patients, with many benefits. This case report presents a 14-year-old male with an unrestorable, decayed mandibular first molar with bifurcation and periapical lesions. After the extraction, the socket was debrided and prepared for an immediate autotransplantation of the immature mandibular third molar. Radiologic and clinical follow-up for 1 year showed periodontal healing with the absence of any complications despite the autotransplantation into an infected site. Thus, third-molar autotransplantation was a good solution to replace an unrestorable first molar with a satisfactory result. Despite the existence of periradicular lesion, the curettage, debridement, and irrigation were enough to perform successful immediate tooth autotransplantation in this case. (Quintessence Int 2023;54:228–233; doi: 10.3290/j.qi.b3631831)

Key words: first mandibular permanent molar, immature mandibular third molar, periradicular lesion, tooth autotransplantation

There are many reasons for missing permanent teeth, such as extractions due to dental caries, periodontal diseases, trauma, or even failed dental treatment. The two main causes of tooth extraction are dental caries and periodontal diseases,[1] and dental trauma is responsible for the loss of many incisors in children and adolescents.[2]

As the first permanent molar erupts early, it is more prone to dental caries, and early extraction may be indicated before adulthood. On the other hand, the early loss offers a great chance to maintain the important, central function of the first permanent molar for normal mastication and dentofacial harmony. Without intervention, early extraction leads to accelerated development and eruption of the second and third molars, decreasing the post-extraction space, and causing lingual tipping and retrusion of incisors, and counterclockwise rotation of the occlusal plane.[3,4]

Besides prosthetic replacement or orthodontic treatment, tooth autotransplantation offers an inexpensive and biologic treatment option, especially in young patients.[5] Tooth autotransplantation is defined as the movement of one tooth from one position to another, within the same person.[6] This could involve the transfer of impacted, embedded, or erupted teeth into extraction sites or surgically prepared sockets.[7]

Autotransplantation of immature third molars as a replacement for decayed first molars was first reported in the 1950s.[8] Since then, autotransplantation of third molars has become an acceptable treatment option for missing posterior teeth, and high success rates have been reported for the autotransplantation of immature third molars.[9]

This case report presents an immediate tooth autotransplantation to replace an unrestorable decayed first mandibular permanent molar in spite of a periradicular lesion, with an immature mandibular third molar.

Case presentation

A 14-year-old male patient was referred to the dental clinic with the chief complaint of pain and discomfort while chewing on the right side of the mandible.

The medical history revealed no general problems. The clinical and radiographic examination showed a severely decayed mandibular right first molar with a bifurcation and peri-

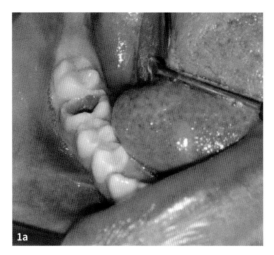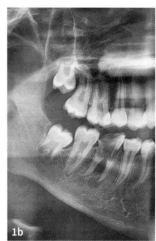

Figs 1a and 1b Clinical and radiographic image of the nonrestorable mandibular first molar where extensive caries led to severe destruction and pulp necrosis in a 14-year-old leading to a periapical lesion. The immature third molar offers the chance for an auto-transplantation as donor tooth, but with only beginning root formation.

apical lesions, without any possibility of performing restorative treatment (Fig 1).

After discussing the treatment options with the parents, it was decided to extract the first molar and perform an auto-transplantation of the immature third molar located in the same quadrant of the mandible.

After local anesthesia with 2% lidocaine and 1:100,000 epinephrine (medicaine 2% with epinephrine, MediS Laboratories), the first molar was extracted, the pathologic tissues were removed by curettage, and the extraction socket was debrided, prepared to fit the donor tooth with preservation of the bony walls intact, and copiously irrigated with saline. After elevating an envelope flap and bone removal, the impacted third molar was atraumatically extracted and quickly repositioned in the recipient site with slight infra-occlusion. The gingival tissue on the mesial and distal aspects of the transplanted molar and the elevated flap were sutured (4/0 silk, SMI) and a radiograph was taken. After the bleeding stopped, the transplanted molar was stabilized with a semirigid splint made of composite resin and orthodontic wire (Fig 2).

Antibiotics (amoxicillin 500 mg every 8 hours for 7 days), nonsteroidal anti-inflammatory drug (ibuprofen 400 mg every 8 hours for 3 days), and mouth rinse (0.12% chlorhexidine gluconate for 10 days) were prescribed along with the according instructions. After 10 days, the splint and sutures were removed and the wound was cleaned with normal saline. After removal of the splint, the tooth already showed good stability.

The patient was evaluated by clinical and radiographic examination at 1, 3, 6, and 12 months, and the success was evaluated according to the primary success criteria of the transplanted tooth of Tsukiboshi et al,[10] which include clinical and radiographic criteria. The clinical criteria include normal mobility, normal percussion sound, no periodontal pocket, no sign of inflammation, and normal function of chewing. The radiographic criteria include normal periodontal space, presence of the lamina dura, and no sign of root resorption. The clinical and radiographic examinations demonstrated the periradicular healing, presence of the lamina dura and periodontal space, the absence of any clinical symptoms, and normal mobility (Fig 3).

Discussion

In general, the ideal treatment option in case of missing permanent teeth are dental implants, but before completion of skeletal growth dental implant placement is not recommended, especially in the posterior mandible, as it leads to progressive infraocclusion of the implant and it may harm adjacent teeth.[11] Thus, implants are contraindicated in young growing patients, and tooth auto-transplantation can be considered a biologic alternative. Besides the low costs, it provides arch space maintenance without alterations to the growing jaw. The formation of a functional periodontal ligament allows eruption of the tooth and promotes alveolar bone development in the receptor area. Afterwards the transplanted teeth can be moved orthodontically and the esthetic results can be superior to prosthetic alternatives. Moreover, it can be performed as a single-step surgical procedure.[12,13]

The success of tooth autotransplantation is related to many factors like the patient, the donor tooth, the recipient site, and the surgical procedure,[14] but it can achieve high success rates when planned and performed properly.[5] The patient in the present case report was healthy and young, with good oral hygiene, which is crucial for the healing process. Good general health and proper postoperative instructions as well as compliance with future appointments and treatment are also important.[15]

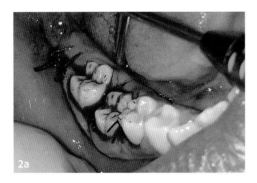
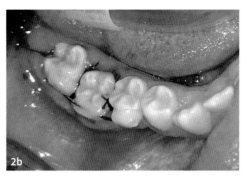
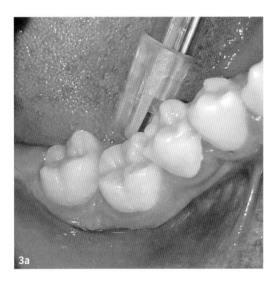
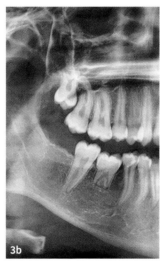

Figs 2a to 2c   Clinical images immediately after autotransplantation and suturing. *(a)* The suturing included the gingival tissue on the mesial and distal aspects of the autotransplanted tooth and the elevated flap. *(b)* Splinting was performed after the bleeding had stopped, with a semirigid splint made using composite resin and orthodontic wire. *(c)* The radiograph taken immediately after autotransplantation shows the third molar fitting well in the socket of the first molar tooth socket. In addition, the large bone defect due to the periapical lesions after the first molar extraction is clearly visible.

Figs 3a and 3b   Clinical and radiographic images of the transplanted third molar at 1-year follow-up with normal appearance of the surrounding soft tissues *(a)*, increased root formation *(b),* periradicular healing as well as the presence of the lamina dura and periodontal space. Thus, the autotransplanted tooth has healed without postoperative complications despite the transplantation into a prior infected site and minimal initial root formation.

The candidate teeth for autotransplantation can be with open or closed apices. Generally, third molars, impacted teeth, premolars, and supernumerary teeth can be excellent donor teeth. The selected tooth for autotransplantation in this case was an immature third molar with beginning root formation, which is quite early and runs the risk of total tooth loss in the case of pulp necrosis as endodontics are not feasible. Donor teeth with one-half to two-thirds complete root formation are more ideal candidates for transplantation due to the existing root part and the potential for further root development with a vital pulp, while endodontic treatment of the transplanted tooth with complete root formation is obligatory.[14,16] The pulp vitality tests in the follow-up periods of the present case showed retained pulp vitality. Waiting for more root development would

have taken about a year, with possible bone loss at the reception site and problems with proper implantation after the complete formation of solid cortical bone. Also, closing of the space would have happened without an adequate space maintainer.

The present patient's recipient site was well debrided to remove the pathologic tissues, prepared to fit the donor tooth along with preserving the bony walls intact, and irrigated with saline. The donor tooth was immediately replanted despite the infection prior to the autotransplantation. Ideally the recipient site should be free from acute infection to receive the transplanted tooth, and in the case of a periapical lesion the tooth autotransplantation should be postponed for 8 to 12 weeks because the residues of inflamed tissue could damage the repair processes of bones and soft tissues after autotransplantation. Postponing the tooth autotransplantation from 8 to 12 weeks will probably result in a site free of inflammation and more comfortable handling of the recipient site due to the immaturity of the osteogenic bone.[16-18] However, in the present case, the good curettage, debridement, and irrigation were enough to perform successful immediate tooth autotransplantation without the need to postpone the autotransplantation procedure to a second, subsequent visit.

The recipient site should have good bone support to receive the transplanted tooth.[16] It was found that lack of a buccal cortex and a narrow recipient site are considered risk factors for the failure of the operation.[19] For accurate dimensioning and optimal locating of the artificial socket relative to the alveolar bone borders and the adjacent teeth roots, a 3D surgical guide and a replica of the transplanted donor tooth were used based on computerized 3D simulations and guidance.[20] In the present case, the bony walls of the recipient site were preserved intact and there was enough space to receive the donor tooth.

The extraction of the third molar was done carefully to preserve the periodontal ligament, and the extracted third molar was immediately replanted in the prepared recipient site. One of the most important factors for the success of the transplanted tooth is preserving the periodontal ligament, so the careful extraction of the donor tooth is very important.[21] Also, the immediate replantation of extracted teeth into a fresh extraction socket is known to have a good prognosis, while transplanted teeth to recipient beds prepared at the same time show a high prevalence of root resorption.[22] The oral surgeon must have considerable skill and patience, and a careful surgical procedure is essential to achieve a successful outcome.[12]

Various techniques for stabilizing transplanted teeth have been described, such as fixation with sutures, ligatures, orthodontic brackets, and composite resins. The period of immobilization varies from 1 to 6 weeks, but short-term flexible splinting for 7 to 10 days appears to be more favorable.[9] In the present case, a semirigid splint for 10 days was selected, and the donor tooth was kept out of occlusal contact to prevent occlusal forces from interfering with the healing of the periodontium.

The present patient was healthy and young, so antibiotics were not prescribed before surgery. The benefit of using antibiotics before surgical and nonsurgical dental procedures is controversial. While systematic reviews suggest that antibiotic prophylaxis may be effective for reducing postoperative complications, more recent investigations with better methodologic quality have failed to find adequate scientific evidence that supports the routine use of antibiotics to prevent infectious complications in healthy patients. Moreover, the immune defenses of young healthy patients are sufficient. Antibiotics are considered pharmacologic adjuvants, and correct management of oral bacterial contamination along with atraumatic surgical techniques are the main factors influencing the success rates of surgical interventions, rather than antibiotic administration. Antibiotic prophylaxis is advisable only in medically compromised patients with a risk of severe infective complications.[23-27]

In the present case, however, amoxicillin was prescribed after surgery because surgery included first molar extraction, removing the pathologic tissues from the extraction socket by curettage and debridement, preparing the extraction socket to fit the donor tooth, elevating a flap, and bone removal to extract the impacted third molar. Postoperative systemic antibiotics therapy is recommended for long-duration surgeries with osteotomy or antibiotic therapies in complicated infections. Commonly, penicillin is considered to be the first-line drug and the gold standard for the treatment of odontogenic infections because of its cost-effectiveness, low incidence of side effects, and appropriate antimicrobial activity. Amoxicillin is a penicillin antibiotic and is commonly considered to be the first line of treatment in nonallergic patients.[27,28]

In other cases, tooth autotransplantation can be accompanied by complications: Most common are root ankylosis, root resorption, and pulp necrosis.[9] Still, the systematic review and meta-analysis by Rohof et al[14] in 2018, found that the survival and success rates of autotransplantation teeth with incomplete root formation were very high (> 95%), and severe complications such as ankyloses (2.0%), root resorption (2.9%), and pulp necrosis (3.3%) were below the failures of implants.[14] No complications were reported in the present case after follow-up for 1 year, indicating an excellent prognosis, especially with the normal root development. ▦

Conclusion

In this case the 1-year follow-up demonstrated good gingival and periodontal healing as well as normal development for a tooth autotransplantation of an immature third molar into the socket of a lost first permanent molar, despite the existence of periradicular lesion at the donor site and only beginning root formation of the third molar. Curettage, debridement, and irrigation were enough to perform successful immediate tooth autotransplantation.

Disclosure

The authors confirm there are no conflicts of interest.

References

1. Chrysanthakopoulos NA. Reasons for extraction of permanent teeth in Greece: a five-year follow-up study. Int Dent J 2011; 61:19–24.

2. Krastl G, Filippi A, Weiger R. Initial management of dental trauma: musts, shoulds, and cans. Quintessence Int 2020;51:763–774.

3. Saber AM, Altoukhi DH, Horaib MF, El-Housseiny AA, Alamoudi NM, Sabbagh HJ. Consequences of early extraction of compromised first permanent molar: a systematic review. BMC Oral Health 2018;18:59.

4. Gill DS, Lee RT, Tredwin CJ. Treatment planning for the loss of first permanent molars. Dent Update 2001;28:304–308.

5. Pecci Lloret MP, Martínez EP, Rodríguez Lozano FJ, et al. Influencing factors in autotransplantation of teeth with open apex: a review of the literature. Appl Sci 2021; 11:4037.

6. Leffingwell CM. Autogenous tooth transplantation: a therapeutic alternative. Dent Surv 1980;56:22–23,26.

7. Northway WM, Konigsberg S. Autogenic tooth transplantation. The "state of the art". Am J Orthod 1980;77:146–162.

8. Apeel H. Autoplasty of enucleated prefunctional third molars. J Oral Surg (Chic) 1950;8:289–296.

9. Dioguardi M, Quarta C, Sovento D, et al. Autotransplantation of the third molar: a therapeutic alternative to the rehabilitation of a missing tooth: a scoping review. Bioengineering (Basel) 2021;8:120.

10. Tsukiboshi M, Andreasen J, Asai Y. Autotransplantation of teeth. Chicago; Quintessence, 2001:10–14,97,152–167.

11. Op Heij DG, Opdebeeck H, van Steenberghe D, Quirynen M. Age as compromising factor for implant insertion. Periodontol 2000 2003;33:172–184.

12. Machado LA, do Nascimento RR, Ferreira DM, Mattos CT, Vilella OV. Long-term prognosis of tooth autotransplantation: a systematic review and meta-analysis. Int J Oral Maxillofac Surg 2016;45:610–617.

13. Yoon Y, Kim YG, Suh JY, Lee JM. The prognosis of autotransplanted tooth on molar region: 5 years follow up cases. Oral Biol Res 2017;41:147–152.

14. Rohof ECM, Kerdijk W, Jansma J, Livas C, Ren Y. Autotransplantation of teeth with incomplete root formation: a systematic review and meta-analysis. Clin Oral Investig 2018;22:1613–1624.

15. Armstrong L, O'Reilly C, Ahmed B. Autotransplantation of third molars: a literature review and preliminary protocols. Br Dent J 2020;228:247–251.

16. Nimčenko T, Omerca G, Varinauskas V, Bramanti E, Signorino F, Cicciù M. Tooth auto-transplantation as an alternative treatment option: A literature review. Dent Res J (Isfahan) 2013;10:1–6.

17. Tsukiboshi M. Autotransplantation of teeth: requirements for predictable success. Dent Traumatol 2002;18:157–180.

18. Arbel Y, Lvovsky A, Azizi H, Hadad A, Averbuch Zehavi E, Via S et al. Autotransplantation after primary bone repair of a recipient site with a large periradicular lesion: a case report. Int Endod J 2019;52:1789–1796.

19. Aoyama S, Yoshizawa M, Niimi K, Sugai T, Kitamura N, Saito C. Prognostic factors for autotransplantation of teeth with complete root formation. Oral Surg Oral Med Oral Pathol Oral Radiol 2012;114(5 Suppl):S216–S228.

20. Ashkenazi M, Shashua D, Kegen S, Nuni E, Duggal M, Shuster A. Computerized three-dimensional design for accurate orienting and dimensioning artificial dental socket for tooth autotransplantation. Quintessence Int 2018;49:663–671.

21. Park JH, Tai K, Hayashi D. Tooth autotransplantation as a treatment option: a review. J Clin Pediatr Dent 2010;35:129–135.

22. Marques-Ferreira M, Rabaça-Botelho MF, Carvalho L, Oliveiros B, Palmeirão-Carrilho EV. Autogenous tooth transplantation: evaluation of pulp tissue regeneration. Med Oral Patol Oral Cir Bucal 2011;16:e984–e989.

23. Lollobrigida M, Pingitore G, Lamazza L, Mazzucchi G, Serafini G, De Biase A. Antibiotics to prevent surgical site infection (SSI) in oral surgery: survey among Italian dentists. Antibiotics (Basel) 2021;10:949.

24. Termine N, Panzarella V, Ciavarella D, et al. Antibiotic prophylaxis in dentistry and oral surgery: use and misuse. Int Dent J 2009;59:263–270.

25. Yanine N, Sabelle N, Vergara-Gárate V, et al. Effect of antibiotic prophylaxis for preventing infectious complications following impacted mandibular third molar surgery. A randomized controlled trial. Med Oral Patol Oral Cir Bucal 2021;26:e703–e710.

26. Chugha A, Patnanaa AK, Kumara P, Chugha VK, Kherab D, Singh S. Critical analysis of methodological quality of systematic reviews and meta-analysis of antibiotics in third molar surgeries using AMSTAR 2. J Oral Biol Craniofac Res 2020;10: 441–449.

27. Buonavoglia A, Leone P, Solimando AG, et al. Antibiotics or no antibiotics, that is the question: an update on efficient and effective use of antibiotics in dental practice. Antibiotics (Basel) 2021;10:550.

28. Ahmadi H, Ebrahimi A, Ahmadi F. Antibiotic therapy in dentistry. Int J Dent 2021;2021:6667624.

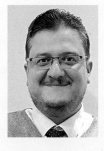

Ahmad Mekari

Ahmad Mekari PhD student, Department of Oral & Maxillofacial Surgery, Damascus University, Damascus, Syria

Abdulkareem Almarrawi Assistant Professor, Department of Oral & Maxillofacial Surgery, Damascus University, Damascus, Syria

Christian H. Splieth Professor and Head of the Department of Preventive and Paediatric Dentistry, University of Greifswald, Greifswald, Germany

Correspondence: Prof Dr Ch H Splieth, Department of Preventive and Pediatric Dentistry, University of Greifswald, Fleischmannstr. 42, 17487 Greifswald, Germany. Email splieth@uni-greifswald.de

First submission: 19 Oct 2022
Acceptance: 19 Nov 2022
Online publication: 29 Nov 2022

PERIODONTOLOGY

Effect of antibiotics as an adjuvant to subgingival instrumentation on systemic inflammation in patients with periodontitis: a randomized clinical trial

Manpreet Kaur, MDS/Rajinder Kumar Sharma, MDS/Shikha Tewari, MDS/Ritika Arora, MDS/
Nishi Tanwar, MDS/Aditi Sangwan, MDS

Objectives: The aim of the present study was to evaluate the effect on systemic inflammation of subgingival instrumentation (SI) with or without antibiotics. Moreover, systemic parameters were compared between periodontally healthy (PH) individuals and periodontitis patients. **Method and materials:** Patients with generalized periodontitis: stage III and PH individuals were recruited. Forty eight periodontitis patients were randomly allocated to each treatment group; systemic antibiotics for seven days after completion of SI (AB group), or SI alone (SI group). Periodontal parameters, serum high-sensitivity C-reactive protein (hsCRP), and hematological parameters were assessed at baseline and at week 8. Multivariate analysis was applied to analyze predictive effect of treatment allocated and improvement in periodontal parameters on change in systemic parameters. **Results:** At baseline, hsCRP, total leukocyte count (TLC), neutrophil, and monocyte count were significantly higher in periodontitis patients. There was comparable reduction in neutrophil count in both treatment groups. At week 8, change in periodontal parameters was similar in treatment groups, except for probing pocket depth (PPD). Improvement in both PPD and clinical attachment level (CAL) and CAL alone was predictive of change in TLC and lymphocyte count, respectively. **Conclusion:** This study failed to demonstrate the significant benefit of systemic antibiotics as an adjuvant to SI on improvement in periodontal inflammation and systemic inflammatory parameters, despite significantly higher reduction in PPDs. (*Quintessence Int 2023;54:460–471; doi: 10.3290/j.qi.b3942249*)

Key words: C-reactive protein, inflammation, lymphocyte count, root planing

Non-communicable diseases (NCDs) are the major cause of mortality, accounting for 74% of the total deaths worldwide.[1] Of all NCD-related mortalities, 43.7% deaths are attributed to cardiovascular diseases (CVDs).[1] Infectious agents are postulated to be either directly involved in the CVD process or increase the systemic inflammation that further mediates its effects.[2] Periodontitis is characterized by microbially infected, host-mediated inflammation that results in loss of periodontal attachment.[3] Periodontitis is detrimental not only to periodontal tissues but also to cardiovascular health.[2] Periodontitis increases the propensity for occurrence of CVDs.[2] This effect is due to involvement of periodontal pathogens in formation and progression of atheromatous plaques.[4] As reported in mice,[5] inflammation induced by periodontal pathogens in vascular walls seems to result in formation of atheromatous plaques. Moreover, in periodontitis patients, periodontal pathogens are isolated from human atheromatous plaques.[6] Additionally, periodontal pathogens entering the systemic circulation stimulate liver to secrete acute phase proteins, such as high-sensitivity C-reactive protein (hsCRP) in circulation. Periodontitis also leads to alterations in total leukocyte count (TLC), differential leukocyte count (DLC), and blood parameters related to platelet activity. Higher blood viscosity due to alterations in TLC, DLC, and platelet parameters associated with periodontitis may be responsible for increased risk of thrombus formation. The altered count of these hematologic parameters due to periodontitis is of concern because of their association with increased risk for CVDs.[2,7-9] Also, serum hsCRP is predictive of

CVDs independent of traditional risk factors.[10] Owing to increased prevalence of severe periodontitis, being the sixth most prevalent condition affecting 11.2% population worldwide,[11] treatment of periodontitis is necessary not only to restore periodontal health but also to attain systemic health.

The periodontal pocket is colonized with anerobic bacteria responsible for chronic nonhealing lesions.[12,13] These morphologic and ecologic alterations are associated with loss of health-associated resilience of normal oral microbiome. It has the potential of creating a vicious cycle of microbially driven periodontal inflammation and more virulent microbial challenge.[14] Subgingival instrumentation (SI) results in resolution of periodontal inflammation as well as reduction in probing pocket depth (PPD). Despite clinical benefits of SI, putative periodontal pathogens cannot be eradicated with SI because of their penetrance into hard tissues of teeth including dentin and cementum,[15] and deeper soft periodontal tissues[16] through ulcerated pocket epithelium. Therefore, systemic antibiotics as an adjuvant to SI may be the treatment of choice. In a review article it was concluded that combination of systemic amoxicillin and metronidazole resulted in greater reduction in the number of periodontal pathogens and better clinical outcomes as compared to SI alone.[17] The suppressive effect of systemic antibiotics on periodontal pathogens was evident even at 12 months posttreatment and resulted in a significantly greater reduction in the number of sites with PPD ≥ 5 mm and a higher percentage of subjects reaching the clinical end point for treatment (≤ four sites with PPD ≥ 5 mm).[18] Furthermore, findings of a meta-analysis revealed that combination of systemic amoxicillin and metronidazole as an adjuvant to SI had an increased effect of about 40% to 50% in PPD reduction, higher percentage of pocket closure, clinical attachment level (CAL) gain, and bleeding on probing (BOP) reduction with maintenance of achieved clinical results up to 12 months of follow-up.[19] The presence of pathogenic bacteria is not only limited to periodontal tissues but is also evident in circulation and atheromatous plaques. Treatment of severe periodontitis with SI and systemic antibiotics,[20] or local drug delivery system[21] has been reported to bear a positive effect on systemic health by reducing systemic inflammation[20,21] and improving endothelial function.[20] However, a meta-analysis revealed that SI resolves systemic inflammation measured in terms of reduction in hsCRP only in patients with other comorbidities.[22]

An additional role of systemic antibiotics as an adjuvant to SI versus SI alone has not been evaluated to date. With this aim, the present randomized trial was conducted to evaluate the effect of combination of systemic amoxicillin and metronidazole as an adjuvant to SI versus SI alone on resolution of systemic inflammation measured in terms of variations in hsCRP, and hematologic parameters including TLC, DLC, platelet count, mean platelet volume (MPV), and platelet distribution width (PDW) in patients with periodontitis.

Method and materials

Study design and ethics statement

The present parallel-design, examiner blinded, randomized clinical trial was conducted in department of Periodontics, Post Graduate Institute of Dental Sciences (PGIDS), Rohtak, Haryana, India. The study protocol was approved by the Biomedical and Health Research Ethics Committee (PGIDS/BHRC/20/13). The study was conducted in accordance with the Declaration of Helsinki 1975, as revised in 2013.

Study population

Individuals aged 35 to 45 years were recruited from the outpatient department of periodontics. The study population included systemically healthy individuals having at least 20 natural teeth excluding third molars. The study population comprised periodontitis patients (25 women and 23 men; mean age 39.67 ± 3.55 years) and periodontally heathy (PH) individuals (10 females, and 8 males; mean age 38.94 ± 3.73 years). Periodontitis criteria included stage III periodontitis[3] with ≥ 30% teeth involved and BOP at > 30% sites.[23] PH individuals were defined as having < 10% bleeding sites with PPD ≤ 3 mm.[23]

Exclusion criteria

Exclusion criteria were as follows:

- history of periodontal treatment in the previous 1 year
- presence of periapical lesions due to caries or periodontitis
- undergoing or requiring an extensive dental or orthodontic treatment
- individuals requiring prophylactic antibiotics prior to dental treatment
- confirmed or assumed allergies or hypersensitivity reactions to amoxicillin and/or metronidazole
- alcohol consumers
- history of systemic medications known to influence periodontal status such as steroids, immunosuppressants, antibiotics, anti-inflammatory drugs, lipid lowering drugs, anti-convulsants, anti-coagulants, anti-hypertensives, or any other host modulatory drugs within 6 months prior to study commencement

- pregnant women or lactating mothers
- current or former users of tobacco in any form
- history of infections within 2 months prior to study commencement.

Individuals meeting the inclusion criteria were explained the purpose of the study, provided with a patient information sheet, and enrolled after obtaining written informed consent.

Sample size calculation

Sample size was estimated using the software G-Power 3.0.10 (Heinrich-Heine University, Dusseldorf, Dusseldorf, Germany). With 80% power and α error of 5%, to detect a difference of 0.5 mg/L in hsCRP between the two treatment groups based on a previous study,[22] for a standard deviation of 0.5 mg/L, the sample size was calculated to be 18 individuals in each group. To compensate for potential drop-outs, 24 individuals were recruited in each treatment group.

Randomization

Patients with periodontitis were randomly allocated to receive one of the two treatments (Fig 1). Randomization was performed by block randomization technique (four-unit block size), with equal allocation between groups by a clinician unrelated to the present study. Allocation sequence was concealed in an opaque envelope. As placebo drug was not allocated, patients were not blinded to the assigned treatment group. However, the researchers (RS) assessing the outcomes of the study, and performing SI (MK) were unaware of treatment allocated.

Periodontal examination

Plaque Index (PI),[24] Gingival Index (GI),[25] BOP, PPD, and CAL were recorded using a periodontal probe (PCP-UNC 15 periodontal probe; Hu-Friedy) at six sites per tooth excluding third molars. Periodontal inflamed surface area (PISA) was calculated.[26] PPD, BOP, CAL, and recession were taken into consideration for calculating the PISA using a freely available spreadsheet (www.parsprototo.info). All periodontal parameters were analyzed at baseline and during the follow-up visit at 8 weeks in both treatment groups. As PH individuals participated only at baseline, periodontal parameters were recorded only at baseline. Periodontal examination was carried out by a single investigator blinded to treatment allocation (RS) to preclude inter-examiner variability. Prior to study commencement, the calibration exercise was performed at two occasions 48 hours apart in ten periodontitis patients not included in the present study. The intraclass correlation coefficient for PPD and CAL was calculated to be 0.92 and 0.90, respectively.

Anthropometric measurement

Body mass index (BMI) was calculated in the study population at baseline.

Evaluation of hsCRP and hematologic parameters

Following overnight fasting, venous blood samples were obtained from all the participants of the study at baseline. Blood samples were again collected at 8 weeks for both treatment groups.

Serum hsCRP was measured using commercial enzyme-linked immunosorbent assay (ELISA) kits (Calbiotech). Assays were carried out according to the manufacturers' recommendations.

Total leukocyte count (TLC), differential leukocyte count (DLC) including neutrophil count, lymphocyte count, monocyte count, eosinophil count, and basophil count; platelet count; MPV; and PDW were assessed. All hematologic parameters were assessed using an automated hematology analyzer (BC-5800, Mindray).

Periodontal treatment

At baseline, after periodontal examination and blood sample collection, oral hygiene instructions were given to periodontitis patients. SI was then performed in various sessions using manual scalers (Hu-Friedy), curettes (Hu-Friedy), and an ultrasonic scaler (EMS, Nylon) by a single researcher (MK), and was completed within 1 week. One treatment group was prescribed amoxicillin (500 mg) and metronidazole (400 mg) thrice daily for 7 days (AB group) at the last session of SI. The SI group received only SI treatment.

Follow-up visits and reevaluation

Patients of both treatment groups were recalled at weeks 4 and 8. Professional plaque control was performed, and reinforcement of oral hygiene instructions was done at week 4. At week 8, periodontal examination was performed. Serum hsCRP and hematologic parameters were again analyzed for both treatment groups.

Fig 1 CONSORT flow diagram of the study population.

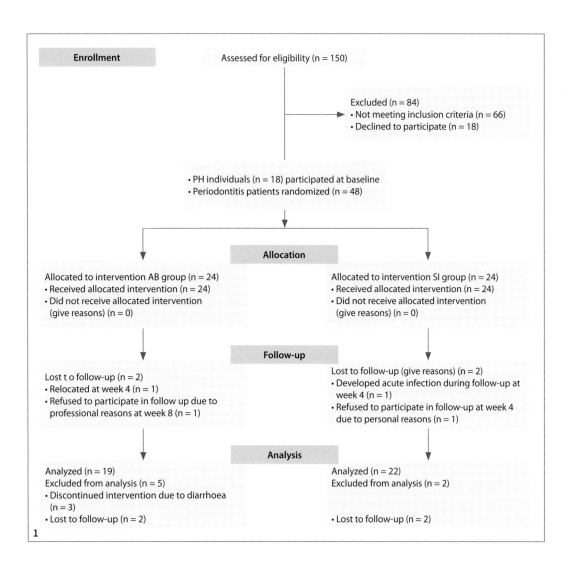

Outcome variables

Change in hsCRP at week 8 was the primary outcome variable, and changes in hematologic parameters were the secondary outcome variables.

Statistical analysis

Statistical analysis was performed using the statistical software program SPSS (v.20, IBM). Normality of data was determined using the Shapiro–Wilk test. Normally distributed and nonnormally distributed continuous data are presented as mean± standard deviation (SD) and median (25th; 75th percentile), respectively. Difference in between groups was assessed using the unpaired Student t test (for normally distributed data) and the Mann–Whitney U test (for nonnormally distributed data). Intragroup comparison at two different time points was done using the paired t test and Wilcoxon signed-rank test for parametric and nonparametric data, respectively. Sex, being a categorical variable, is presented as number (percentage), and was analyzed using the chi-squared test. Spearman rank correlation coefficient was calculated to determine the association between the improvement in periodontal parameters and the change in systemic parameters at week 8. Parameters having significant correlations were further analyzed using multivariate linear regression to assess whether treatment group and improvement in periodontal parameters predicted change in systemic parameters. Statistical significance was set at $P<.05$.

Results

Study sample

The PH group included 18 patients. In total, 24 periodontitis patients were enrolled in each treatment group (Fig 1). However, 19 patients in the AB group and 22 patients in the SI group completed the 8-week follow-up. Details of recruitment and drop-outs of the study population are shown in the CONSORT flow diagram (Fig 1). The actual study start date was 26 November 2021, and the study was completed on 10 June 2022.

Demographic and anthropometric variables

There were no statistically significant differences in any of the variables between periodontitis patients and PH individuals ($P > .05$; Table 1) at baseline. Variables were also comparable between the AB and SI groups ($P > .05$; Table 1).

Periodontal parameters

All the periodontal parameters were significantly higher in patients with periodontitis than in PH individuals at baseline ($P = .000$; Table 1). At baseline, all periodontal parameters were comparable in both the treatment groups ($P > .05$; Table 1), except for a significantly higher PPD in the AB group than in the SI group ($P = .018$; Table 1).

At 8 weeks after periodontal treatment, both treatments (AB and SI) led to significant improvement/change [Δ] in periodontal parameters ($P = .000$; Table 1). ΔPI, ΔGI, ΔBOP, ΔCAL, and ΔPISA were comparable in both the AB group and the SI group, apart from a significantly higher ΔPPD in the AB group than in the SI group ($P = .043$; Table 1).

hsCRP and hematologic parameters

At baseline, compared to PH individuals, periodontitis patients had a significantly higher hsCRP, TLC, neutrophil count, and monocyte count ($P < .05$; Table 2). However, lymphocyte count, eosinophil count, basophil count, platelet count, MPV, and PDW were comparable in periodontitis patients and PH individuals ($P > .05$; Table 2).

At baseline and at week 8, there was no significant difference in hsCRP and other hematologic parameters in both the AB and the SI groups ($P > .05$; Table 2). The effect size for ΔhsCRP was −0.608 with 95% confidence interval (CI) of −1.999 to 1.611. There was a significant decrease in neutrophil count in both the treatment groups at week 8 ($P < .05$; Table 2); however, Δneutrophil count was comparable in the AB group and SI group ($P > .05$; Table 2) with effect size (95% CI) of 0.199 (−0.342 to 0.656). Effect sizes (95% CI) for ΔTLC, Δlymphocyte count, Δmonocyte count, Δeosinophil count, and Δbasophil count were 0.048 (−0.789 to 0.918), −0.130 (−0.516 to 0.340), 0.042 (−0.088 to 0.101), −0.123 (−0.105 to 0.071), and 0.433 (−0.003 to 0.015), respectively. ΔPlatelet count, ΔMPV, and ΔPDW had effect sizes (95% CI) of 0.005 (−31.488 to 31.966), −0.524 (−1.052 to 0.100), and −0.348 (−1.130 to 0.328), respectively.

Correlation and multivariate analysis between Δperiodontal parameters and Δsystemic parameters

A significant positive correlation was observed in the following parameters: ΔPPD/Δbasophil count (rho = 0.437, $P = .004$), ΔCAL/Δbasophil count (rho = 0.439, $P = .004$) (Table 3). A significant negative correlation existed between the following parameters: ΔBOP/Δeosinophil count (rho = −0.323, $P = .039$), ΔPPD/Δeosinophil count (rho = −0.328, $P = .036$), ΔCAL/ΔTLC (rho = −0.316, $P = .044$), ΔCAL/Δlymphocyte count (rho = −0.374, $P = .016$), ΔCAL/Δmonocyte count (rho = −0.374, $P = .016$), ΔCAL/Δeosinophil count (rho = −0.360, $P = .021$), and ΔPISA/Δeosinophil count (rho = −0.374, $P = .016$) (Table 3). However, ΔhsCRP, Δneutrophil count, Δplatelet count, ΔMPV, and ΔPDW had no association with Δperiodontal parameters ($P > .05$, Table 3).

Multivariate analysis revealed that treatment intervention (AB or SI group) did not predict Δhematologic parameters at week 8 ($P > .05$; Table 4). ΔPPD was a positive predictor whereas ΔCAL was a negative predictor for ΔTLC ($P = .041$, $P = .007$, respectively, Table 4). ΔCAL was a significant negative predictor for Δlymphocyte count ($P = .020$; Table 4).

Discussion

The degree of periodontal inflammation, periodontal destruction, measured in terms of PISA and CAL, respectively, as well as the amount of plaque were comparable in AB and SI groups at baseline. Similar improvement in periodontal parameters was evident in both the treatment groups at week 8. However, in the AB group, a significantly greater improvement in PPD was found than in the SI group, which may be due to a higher PPD at baseline in the AB group, as sites with deeper periodontal pockets undergo better healing than sites with shallower PPD.[27]

In agreement with previous studies,[28,29] serum hsCRP levels were significantly higher in periodontitis patients (mean ± SD 3.36 ± 3.27 mg/L) than in PH individuals (1.01 ± 1.08 mg/L). There

Table 1 Characteristics of study population at baseline, at week 8, and improvement (Δ) in periodontal parameters at week 8 compared to baseline

Variable			PH (n = 18)	Periodontitis patients (n = 41) AB (n = 19)	SI (n = 22)	P value
Demographic characteristics	Age (y)	Baseline	38.50 (35.75;42.50)	40.00 (36.00;44.00)		.342†
		Baseline	NA	37.00 (36.00;42.00)	40.00 (36.75;45.00)	.202†
	Sex (M:F), n (%)	Baseline	8 (44.44):10 (55.56)	16 (39.02):25 (60.98)		.696‖
		Baseline	NA	8 (42.11):11 (57.89)	8 (36.36):14 (63.64)	.707‖
Anthropometric parameter	BMI (kg/m²)	Baseline	24.59±3.22	25.34±3.86		.473‡
		Baseline	NA	26.50±2.60	24.33±4.50	.072‡
Periodontal parameters	Mean PI	Baseline	0.09 (0.06;0.20)	1.97 (1.71;2.26)		.000†*
		Baseline	NA	1.97 (1.77;2.24)	1.99 (1.64;2.32)	.855†
		Week 8	NA	0.17 (0.07;0.44)	0.28 (0.17;0.56)	.154†
		Δ	NA	1.73 (1.45;1.93)	1.57 (1.30;1.78)	.205†
		P value	NA	.000§*	.000§*	NA
	Mean GI	Baseline	0.05 (0.01;0.06)	1.32 (1.19;1.46)		.000†*
		Baseline	NA	1.35 (1.20;1.48)	1.30 (1.16;1.42)	.340†
		Week 8	NA	0.15 (0.04;0.32)	0.11 (0.05;0.22)	.656†
		Δ	NA	1.22 (1.01;1.33)	1.17 (1.06;1.21)	.556†
		P value	NA	.000§*	.000§*	NA
	Mean BOP (%)	Baseline	3.94 (2.98;6.45)	66.07 (55.93;78.87)		.000†*
		Baseline	NA	67.33 (57.69;79.76)	64.51 (53.72;78.72)	.583†
		Week 8	NA	10.67 (6.79;28.57)	13.03 (8.74;18.16)	.754†
		Δ	NA	50.64 (47.43;63.09)	53.09 (40.40;62.63)	.937†
		P value	NA	.000§*	.000§*	NA
	Mean PPD (mm)	Baseline	1.49 (1.19;1.77)	4.01 (3.68;4.57)		.000†*
		Baseline	NA	4.32 (4.01;4.61)	3.87 (3.63;4.14)	.018†*
		Week 8	NA	2.90 (2.58;3.84)	3.09 (2.69;3.32)	.714†
		Δ	NA	1.18 (0.93;1.64)	0.91 (0.50;1.36)	.043†*
		P value	NA	.000§*	.000§*	NA
	Mean CAL (mm)	Baseline	0.00 (0.00;0.05)	4.49 (4.18;4.95)		.000†*
		Baseline	NA	4.62 (4.24;5.09)	4.38 (4.02;4.75)	.261†
		Week 8	NA	3.34 (3.04;4.25)	3.55 (3.28;4.11)	.574†
		Δ	NA	1.00 (0.88;1.28)	0.91(0.40;1.37)	.308†
		P value	NA	.000§*	.000§*	NA
	Mean PISA (mm²)	Baseline	40.20 (31.78;72.83)	2,021.04 (1,422.48;2,295.86)		.000†*
		Baseline	NA	2,086.97 (1,528.48;2,412.38)	1,684.31 (1,385.78;2,291.70)	.219†
		Week 8	NA	237.94 (102.96;384.21)	283.18 (207.33;413.19)	.548†
		Δ	NA	1,748.43 (1,202.35;2,043.02)	1,394.32 (1,082.96;1,848.49)	.239†
		P value	NA	.000§*	.000§*	NA

Parametric and nonparametric data are presented as mean ± SD or median (25th; 75th percentile), respectively.
*Statistical significance (P < .05).
†Difference between groups at each time point was assessed by the Mann–Whitney U test (nonparametric data)
‡Difference between groups at each time point was assessed by the unpaired Student t test (parametric data).
§Intragroup difference over time was analyzed using Wilcoxan signed-rank test (nonparametric data).
‖Sex was compared between groups using chi-squared test.
BMI, body mass index; BOP, bleeding on probing; CAL, clinical attachment level; F, female; GI, gingival index; M, male; NA, not applicable; PI, Plaque Index; PISA, periodontal inflamed surface area; PPD, probing pocket depth.

are contradictory findings on the effect of SI on hsCRP,[29-32] and a meta-analysis[22] reported no effect of SI on hsCRP in systemically healthy individuals. Similarly, the present study reported no change in hsCRP levels in periodontitis patients treated with SI. Treatment with antibiotics as an adjuvant also had no effect on reduction of hsCRP, although previous studies reported that periodontal treatment with SI and systemic[20] or local antibiotics[21] resulted in a decrease in hsCRP.[20,21] However, a recent meta-analysis supports the findings of the present study that SI alone or with local or systemic antibiotics has no advantage in

Table 2 Serum inflammatory marker and hematologic parameters at baseline and at week 8, and their improvement (Δ) at week 8 in the study population

Variables			PH (n = 18)	Periodontitis patients (n = 41) AB (n = 19)	SI (n = 22)	P value
Serum inflammatory marker	hsCRP (mg/L)	Baseline	0.41 (0.29;1.74)	2.59 (1.10;4.33)		.001†*
		Baseline	NA	3.21 (1.34;5.17)	2.14 (0.67;3.56)	.229†
		Week 8	NA	3.57 (1.39;5.61)	1.59 (0.81;5.53)	.272†
		Δ	NA	0.49 (−0.84;1.52)	−0.10 (−1.70;1.78)	.794†
		P value	NA	.687§	.935§	NA
Hematologic parameters	TLC (× 10⁹/L)	Baseline	5.27 (4.46;6.63)	6.32 (5.33;7.59)		.024†*
		Baseline	NA	6.55 (5.35;7.54)	6.30 (5.23;7.68)	.410†
		Week 8	NA	5.63 (5.21;7.96)	6.00 (5.06;7.25)	.629†
		Δ	NA	0.38 (−0.67;1.32)	0.20 (−0.66;1.58)	.927†
		P value	NA	.165§	.205§	NA
	Neutrophil count (× 10⁹/L)	Baseline	2.92 ± 1.02	3.82 ± 1.01		.003‡*
		Baseline	NA	3.99 ± 0.92	3.66 ± 1.08	.302‡
		Week 8	NA	3.46 ± 0.97	3.29 ± 1.14	.608‡
		Δ	NA	0.54 ± 0.77	0.38 ± 0.80	.528‡
		P value	NA	.007¶*	.038¶*	NA
	Lymphocyte count (× 10⁹/L)	Baseline	2.12 (1.59;2.39)	2.02 (1.64;2.53)		.974†
		Baseline	NA	1.96 (1.65;2.32)	2.06 (1.58; 2.67)	.744†
		Week 8	NA	2.12 (1.71;2.28)	2.00 (1.43;2.61)	.548†
		Δ	NA	−0.01(−0.34;0.25)	0.19(−0.36;0.56)	.513†
		P value	NA	.615§	.721§	NA
	Monocyte count (× 10⁹/L)	Baseline	0.33 ± 0.13	0.41 ± 0.14		.036‡*
		Baseline	NA	0.42 ± 0.15	0.41 ± 0.14	.692‡
		8th week	NA	0.40 ± 0.10	0.39 ± 0.13	.752‡
		Δ	NA	0.03 ± 0.15	0.02 ± 0.15	.895‡
		P value	NA	.451¶	.554¶	NA
	Eosinophil count (× 10⁹/L)	Baseline	0.13 (0.07;0.24)	0.16 (0.10;0.34)		.378†
		Baseline	NA	0.18 (0.09;0.34)	0.15 (0.10;0.34)	.875†
		Week 8	NA	0.18 (0.14;0.35)	0.15 (0.10;0.34)	.417†
		Δ	NA	−0.02 (−0.07;0.02)	−0.01 (−0.06;0.05)	.556†
		P value	NA	.276§	.782§	NA
	Basophil count (× 10⁹/L)	Baseline	0.02(0.02;0.03)	0.02(0.01;0.02)		.171†
		Baseline	NA	0.02 (0.01;0.03)	0.02 (0.010;.02)	.425†
		Week 8	NA	0.02 (0.01;0.02)	0.02 (0.01;0.03)	.639†
		Δ	NA	0.00 (−0.01;0.01)	0.00 (−0.01;0.00)	.205†
		P value	NA	.719§	.173§	NA
	Platelet count (× 10⁹/L)	Baseline	229.50 (209.50;284.75)	231.00 (183.50;277.50)		.425†
		Baseline	NA	243.00 (190.00;294.00)	220.50 (176.50;274.00)	.565†
		Week 8	NA	251.00 (219.00;320.00)	259.00 (187.50;278.75)	.705†
		Δ	NA	−9.00 (−58.00;18.00)	−7.50 (−34.25;4.50)	.814†
		P value	NA	.286§	.104§	NA
	MPV (fL)	Baseline	9.50 (8.83;9.88)	9.30 (8.05;10.75)		.993†
		Baseline	NA	8.90 (8.00;9.70)	9.70 (8.60;11.45)	.102†
		Week 8	NA	8.70 (8.00;10.20)	9.80 (8.58;10.55)	.301†
		Δ	NA	0.10 (−0.70;0.40)	0.30(−0.23;0.78)	.158†
		P value	NA	.663§	.127§	NA
	PDW (%)	Baseline	16.00 (15.78;16.15)	16.10 (15.70;16.65)		.265†
		Baseline	NA	16.10 (15.40;16.50)	16.15 (15.78;16.80)	.307†
		Week 8	NA	15.90 (15.60;16.80)	16.10 (15.77;16.80)	.394†
		Δ	NA	0.00 (−0.20;0.30)	−0.05 (−0.23;0.30)	.896†
		P value	NA	.793§	.970§	NA

Parametric and nonparametric data are presented as means ± SD or median (25th;75th percentile), respectively.
*Statistically significant (P <.05).
†Difference between groups at each time point was assessed by the Mann–Whitney U-test (nonparametric data).
‡Difference between groups at each time point was assessed by the unpaired Student t test (parametric data).
§Intragroup difference over time was analyzed using Wilcoxon signed-rank test (nonparametric data).
¶Intragroup difference over time was analyzed using paired t test (parametric data).
hsCRP, high-sensitivity C-reactive protein; MPV, mean platelet volume; PDW, platelet distribution width, TLC, total leukocyte count.

Table 3 Correlation between improvement (Δ) in periodontal parameters and change (Δ) in systemic parameters at week 8 with respect to baseline

Parameters		ΔPI	ΔGI	ΔBOP	ΔPPD	ΔCAL	ΔPISA
ΔhsCRP (mg/L)	rho	0.103	0.067	−0.145	0.080	0.103	−0.113
	P value	.520	.677	.365	.619	.523	.482
ΔTLC (×10⁹/L)	rho	−0.127	−0.090	−0.220	−0.196	−0.316	−0.209
	P value	.429	.576	.168	.220	.044*	.190
ΔNeutrophil count (×10⁹/L)	rho	0.001	0.150	−0.122	−0.010	−0.100	−0.136
	P value	.993	.349	.449	.948	.533	.397
ΔLymphocyte count (×10⁹/L)	rho	−0.132	−0.200	−0.223	−0.281	−0.374	−0.186
	P value	.411	.210	.161	.075	.016*	.245
ΔMonocyte count (×10⁹/L)	rho	0.034	−0.007	−0.218	−0.289	−0.374	−0.182
	P value	.834	.967	.172	.067	.016*	.254
ΔEosinophil count (×10⁹/L)	rho	−0.165	−0.297	−0.323	−0.328	−0.360	−0.374
	P value	.303	.059	.039*	.036*	.021*	.016*
ΔBasophil count (×10⁹/L)	rho	0.054	0.068	0.186	0.437	0.439	0.298
	P value	.737	.671	.243	.004*	.004*	.059
ΔPlatelet count (×10⁹/L)	rho	−0.057	0.088	−0.081	−0.171	−0.199	−0.187
	P value	.726	.584	.616	.285	.213	.242
ΔMPV (fL)	rho	−0.108	−0.202	−0.218	−0.055	0.041	−0.120
	P value	.502	.205	.171	.731	.797	.457
ΔPDW (%)	rho	−0.141	−0.247	−0.252	−0.072	−0.021	−0.162
	P value	.380	.120	.112	.654	.897	.312

*Statistically significant ($P<.05$).
BOP, bleeding on probing; CAL, clinical attachment level; GI, Gingival Index; hsCRP, high-sensitivity C-reactive protein; MPV, mean platelet volume; PDW, platelet distribution width; PI, Plaque Index; PISA, periodontal inflamed surface area; PPD, probing pocket depth; TLC, total leukocyte count.

reducing hsCRP among systemically healthy individuals.[33] Due to the antibacterial and anti-inflammatory effect of systemic antibiotics, their utility in the secondary prevention of CVDs has been assessed in a recent meta-analysis.[34] However, antibiotics do not seem to be beneficial in combating risk associated with CVDs.[34]

Increased TLC, although within normal range, is associated with CVD.[35] Moreover, the increased TLC at or above $7.0×10^9$/L as compared to TLC below $4.8×10^9$/L predicts the risk for occurrence of CVD and its associated mortality.[36] Relatively higher TLC due to periodontitis,[28,37-39] although within normal range, may raise a concern for its impact on systemic health. In the present study, there was significantly higher mean TLC in periodontitis patients ($6.62±1.67×10^9$/L) as compared to PH individuals ($5.58±1.52×10^9$/L). Relatively higher TLC is attributed to an increase in neutrophil count among periodontitis patients as TLC are majorly constituted of neutrophils. In the present study, increased neutrophil and monocyte count, although within normal range, in periodontitis patients contributed to a comparative increase in TLC. In the current study, lymphocyte count did not contribute to any alteration in TLC as its level was

similar in both periodontitis patients and PH individuals. In previous studies, increased neutrophil count[28,37-39] and increased lymphocyte count,[37] both within normal range, are responsible for a relative increase in TLC in periodontitis patients. However, no change in lymphocyte count[40] and decreased lymphocyte count[28,39] in periodontitis patients are also reported. The alterations in DLC may have important systemic health implications, as increased neutrophil count and monocyte count as well as decreased lymphocyte count are independent predictors for risk of CVD[7,41] and its associated mortality.[7] Effect of SI on TLC is equivocal with either similar TLC and neutrophil count[32] or a decrease in their count[42] from elevated levels. In the present study, TLC was not reduced at week 8 on treatment with either SI alone or SI with systemic antibiotics. However, treatment with SI and systemic antibiotics in previous studies presented conflicting results.[20,43] In one study, despite improved endothelial function and decrease in hsCRP, there was no effect of SI and systemic antibiotics on TLC.[20] From these findings, it is concluded that further studies with similar research methodology are needed to assess the effect of systemic antibiotics on TLC. In the present study, irrespective

Table 4 Multivariate linear regression analysis evaluating change (Δ) in hematologic parameters (dependent variable), based on improvement (Δ) in periodontal parameters (independent predictor variables) and treatment group (AB/SI)

Blood parameters	Variable	B	SE	95% CI Lower	95% CI Upper	Partial η^2	P value
ΔTLC (× 10^9 L)	Intercept	1.378	0.678	0.002	2.755	0.106	.050
	ΔBOP	−0.006	0.022	−0.051	0.038	0.002	.770
	ΔPPD	2.958	1.398	0.121	5.796	0.113	.041*
	ΔCAL	−4.286	1.501	−7.333	−1.238	0.189	.007*
	ΔPISA	0.000	0.001	−0.001	0.002	0.008	.603
	AB (SI reference)	−0.285	0.456	−1.211	0.642	0.011	.537
ΔLymphocyte count (× 10^9 L)	Intercept	0.612	0.332	−0.062	1.286	0.088	.074
	ΔBOP	−0.010	0.011	−0.032	0.012	0.025	.353
	ΔPPD	0.979	0.684	−0.409	2.368	0.055	.161
	ΔCAL	−1.788	0.735	−3.280	−0.297	0.145	.020*
	ΔPISA	0.000	0.000	0.000	0.001	0.045	.207
	AB (SI reference)	−0.181	0.223	−0.635	0.272	0.018	.423
ΔMonocyte count (× 10^9 L)	Intercept	0.179	0.078	0.022	0.336	0.132	.027*
	ΔBOP	−0.002	0.002	−0.007	0.003	0.018	.424
	ΔPPD	0.053	0.160	−0.272	0.377	0.003	.743
	ΔCAL	−0.199	0.172	−0.547	0.150	0.037	.255
	ΔPISA	0.000	0.000	0.000	0.000	0.013	.505
	AB (SI reference)	0.014	0.052	−0.092	0.120	0.002	.784
ΔEosinophil count (× 10^9 L)	Intercept	0.104	0.077	−0.053	0.261	0.049	.187
	ΔBOP	−0.003	0.002	−0.008	0.002	0.030	.309
	ΔPPD	0.126	0.159	−0.197	0.449	0.018	.434
	ΔCAL	−0.182	0.171	−0.529	0.165	0.031	.295
	ΔPISA	0.000	0.000	0.000	0.000	0.016	.452
	AB (SI reference)	−0.037	0.052	−0.143	0.068	0.015	.476
ΔBasophil count (× 10^9 L)	Intercept	−0.016	0.007	−0.031	−0.001	0.122	.034*
	ΔBOP	0.000	0.000	−0.001	0.000	0.005	.692
	ΔPPD	−0.005	0.015	−0.036	0.027	0.002	.769
	ΔCAL	0.016	0.016	−0.017	0.050	0.027	.332
	ΔPISA	0.000	0.000	0.000	0.000	0.010	.549
	AB (SI reference)	0.004	0.005	−0.006	0.015	0.022	.381

*Statistically significant (P<.05).
BOP, bleeding on probing; CAL, clinical attachment level; η^2, eta-squared; PISA, periodontal inflamed surface area; PPD, probing pocket depth; TLC, total leukocyte count.

of treatment group (AB or SI group), improvement in PPD predicted a decrease in TLC, thereby implicating a positive effect of periodontal treatment on cardiovascular health. Treatment with locally delivered minocycline along with SI resulted in a significant decrease in TLC at week 8.[21] This may be due to the pronounced effect of local delivery of antibiotics in comparison with systemic antibiotics on diseased periodontal pockets.

In the present study, there was a significant decrease in neutrophil count in both the AB and SI groups. However, the improvement in neutrophil count was similar in both the treat-

ment groups. Similar improvement in periodontal inflammation measured in terms of PISA may be responsible for comparable findings in both groups. A previous study reported a similar finding of reduction in neutrophil count on treatment with systemic antibiotics and SI.[43] Greater improvement in neutrophil count (16.87%) in a previous study compared to the AB group of the present study (13.28%) further suggests a significant decrease in TLC in the previous study.[43]

In the present study, similar eosinophil and basophil counts were found in periodontitis patients and PH individuals. This finding is similar to the finding previously reported.[37] In the present study, change in lymphocyte count, monocyte count, eosinophil count, and basophil count at week 8 was not evident in both the groups. Similar results are reported after treatment with SI.[32] In the present study, despite no change in lymphocyte count at week 8, improvement in CAL due to SI with or without systemic antibiotics was found to be a negative predictor for change in lymphocyte count. This association might have contributed to negative predictability of improvement in CAL for change in TLC. The proportional increase in lymphocyte count due to improvement in CAL may have some implication in reducing risk for CVDs, but needs to be confirmed by conducting long-term follow-ups.

MPV and PDW are related to the degree of platelet activation. Due to the association of increased platelet activation with CVDs, it is intriguing to evaluate the impact of both treatment modalities on parameters of platelets. In the present study, platelet count, MPV, and PDW were similar in periodontitis patients and PH individuals. Previous study reported similar platelet count,[43,44] but decreased[43] to similar MPV[44] and increased PDW[44] in periodontitis patients compared with PH individuals. Contrary findings with similar platelet count[39,40] and MPV[39] as well as decreased platelet count[38] and decreased MPV[38] have been reported in patients with aggressive periodontitis as compared to PH individuals. SI has been reported to result in a decrease in platelet count in generalized aggressive periodontitis patients; however, its value at baseline was not compared with platelet count in PH individuals.[42] This finding[42] hints towards the importance of periodontal treatment, as increased platelet count is associated with increased incident for CVDs and its associated mortality.[9] However, in the present study, neither the AB group nor the SI group presented with a change in platelet count. Furthermore, there was no change in MPV or PDW in either treatment group. This finding is in contrast to a previous study that reported an increase in MPV at 1 month after treatment with SI and antibiotics in severe periodontitis patients, despite no change in platelet count.[43] Moreover, an increase in MPV is also correlated with improvement in PPD.[43] As association of increased MPV with risk for CVD is due to increased thrombotic potential of large-sized platelets, increase in MPV after periodontal therapy in severe periodontitis patients[43] represents a contradictory finding. Increased utilization of platelets in severe periodontitis is responsible for decreased MPV (although within normal range) in severe periodontitis, and this number increased within normal range after periodontal treatment.[43] Hence, increase in MPV beyond normal values may hold importance when comparing its association with both CVD and periodontitis rather than comparison within normal ranges.

As increased BMI is associated with risk for CVDs.[45] Comparable BMI among groups, strict well-defined inclusion and exclusion criteria, assessment of periodontal inflammation measured in terms of PISA as well as its correlation with systemic parameters, and consistency of blood collection with regards to fasting status, were the potential strengths of the present study. Dosage and duration of amoxicillin and metronidazole delivered to the AB group was based on meta-analysis.[46] The duration of combination therapy with amoxicillin and metronidazole for 7 days and 14 days was evaluated in this meta-analysis.[46] It was suggested that administration of antibiotics (400/500 mg or 500/500 mg combinations of amoxicillin and metronidazole, respectively) for 7 days seems appropriate as comparable improvement in periodontal parameters is observed in both regimens.

Post intervention time point of assessment at week 8 in the present study was based on the findings of continued periodontal healing till 8 weeks after nonsurgical periodontal intervention.[47] However, the impact of systemic antibiotics as an adjuvant to SI on systemic inflammation would merit evaluation at multiple timepoints so that immediate and long-term effects may be assessed. Another limitation of the study was noninclusion of microbiologic assessment in the study design. Longitudinal studies on patients with varying staging of periodontitis, assessment at multiple time points, and inclusion of other hard endpoints of CVD such as endothelial function, and carotid intima media thickness, would benefit the present study. ▦

Conclusions

Within the limits of the present study, the following conclusions can be drawn. Irrespective of the adjunctive use of systemic antibiotics, change in hematologic parameters is accompanied by improvement in periodontal parameters. SI with or without antibiotics had a marked effect on the reduction of neutrophil count. Change in lymphocyte count is correlated with improvement in CAL. Therefore, systemic antibiotics did not have an additive beneficial effect on the reduction of systemic inflammation.

Disclosure

The authors state explicitly that there are no conflicts of interest in connection with this article. There were no external sources of funding.

References

1. World Health Organization. Noncommunicable diseases: Key facts. 2021;https://www.who.int/news-room/fact-sheets/detail/noncommunicable-diseases. Accessed: 8 July 2021.

2. Sedghi L, DiMassa V, Harrington A, Lynch SV, Kapila YL. The oral microbiome: Role of key organisms and complex networks in oral health and disease. Periodontol 2000 2021; 87:107–131.

3. Tonetti MS, Greenwell H, Kornman KS. Staging and grading of periodontitis: Framework and proposal of a new classification and case definition. J Periodontol 2018;89 (Suppl 1):S159–S172.

4. Reyes L, Herrera D, Kozarov E, Roldán S, Progulske-Fox A. Periodontal bacterial invasion and infection: contribution to atherosclerotic pathology. J Clin Periodontol 2013;40(Suppl 14):S30–S50.

5. Kobayashi R, Hashizume-Takizawa T, Kurita-Ochiai T. Lactic acid bacteria prevent both periodontitis and atherosclerosis exacerbated by periodontitis in spontaneously hyperlipidemic mice. J Periodontal Res 2021;56:753–760.

6. Zaremba M, Górska R, Suwalski P, Kowalski J. Evaluation of the incidence of periodontitis-associated bacteria in the atherosclerotic plaque of coronary blood vessels. J Periodontol 2007;78:322–327.

7. Horne BD, Anderson JL, John JM, et al. Which white blood cell subtypes predict increased cardiovascular risk? J Am Coll Cardiol 2005;45:1638–1643.

8. He S, Lei W, Li J, et al. Relation of platelet parameters with incident cardiovascular disease (The Dongfeng-Tongji Cohort Study). Am J Cardiol 2019;123:239–248.

9. Patti G, Di Martino G, Ricci F, et al. Platelet indices and risk of death and cardiovascular events: results from a large population-based cohort study. Thromb Haemost 2019; 119:1773–1784.

10. Wang Z, Hoy WE. C-reactive protein: an independent predictor of cardiovascular disease in Aboriginal Australians. Aust N Z J Public Health 2010;34(Suppl 1):S25–S29.

11. Kassebaum NJ, Bernabé E, Dahiya M, Bhandari B, Murray CJ, Marcenes W. Global burden of severe periodontitis in 1990–2010: a systematic review and meta-regression. J Dent Res 2014;93:1045–1053.

12. Wade WG. Resilience of the oral microbiome. Periodontol 2000 2021;86:113–122.

13. Darveau RP, Curtis MA. Oral biofilms revisited: A novel host tissue of bacteriological origin. Periodontol 2000 2021;86:8–13.

14. Joseph S, Curtis MA. Microbial transitions from health to disease. Periodontol 2000 2021;86:201–209.

15. Giuliana G, Ammatuna P, Pizzo G, Capone F, D'Angelo M. Occurrence of invading bacteria in radicular dentin of periodontally diseased teeth: microbiological findings. J Clin Periodontol 1997;24:478–485.

16. Baek K, Ji S, Choi Y. Complex intratissue microbiota forms biofilms in periodontal lesions. J Dent Res 2018;97:192–200.

17. Belibasakis GN, Belstrøm D, Eick S, Gursoy UK, Johansson A, Könönen E. Periodontal microbiology and microbial etiology of periodontal diseases: Historical concepts and contemporary perspectives (Epub ahead of print, 20 Jan 2023). Periodontol 2000 doi: 10.1111/prd.12473.

18. Faveri M, Retamal-Valdes B, Mestnik MJ, et al. Microbiological effects of amoxicillin plus metronidazole in the treatment of young patients with Stages III and IV periodontitis: A secondary analysis from a 1-year double-blinded placebo-controlled randomized clinical trial (Epub ahead of print, 23 Jul 2022). J Periodontol doi: 10.1002/JPER.21-0171.

19. Teughels W, Feres M, Oud V, Martín C, Matesanz P, Herrera D. Adjunctive effect of systemic antimicrobials in periodontitis therapy: A systematic review and meta-analysis. J Clin Periodontol 2020;47(Suppl 22):257–281.

20. Seinost G, Wimmer G, Skerget M, et al. Periodontal treatment improves endothelial dysfunction in patients with severe periodontitis. Am Heart J 2005;149:1050–1054.

21. D'Aiuto F, Parkar M, Nibali L, Suvan J, Lessem J, Tonetti MS. Periodontal infections cause changes in traditional and novel cardiovascular risk factors: results from a randomized controlled clinical trial. Am Heart J 2006;151:977–984.

22. Teeuw WJ, Slot DE, Susanto H, et al. Treatment of periodontitis improves the atherosclerotic profile: a systematic review and meta-analysis. J Clin Periodontol 2014;41:70–79.

23. Chapple ILC, Mealey BL, Van Dyke TE, et al. Periodontal health and gingival diseases and conditions on an intact and a reduced periodontium: Consensus report of workgroup 1 of the 2017 World Workshop on the Classification of Periodontal and Peri-Implant Diseases and Conditions. J Periodontol 2018;89(Suppl 1):S74–S84.

24. Silness J, Loe H. Periodontal disease in pregnancy. II. Correlation between oral hygiene and periodontal condition. Acta Odontol Scand 1964;22:121–135.

25. Loe H, Silness J. Periodontal disease in pregnancy. I. Prevalence and severity. Acta Odontol Scand 1963;21:533–551.

26. Nesse W, Abbas F, van der Ploeg I, Spijkervet FK, Dijkstra PU, Vissink A. Periodontal inflamed surface area: quantifying inflammatory burden. J Clin Periodontol 2008;35:668–673.

27. Hung HC, Douglass CW. Meta-analysis of the effect of scaling and root planing, surgical treatment and antibiotic therapies on periodontal probing depth and attachment loss. J Clin Periodontol 2002;29:975–986.

28. Gaddale R, Mudda JA, Karthikeyan I, Desai SR, Shinde H, Deshpande P. Changes in cellular and molecular components of peripheral blood in patients with generalized aggressive periodontitis. J Investig Clin Dent 2016;7:59–64.

29. Shimada Y, Komatsu Y, Ikezawa-Suzuki I, Tai H, Sugita N, Yoshie H. The effect of periodontal treatment on serum leptin, interleukin-6, and C-reactive protein. J Periodontol 2010;81:1118–1123.

30. Ide M, McPartlin D, Coward PY, Crook M, Lumb P, Wilson RF. Effect of treatment of chronic periodontitis on levels of serum markers of acute-phase inflammatory and vascular responses. J Clin Periodontol 2003;30:334–340.

31. D'Aiuto F, Parkar M, Andreou G, et al. Periodontitis and systemic inflammation: control of the local infection is associated with a reduction in serum inflammatory markers. J Dent Res 2004;83:156–160.

32. Marcaccini AM, Meschiari CA, Sorgi CA, et al. Circulating interleukin-6 and high-sensitivity C-reactive protein decrease after periodontal therapy in otherwise healthy subjects. J Periodontol 2009;80:594–602.

33. Orlandi M, Muñoz Aguilera E, Marletta D, Petrie A, Suvan J, D'Aiuto F. Impact of the treatment of periodontitis on systemic health and quality of life: A systematic review. J Clin Periodontol 2022;49(Suppl 24): 314–327.

34. Sethi NJ, Safi S, Korang SK, et al. Antibiotics for secondary prevention of coronary heart disease. Cochrane Database Syst Rev 2021;2:CD003610.

35. Ates AH, Canpolat U, Yorgun H, et al. Total white blood cell count is associated with the presence, severity and extent of coronary atherosclerosis detected by dual-source multislice computed tomographic coronary angiography. Cardiol J 2011; 18:371–377.

36. Lee CD, Folsom AR, Nieto FJ, Chambless LE, Shahar E, Wolfe DA. White blood cell count and incidence of coronary heart disease and ischemic stroke and mortality from cardiovascular disease in African-American and White men and women: atherosclerosis risk in communities study. Am J Epidemiol 2001;154:758–764.

37. Nibali L, D'Aiuto F, Griffiths G, Patel K, Suvan J, Tonetti MS. Severe periodontitis is associated with systemic inflammation and a dysmetabolic status: a case-control study. J Clin Periodontol 2007;34:931–937.

38. Zhan Y, Lu R, Meng H, Wang X, Hou J. Platelet activation and platelet-leukocyte interaction in generalized aggressive periodontitis. J Leukoc Biol 2016;100:1155–1166.

39. Shi D, Meng H, Xu L, et al. Systemic inflammation markers in patients with aggressive periodontitis: a pilot study. J Periodontol 2008;79:2340–2346.

40. Lu R, Li W, Wang X, Shi D, Meng H. Elevated neutrophil-to-lymphocyte ratio but not platelet-to-lymphocyte ratio is associated with generalized aggressive periodontitis in a Chinese population. J Periodontol 2021;92:507–513.

41. Kim JH, Lee YJ, Park B. Higher monocyte count with normal white blood cell count is positively associated with 10-year cardiovascular disease risk determined by Framingham risk score among community-dwelling Korean individuals. Medicine (Baltimore) 2019;98:e15340.

42. Christan C, Dietrich T, Hägewald S, Kage A, Bernimoulin JP. White blood cell count in generalized aggressive periodontitis after non-surgical therapy. J Clin Periodontol 2002;29:201–206.

43. Wang X, Meng H, Xu L, Chen Z, Shi D, Lv D. Mean platelet volume as an inflammatory marker in patients with severe periodontitis. Platelets 2015;26:67–71.

44. Temelli B, Yetkin Ay Z, Aksoy F, et al. Platelet indices (mean platelet volume and platelet distribution width) have correlations with periodontal inflamed surface area in coronary artery disease patients: A pilot study. J Periodontol 2018;89:1203–1212.

45. Khan SS, Ning H, Wilkins JT, et al. Association of body mass index with lifetime risk of cardiovascular disease and compression of morbidity. JAMA Cardiol 2018;3:280–287.

46. McGowan K, McGowan T, Ivanovski S. Optimal dose and duration of amoxicillin-plus-metronidazole as an adjunct to non-surgical periodontal therapy: A systematic review and meta-analysis of randomized, placebo-controlled trials. J Clin Periodontol 2018;45:56–67.

47. Segelnick SL, Weinberg MA. Reevaluation of initial therapy: when is the appropriate time? J Periodontol 2006;77:1598–1601.

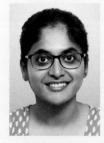

Manpreet Kaur

Manpreet Kaur   Senior Resident, Department of Periodontics, Post Graduate Institute of Dental Sciences, Rohtak, Haryana, India

Rajinder Kumar Sharma   Senior Professor and Head, Department of Periodontics, Post Graduate Institute of Dental Sciences, Rohtak, Haryana, India

Shikha Tewari   Senior Professor, Department of Periodontics, Post Graduate Institute of Dental Sciences, Rohtak, Haryana, India

Ritika Arora   Associate Professor, Department of Periodontics, Post Graduate Institute of Dental Sciences, Rohtak, Haryana, India

Nishi Tanwar   Professor, Department of Periodontics, Post Graduate Institute of Dental Sciences, Rohtak, Haryana, India

Aditi Sangwan   Associate Professor, Department of Periodontics, Post Graduate Institute of Dental Sciences, Rohtak, Haryana, India

Correspondence: Dr Rajinder Kumar Sharma, Senior Professor and Head, Department of Periodontics, Post Graduate Institute of Dental Sciences, Rohtak, Haryana, India. Email: rksharmamds@yahoo.in. ORCID: 0000-0001-7839-1097

First submission: 11 Jan 2023
Acceptance: 25 Feb 2023
Online publication: 6 Mar 2023

The role of home care therapy in periodontal disease treatment and management

Tae H. Kwon, DDS, MMSc/Daliah M. Salem, DMD, MMSc/Liran Levin, DMD, FRCD(C), FIADT, FICD

Home care therapy is indispensable to manage periodontal disease successfully. Often, during and following initial periodontal treatment, it is unclear how much of the clinical improvement was due to patients' home care or to professional intervention, as these two therapeutic components are often amalgamated in clinical practice as well as in studies. In this case series, four patients with periodontal disease received education on using oral hygiene devices and used them competently prior to initiation of professional periodontal treatment. The changes in their clinical presentations, solely attributed to their home care therapy, were documented. The rationale and suggested clinical guidelines are also presented. **Conclusion:** Home care therapy is an indispensable but often overlooked step in the successful management of periodontal diseases. Ideally, this step should be solidified prior to proceeding with any professional treatment. By motivating patients to participate in the treatment more actively, clinicians can significantly improve the outcome and longevity of their professional interventions. *(Quintessence Int 2023;54:288–295; doi: 10.3290/j.qi.b3773959)*

Key words: bone loss, caries, dental plaque, gingivitis, oral hygiene, periodontitis

Optimizing oral hygiene is an important component not only of phase I periodontal therapy but also of cause-related therapy.[1] Cause-related therapy is achieved by therapeutic interventions that suppresses the etiologic factors and by the constant review of home care therapy with the patient.[1,2] The primary etiology of the two most common diseases of the oral cavity, dental caries and periodontal disease, is plaque bacteria on a susceptible host.[3] In cases of periodontal disease, insufficient removal of dental plaque leads to a microbiologic shift of the predominant "red complex" bacteria triggering a pro-inflammatory cascade.[4-6] Consequently, irreversible periodontal attachment loss occurs.[5-7]

Optimal oral hygiene is not only a necessary component in cause-related therapy, but it is also prerequisite before performing periodontal surgeries. Undergoing scaling and root planing and oral hygiene instructions leads to a reduction in periodontal pathogens and a change in the microbiome.[8,9] This results in an improved oral environment preceding surgical intervention, leading to a more optimal healing response.[1,8,9] Furthermore, good oral hygiene is needed for the long-term success of periodontal treatment.[10,11] Unfortunately, a recent study reported that the oral hygiene phase was variable in length and content, variable in the consequential result, insufficiently instructed, and invariably amalgamated with the scaling and root planing, which is the intervention or part of an intervention.[12] Thus, the aim of the present case series was to report the improvement of periodontal conditions solely from patients' home care therapy prior to initiating any active professional intervention.

Case 1

A 46-year-old man was referred to the clinic for evaluation of gingival overgrowth and persistent halitosis. His medical history revealed hypertension for which he was taking a calcium channel blocker (nifedipine). A comprehensive periodontal evaluation revealed generalized marginal gingival erythema, gingival hyperplasia, periodontal probing depth of 3 to 7 mm, and gener-

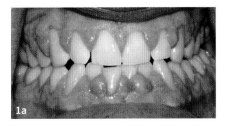 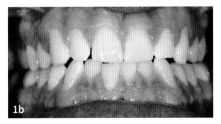 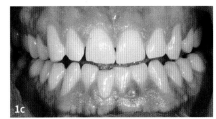

Fig 1a Initial presentation: Generalized marginal gingival erythema and gingival hyperplasia were noted, and they were more pronounced in the interproximal sites and the mandibular anterior sextant.

Fig 1b Two-week follow-up. Generalized reduction in marginal gingival erythema and gingival hyperplasia were noted at 2 weeks following home care therapy initiation.

Fig 1c 12-week follow-up: Further reduction in marginal gingival erythema and gingival hyperplasia were noted at 12 weeks. Mild gingival erythema and hyperplasia were noted on mandibular anterior sextant while a complete resolution was noted at the rest of the oral cavity.

alized bleeding on probing, with no radiographic evidence of apparent alveolar bone loss. The gingival hyperplasia appeared more pronounced in interproximal sites and the mandibular anterior sextant (Fig 1a). There were moderate deposits of supragingival and subgingival dental plaque. His halitosis appeared to be associated with the chronic presence of dental plaque in the pseudo periodontal pockets.

Periodontal diagnosis of generalized biofilm-induced gingivitis with generalized moderate drug-influenced gingival enlargements was made.[13,14]

The patient was recommended intensive home care therapy in combination with repeated professional nonsurgical periodontal debridement, followed by reevaluation, and when appropriate, maintenance visits every 3 months. Medical consultation was conducted with his treating physician for switching his anti-hypertensive medication to another class, for which the physician agreed. He was prescribed an angiotensin II receptor antagonist (losartan), which was as effective as the calcium channel blocker in managing his hypertension. Prior to proceeding with nonsurgical periodontal debridement, an intensive home care therapy was executed. Based on the principles of cause-related therapy, the patient was specifically informed about the dental plaque as the primary etiologic factor for his periodontal disease. The modified bass technique was demonstrated. He was recommended to spend 4 seconds on each surface of the teeth (ie, buccal, lingual, and occlusal) throughout his oral cavity using an oscillating electric toothbrush twice daily. In addition to daily flossing, the patient was recommended to use a rubber tip stimulator three times

a day. He was instructed to insert a rubber tip stimulator interproximally until resistance was felt, then massage the interproximal gingiva with circular motions applying firm apical pressure until his gingiva blanched. After 12 weeks of home care therapy (Figs 1b and 1c), a significant resolution of the marginal gingival erythema and gingival overgrowth was noted. Throughout this period, the patient was fully compliant with the suggested home care therapy with minimally visible residual dental plaque. Furthermore, significant reduction in probing depth was achieved, with all sites exhibiting 3 to 5 mm with minimal to no bleeding on probing.

Case 2

A 27-year-old man was referred to the clinic for evaluation of his periodontal condition. His medical history revealed schizophrenia for which he was taking haloperidol (Hadol decanoate), lithium, and quetiapine (Seroquel). A comprehensive periodontal evaluation revealed generalized marginal gingival erythema and gingival edema, which were more pronounced in the maxillary and mandibular anterior sextants (Fig 2a). There were generalized periodontal probing depths of 3 to 6 mm, with a localized probing depth of 9 mm on the mandibular right first molar, with generalized bleeding on probing, generalized mild horizontal bone loss, and localized vertical bone loss on the mandibular right first molar. There were moderate deposits of supragingival and subgingival dental plaque. Periodontal diagnosis of localized stage III grade C periodontitis with mucogingival defects, recession type 2 (RT2), was determined for the patient.[15,16]

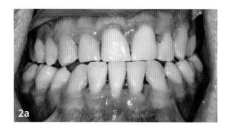
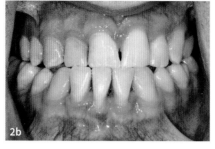
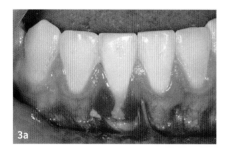
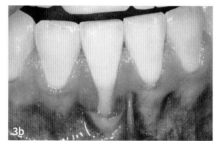

Fig 2a Generalized marginal gingival erythema and gingival edema were more pronounced in the maxillary and mandibular anterior sextants.

Fig 2b Generalized reduction in marginal gingival erythema and edema were noted at 2 weeks following home care therapy.

Fig 3a Marginal gingival erythema and gingival edema around the mandibular right central incisor were noted, with bleeding on probing and moderate deposits of supragingival and subgingival dental plaque. Furthermore, there was mucogingival deformity with lack of attached gingiva and buccal gingival recession.

Fig 3b A significant resolution of gingival erythema and edema were noted following 2 weeks of home care therapy. There was minimally visible dental plaque, suggesting effective plaque removal by the patient.

He was recommended intensive home care therapy in combination with scaling and root planing as part of the initial periodontal therapy. After explaining the importance of removing dental plaque, which was the main etiologic factor for his periodontal disease, home care therapy techniques were reviewed in a similar manner as described in Case 1. After 2 weeks of home care therapy, a significant resolution of marginal gingival erythema and gingival overgrowth was noted in the maxillary and mandibular anterior sextants (Fig 2b). Throughout this period, the patient was compliant with the suggested home care therapy, resulting in minimally visible residual dental plaque. Thereafter, the patient's periodontal disease was controlled and maintained through scaling and root planing, followed by reevaluation and surgical periodontal treatment and maintenance therapy.

Case 3

A 19-year-old woman was referred to the clinic for evaluation of her gingival recession on the mandibular right central incisor. Her medical history was noncontributory. A comprehensive periodontal evaluation revealed localized marginal gingival erythema and gingival edema around the mandibular right central incisor with periodontal probing depth of 4 to 5 mm, bleeding on probing, and moderate deposits of supragingival and subgingival dental plaque. Furthermore, the mandibular right central incisor exhibited 5 mm buccal gingival recession with a complete lack of attached gingiva (Fig 3a). Periodontal diagnosis of gingival health on a reduced periodontium with mucogingival deformity on the mandibular right central incisor, RT1, and lack of keratinized gingiva was made.[13,16]

The patient was recommended an intensive home care therapy regimen to significantly resolve the severe gingival inflammation around the mandibular right central incisor prior to proceeding with mucogingival surgery.

After explaining the importance of removing dental plaque, which was the main etiologic factor for her periodontal disease, home care therapy techniques were reviewed with an emphasis on performing gingival line toothbrushing around the receded marginal gingiva with her right hand while retracting her lower lip with her left hand. This allowed her to visualize and gain better access to the receded gingiva while brushing. After 2 weeks of home care therapy, a significant resolution of marginal gingival erythema and edema were noted in the mandibular right central incisor, with minimally visible residual dental plaque (Fig 3b). Thereafter, it was determined that she was ready to proceed with her gingival graft surgery to correct the mucogingival deformity on the mandibular right central incisor.

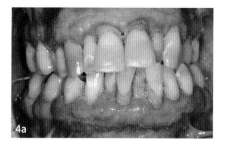
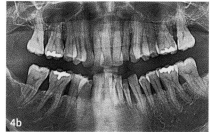
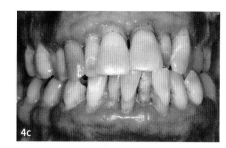
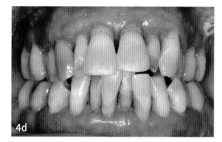
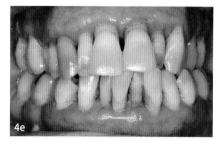

Fig 4a Generalized marginal gingival erythema and marginal gingival edema were noted. There were heavy deposits of supragingival and subgingival dental plaque.

Fig 4b Radiographically, there was generalized moderate to severe alveolar bone loss.

Fig 4c A reduction in gingival erythema and edema was noted 2 weeks after home care therapy initiation.

Fig 4d A continuous reduction in gingival erythema and edema was noted 5 weeks after home care therapy initiation.

Fig 4e A significant resolution of gingival erythema and edema was noted 9 weeks after home care therapy initiation. Although supragingival calculus was present, there were minimal deposits of soft dental plaque, suggesting effective home care by the patient.

Case 4

A 47-year-old man was referred to the clinic for evaluation of periodontal disease. His medical history was noncontributory. A full periodontal evaluation revealed generalized marginal gingival erythema, marginal gingival edema, periodontal probing depth of 5 to 9 mm, generalized bleeding on probing, and radiographic evidence of moderate to severe alveolar bone loss (Figs 4a and 4b). There were heavy deposits of supragingival and subgingival dental plaque. A periodontal diagnosis of generalized stage III, grade B periodontitis with mucogingival defects, RT 2, was made.[15,16]

The patient was recommended initial periodontal therapy, including intensive home care therapy in combination with scaling and root planing. Home care therapy techniques were reviewed in a similar manner as described in Case 1. The patient was recalled for home care therapy review at 2 weeks, 5 weeks, and 9 weeks (Figs 4c to 4e). Throughout this period, a continuous reduction in marginal gingival erythema and edema were noted. The patient was fully compliant with the suggested home care therapy as evident by minimally visible dental plaque in 9 weeks. Thus, it was decided that adequate home care was achieved and that he was ready for scaling and root planing followed by reevaluation.

Discussion

Successful long-term management of periodontal disease requires behavioral changes of patients to attain and sustain a high level of daily plaque removal, life long.[17] Treating clinicians should educate and help their patients develop good oral hygiene habits, predominantly toothbrushing and interproximal cleaning, prior to initiating any professional intervention.[18] Not only does it lead to a more optimal healing response,[1,8,9] but it is also needed for long-term success of periodontal treatment and oral health.[10,11,19] Patients with poor oral hygiene exhibited further attachment loss regardless of receiving surgical or nonsurgical treatment.[20,21] Furthermore, maintaining low plaque levels may help reduce the severity and recurrence rate of gingival hyperplasia in patients with medication-induced gingival hyperplasia, such as in Case 1.[22]

The literature suggests that a power-driven toothbrush was more effective than manual toothbrush, especially in reducing Plaque Index and Gingival Index.[23-25] In addition, a recent meta-analysis suggested that an oscillating-rotating power-driven toothbrush was more effective than other electric toothbrushes as measured in whole-mouth Plaque Index, Interproximal Plaque Index, and the number of sites with bleeding.[26] For patients with periodontal disease, a common 2-minute brushing technique may not be long enough.[17]

Table 1 Oral hygiene recommended devices and the suggested techniques

Devices	Instructions	Notes and examples
Oscillating electric toothbrush	Place or park the brush head around the buccal surface of each tooth, leave it for 4 seconds, and move it to another tooth. Place the lower half of the brush head on the gingiva and the upper half in the cervical third of the tooth. When the buccal surfaces are completed, repeat the same process for the lingual surface of each tooth in the same manner. Lastly, place or park the brush head on the biting/occlusal surface of each tooth, apply apical pressure, leave the brush head for 4 seconds, move to another tooth, and repeat the same technique until completion of all occlusal surfaces.	Perform twice a day. Three time daily for severe periodontal patients or high caries risk patients.
Floss	Once passing the interproximal contact, hug/wrap around the distal side of the anterior tooth, slide the floss apically until the floss disappears 2–3 mm subgingivally. Move the floss coronally and apically 2–3 times. Repeat the same on the mesial side of the posterior tooth. When completed, slide the floss out by pulling it buccally. Repeat the same technique for all interproximal contacts.	Perform twice a day. Suitable for patients with healthy periodontium or low caries risk as well as for patients with periodontitis, who have very high dexterity skills and motivation.
Rubber tip stimulator	Place the pointy tip interproximally from the buccal side. Press lingually until the tip is fully engaging. Then, draw 5 circles especially with apical pressure until the gingiva blanches. Repeat the same technique for all interproximal surfaces. Once completed, repeat the same from the lingual side.	For patients with healthy periodontium or gingivitis, perform once a day. Excessive use may induce interproximal recession. For patients with periodontitis, perform 2–3 times a day.
Interdental brush/triangular-shaped wooden toothpick	Place the brush/toothpick between the two teeth from the buccal aspect. Gently push and pull five times from the buccal to the lingual aspect. Ensure the brush/toothpick completely passes through the buccal embrasure to the lingual embrasure. For the toothpick, the apex or the tip of the triangle should be pointing occlusally while the base of the triangle should be in contact with interproximal papilla.	Perform twice a day. Suitable for patients with periodontitis, who have difficulty with effective flossing. Help patients identify the size that fits their embrasures.

For interproximal cleaning, oral hygiene education should be tailored to the patient depending on the motivation level, dexterity, and anatomical factors such as embrasure size.[27] In general, for patients who are less motivated, who do not have good manual dexterity, or who have open interproximal embrasures, an interdental brush or a triangular-shaped wooden toothpick should be used instead of floss.[17,27] The interdental area can be further strengthened by means of gingival stimula-

Table 2 Commonly asked questions from patients and the suggested answers

Commonly asked questions	Suggested answers
"I noticed bleeding while performing my home care therapy. I stopped as I thought that I was damaging my gums making them bleed."	Bleeding is a reliable sign, suggesting the presence of inflammation and disease around your gums. With proper home care therapy techniques, healthy gums should not bleed.
	Thus, instead of avoiding home care in the bleeding sites, I want you to focus more on these sites while performing home care even if it bleeds. In 7–10 days, you will notice the resolution of bleeding in these sites, suggesting the resolution of inflammation or disease.
"How much pressure should I apply while using an electric toothbrush?"	Oscillating-rotating electric toothbrush already has a set torque. Thus, there is no need to apply too much pressure. Instead, park and hold the brush against the teeth/gums and let the brush head remove the plaque. Some electric toothbrush systems come with pressure sensitive heads while brushing that notifies you when you apply too much pressure, which may be helpful as well.
"I rinse my mouth multiple times a day; however, my mouth doesn't seem to be getting better."	Bacteria in the oral cavity live on your tooth surfaces, and are known as biofilm. The biofilm adheres to your teeth strongly. Thus, vigorous swishing or rinsing will not be effective enough to dislodge the biofilm. Instead, the biofilm needs to be mechanically dislodged or removed using toothbrush and interproximal cleaning tools. Furthermore, the antimicrobial ingredients in your mouthwash won't reach bacteria in biofilm effectively as the biofilm creates a wall or barrier through which the antimicrobial ingredients cannot effectively cross.
"I am afraid of brushing my gums, which can cause gum recession."	As long as you brush gently, but thoroughly, gum line brushing would not result in gingival recession. When instructed to brush gently, patients often brush less effectively around their gums, leaving dental plaque behind. The remanent of dental plaque can initiate gum disease, which can result in a further initiation or worsening of gingival recession. Thus, please hold your toothbrush lightly and use a repeated circular motion over the gum line. This would ensure a more effective removal of the dental plaque, which will help you maintain healthier gum.
"I cannot floss well. Is there any other tool that is easier to use on my hands?"	Interdental brush or a triangular-shaped wooden toothpick can be used instead of floss. It can be as effective as floss or, in certain cases, even better in removing dental plaque between the teeth. Patients with limited dexterity may find it easier to use an interproximal brush or a triangular-shaped wooden toothpick than floss.
"Should I use an electric or manual toothbrush? If so, which kind?"	The literature suggest that an electric toothbrush is more effective than a manual toothbrush in removing dental plaque. Particularly, an oscillating-rotating electric toothbrush is more effective than other electric toothbrushes in removing dental plaque and reducing gingival bleeding.

tion using a device such as rubber tip stimulator. The gingival stimulation may help maintain adequate blood circulation and produce surface keratinization.[28,29] Care should be taken for patients without periodontitis as a prolonged or forceful gingival stimulation can result in interproximal soft tissue recession.[28]

Table 1 presents the recommended oral hygiene devices and the suggested techniques.

During patient education, clinicians should encourage them to participate actively. This can be achieved by demonstrating the home care techniques to patients using various aids such as a teeth model or a video, letting patients demonstrate their techniques back to the clinicians for calibration, and repeating these processes in several visits.[1,2,30] Furthermore, instead of using the terminology "oral hygiene instruction," clinicians are suggested to use a more active terminology such as "home care therapy." This would help patients understand that what they perform at home is indeed therapeutic in nature and encourage them to take a more active role in the

management of their periodontal diseases.[31] Table 2 presents commonly asked questions by patients and the suggested answers, which clinicians can utilize for establishing more effective communication with their patients.

Often, home care therapy is done simultaneously with scaling and root planing in clinical trials or clinical settings.[12] This unfortunately makes it difficult to isolate the magnitude of clinical improvement solely attributed to home care therapy.

In the present case series, all of the noted clinical improvements were strictly from patients' home care therapy without any professional intervention.

Furthermore, completing home care therapy prior to active scaling and root planing can significantly reduce gingival erythema, edema, bleeding, and potentially periodontal pocket depths, all of which can make the professional debridement more effective, easier, and with less side effects.[32-34] The advantage of completing home care therapy prior to scaling and root planing was particularly evident in Case 4. ▦

Conclusion

Home care therapy is an indispensable but often overlooked step in the successful management of periodontal diseases. Ideally, this step should be solidified prior to proceeding with any professional treatment. By motivating patients to participate in the treatment more actively, clinicians can significantly improve the outcome and longevity of their professional interventions.

Disclosure

The authors declare no conflict of interest.

References

1. Kwon T, Levin L. Cause-related therapy: a review and suggested guidelines. Quintessence Int 2014;45:585–591.

2. Kwon T, Salem DM, Levin L. Nonsurgical periodontal therapy based on the principles of cause-related therapy: rationale and case series. Quintessence Int 2019;50:370–376.

3. Axelsson P, Lindhe J. Effect of controlled oral hygiene procedures on caries and periodontal disease in adults. J Clin Periodontol 1978;5:133–151.

4. Socransky SS, Haffajee AD, Cugini MA, Smith C, Kent RL. Microbial complexes in subgingival plaque. J Clin Periodontol 1998;25:134–144.

5. Taubman MA, Valverde P, Han X, Kawai T. Immune response: the key to bone resorption in periodontal disease. J Periodontol 2005;76:2033–2041.

6. Page RC. The role of inflammatory mediators in the pathogenesis of periodontal disease. J Periodontal Res 1991;26:230–242.

7. Kwon T, Lamster IB, Levin L. Current concepts in the management of periodontitis. Int Dent J 2021;71:462–476.

8. Aljateeli M, Koticha T, Bashutski J, et al. Surgical periodontal therapy with and without initial scaling and root planing in the management of chronic periodontitis: a randomized clinical trial. J Clin Periodontol 2014;41:693–700.

9. Rawlinson A, Walsh TF. Rationale and techniques of non-surgical pocket management in periodontal therapy. Br Dent J 1993; 174:161–166.

10. Nyman S, Rosling B, Lindhe J. Effect of professional tooth cleaning on healing after periodontal surgery. J Clin Periodontol 1975;2:80–86.

11. Lindhe J, Nyman S. The effect of plaque control and surgical pocket elimination on the establishment and maintenance of periodontal health. A longitudinal study of periodontal therapy in cases of advanced disease. J Clin Periodontol 1975;2:67–79.

12. Preus HR, Maharajasingam N, Rosic J, Baelum V. Oral hygiene phase revisited: How different study designs have affected results in intervention studies. J Clin Periodontol 2019;46:548–551.

13. Trombelli L, Farina R, Silva CO, Tatakis DN. Plaque-induced gingivitis: Case definition and diagnostic considerations. J Periodontol 2018;89(Suppl 1):S46–S73.

14. Murakami S, Mealey BL, Mariotti A, Chapple ILC. Dental plaque-induced gingival conditions. J Clin Periodontol 2018;45 (Suppl 20):S17–S27.

15. Papapanou PN, Sanz M, Buduneli N, et al. Periodontitis: Consensus report of workgroup 2 of the 2017 World Workshop on the Classification of Periodontal and Peri-Implant Diseases and Conditions. J Periodontol 2018;89(Suppl 1):S173–S182.

16. Cairo F, Pagliaro U, Nieri M. Treatment of gingival recession with coronally advanced flap procedures: a systematic review. J Clin Periodontol 2008;35(8 Suppl):136–162.

17. Chapple ILC, Van der Weijden F, Doerfer C, et al. Primary prevention of periodontitis: managing gingivitis. J Clin Periodontol 2015; 42(Suppl 16):S71–S76.

18. Sälzer S, Graetz C, Dörfer CE, Slot DE, Van der Weijden FA. Contemporary practices for mechanical oral hygiene to prevent periodontal disease. Periodontol 2000 2020; 84:35–44.

19. Levin L, Einy S, Zigdon H, Aizenbud D, Machtei EE. Guidelines for periodontal care and follow-up during orthodontic treatment in adolescents and young adults. J Appl Oral Sci 2012;20:399–403.

20. Axelsson P, Lindhe J. The significance of maintenance care in the treatment of periodontal disease. J Clin Periodontol 1981;8: 281–294.

21. Lindhe J, Westfelt E, Nyman S, Socransky SS, Haffajee AD. Long-term effect of surgical/non-surgical treatment of periodontal disease. J Clin Periodontol 1984;11:448–458.

22. Mawardi H, Alsubhi A, Salem N, et al. Management of medication-induced gingival hyperplasia: a systematic review. Oral Surg Oral Med Oral Pathol Oral Radiol 2021;131: 62–72.

23. Heanue M, Deacon SA, Deery C, et al. Manual versus powered toothbrushing for oral health. Cochrane Database Syst Rev 2003;1:CD002281.

24. Sicilia A, Arregui I, Gallego M, Cabezas B, Cuesta S. A systematic review of powered vs manual toothbrushes in periodontal cause-related therapy. J Clin Periodontol 2002; 29(Suppl 3):39–54.

25. Yaacob M, Worthington HV, Deacon SA, et al. Powered versus manual toothbrushing for oral health. Cochrane Database Syst Rev 2014;2014:CD002281.

26. Clark-Perry D, Levin L. Systematic review and meta-analysis of randomized controlled studies comparing oscillating-rotating and other powered toothbrushes. J Am Dent Assoc 2020;151:265–275.e6.

27. Liang P, Ye S, McComas M, Kwon T, Wang CW. Evidence-based strategies for interdental cleaning: a practical decision tree and review of the literature. Quintessence Int 2021;52:84–95.

28. Hirschfeld I. Gingival massage. J Am Dent Assoc 1951;43:290–304.

29. Wada-Takahashi S, Hidaka KI, Yoshino F, et al. Effect of physical stimulation (gingival massage) on age-related changes in gingival microcirculation. PLoS One 2020;15: e0233288.

30. Harnacke D, Beldoch M, Bohn GH, Seghaoui O, Hegel N, Deinzer R. Oral and written instruction of oral hygiene: a randomized trial. J Periodontol 2012;83: 1206–1212.

31. Kwon T, Wang JCW, Levin L. Home care is therapeutic. should we use the term "home-care therapy" instead of "instructions"? Oral Health Prev Dent 2020;18:397–398.

32. Stambaugh RV, Dragoo M, Smith DM, Carasali L. The limits of subgingival scaling. Int J Periodontics Restorative Dent 1981;1:30–41.

33. Waerhaug J. Healing of the dento-epithelial junction following subgingival plaque control. II: As observed on extracted teeth. J Periodontol 1978;49:119–134.

34. Rabbani GM, Ash MM, Caffesse RG. The effectiveness of subgingival scaling and root planing in calculus removal. J Periodontol 1981;52:119–123.

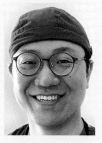

Tae H. Kwon

Tae H. Kwon   Private practice, Keene, NH, USA

Daliah M. Salem   Clinical Assistant Professor, Department of General Dentistry, Goldman School of Dental Medicine, Boston, MA, USA

Liran Levin   Professor of Periodontology, Faculty of Medicine and Dentistry, University of Alberta, Canada

Correspondence: Dr Tae H. Kwon, Monadnock Perio & Implant Center, 819 Court Street, Unit A, Keene, NH 03431, USA.
Email: tkwon3@gmail.com

First submission: 25 Dec 2022
Acceptance: 2 Jan 2023
Online publication: 9 Jan 2023

THE BIG PICTURE

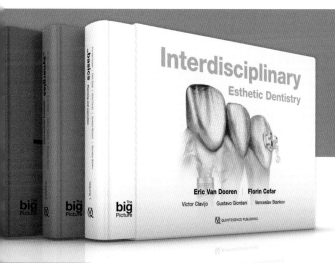

Eric Van Dooren | Florin Cofar | Victor Clavijo
Gustavo Giordani | Venceslav Stankov

Interdisciplinary Esthetic Dentistry

The Big Picture

Hardcover; Three-volume book with slipcase
1,276 pages, 2,300 illus; ISBN 978-2-36615-080-3
€360

Eric Van Dooren and Florin Cofar's new book, produced in collaboration with Victor Clavijo, Gustavo Giordani, and Venceslav Stankov, explores the intersection between conventional esthetic dentistry and the digital world. Eric Van Dooren, regarded as one of the world's leading periodontists, shares the knowledge he has accumulated over the course of his career and highlights the digital protocols that improve and enhance esthetic treatment results. The book examines the fields of fixed prosthetics, implantology, and periodontics from an esthetic point of view. The authors provide keys to simple and complex esthetic treatments, whether performed with analog or digital protocols.

www.quint.link/big-picture

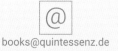

books@quintessenz.de

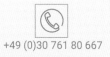

+49 (0)30 761 80 667

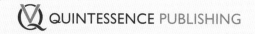

QUINTESSENCE PUBLISHING

The effect of systemic antibiotics on periodontal regeneration: a systematic review and meta-analysis of randomized controlled trials

Lan-Lin Chiou, DDS, MSD/Brandi Herron, DDS/Glendale Lim, DDS, MS/Yusuke Hamada, DDS, MSD

Objective: The aim of this systematic review and meta-analysis was to evaluate the clinical efficacy of the use of systemic antibiotics in regenerative periodontal surgery for treating teeth affected by periodontitis. **Data sources:** Electronic (MEDLINE, EMBASE, LILACS, Scopus, and Cochrane) and manual literature searches for human randomized controlled trial studies published up to November 2022 were conducted by two reviewers. Meta-analysis was performed to assess probing pocket depth (PPD) reduction and clinical attachment level (CAL) gain in groups receiving systemic antibiotics compared to those not receiving systemic antibiotics. A total of eight studies were included. While treated sites were intrabony defects in six papers, two studies focused on furcation defects. For intrabony defects, the weighted mean difference (WMD) of 0.30 mm (95% CI −0.18 to 0.78) and 0.27 mm (95% CI −0.13 to 0.66) was calculated for PPD reduction and CAL gain, respectively. The differences between antibiotics and non-antibiotics groups for PPD and CAL were not statistically significant. Quantitative analysis could not be performed for furcation defects due to the limited number of studies. However, regardless of the membrane type selection, the existing evidence indicated that antibiotics did not lead to superior clinical outcomes for furcation defects at 9 to 12 months after the regenerative procedures. **Conclusion:** Based on this meta-analysis study's findings, the use of adjunct systemic antibiotics in regenerative periodontal surgery did not appear to achieve more favorable clinical outcomes. Thus, the use of adjunct systemic antibiotics as part of the regenerative periodontal therapy might not be justifiable and should be reconsidered. *(Quintessence Int 2023;54: 210–219; doi: 10.3290/j.qi.b3648957)*

Key words: periodontal regeneration, periodontitis, periodontology, surgical procedure, systematic review, systemic antibiotics

Periodontitis, defined by loss of periodontal tissue support around natural dentition, is a multifactorial disease affecting more than 40% of the adult US population.[1,2] Microbiota dysbiosis with a host inflammatory response has been recognized as the primary factor in the pathogenesis of periodontal disease.[3] For treating sites affected by periodontal disease, while the clinical efficacy of scaling and root planing (SRP) and flap surgery with or without osseous recontouring has been demonstrated in longitudinal studies,[4] regenerative therapy is a popular treatment option nowadays.

Regenerative therapies, including the use of bone grafts, barrier membranes, biologics, or combination therapies, for periodontally involved teeth have been well documented for both intrabony and furcation defects.[5,6] Compared to open flap debridement (OFD), the benefits of intrabony defects treated with regenerative therapy has been evidenced by more probing pocket depth (PPD) reduction, clinical attachment level (CAL) gain, and lower incidence of tooth loss.[7] A systematic review and meta-analysis showed that teeth with furcation involvement are 20.9 times more likely to have improved furcation status after regenerative therapy than OFD.[8]

As microbial infection plays a critical role in periodontal disease, it has been suggested that antimicrobial agents may be indicated in periodontal therapy, particularly for recalcitrant or refractory cases or patients with acute periodontal infection.[9,10] The efficacy of systemic or locally delivered antibiotics as an adjunct to nonsurgical periodontal therapy has been investigated in the literature. Recent systematic reviews revealed that SRP with the use of systemic or locally delivered antimicrobials results in statistically higher PPD reduction and CAL gain compared to that without administration of systemic or locally delivered antibiotics in short-term studies,[11,12] although the clinical significance is still a matter of debate. On the other hand, Mombelli et al[13,14] demonstrated that long-term clinical and microbiologic outcomes were similar between administering systemic antibiotics during the nonsurgical and surgical periodontal therapy.

Based on survey research, 73% of periodontists would prescribe antibiotics for guided tissue regeneration (GTR). The prevention of postoperative infections is one of the most common reasons for the use of antibiotics[15] regardless of the low incidence rate of postsurgical infection, with no differences found with and without the use antibiotics reported in the literature.[16] Additionally, a review paper by Herrera et al[17] pointed out that there is not enough evidence to support using systemic antimicrobials as an adjunct to regenerative periodontal surgery.

Despite the increasing concerns about the overuse of antibiotics, guidelines for prescribing antibiotics in periodontal therapy have not been fully established. Moreover, the roles and benefits of postoperative antibiotics coverage adjunct with the regenerative periodontal therapy remain unclear. Therefore, the aim of this systematic review with meta-analysis was to assess the clinical efficacy of the use of systemic antibiotics in regenerative periodontal surgery.

Method and materials

This systematic review with meta-analysis was conducted by following the Preferred Reporting Items for Systematic Review and Meta-Analysis (PRISMA) recommendations and statement.[18] The review was registered in the International Prospective Register of Systematic Reviews (PROSPERO) (ID: CRD42022297809). This review was to answer the following focused question: What is the clinical efficacy of the use of systemic antibiotics in regenerative periodontal surgery in terms of PPD reduction and CAL gain?

Eligibility criteria

- Population (P): Systemically healthy adult patients diagnosed with periodontitis having one, two, three wall, or a combination of intrabony defects or Glickman Grade II furcation defects with more than 5 mm of PPD around natural dentition after nonsurgical periodontal therapy.
- Intervention (I): The test group received systemic antibiotics during and/or after the regenerative periodontal surgery, including monotherapy (GTR with resorbable or nonresorb-

able membranes, bone substitutes graft, or enamel matrix derivatives), or combination approach of those materials.
- Comparison (C): The control group underwent regenerative periodontal surgery, either monotherapy or combination approach, with placebo or without the use of systemic antibiotics during and after the surgical procedure.
- Outcome (O): The outcomes evaluated were PPD reduction and CAL gain of teeth treated.
- Study design (S): Human randomized clinical trials (RCTs) with a minimum of 6 months follow-up time with a total of at least 10 subjects were included.

Additionally, only English-language publications were included. Studies including subjects with systemic diseases such as diabetes mellitus, HIV, or immunosuppression were excluded. In case of studies reporting outcomes on the same subjects, the study which provided the longest follow-up data was selected.

Literature search

Electronic database search was conducted through November 2022 with MEDLINE, EMBASE, LILACS, Scopus, and Cochrane controlled Clinical Trial Register (CENTRAL). The search strategies used for the databases were as follows:

1. for MEDLINE: (periodontal regeneration [All Fields] OR periodontal attachment loss / therapy [MeSH Terms] OR alveolar bone loss / surgery [MeSH Terms] OR guided tissue regeneration, periodontal [MeSH Terms] OR bone substitutes [MeSH Terms] OR bone graft [All Fields] OR enamel matrix derivative [All Fields] OR platelet derived growth factor [All Fields] OR platelet rich fibrin [All Fields] OR bone morphogenic protein [All Fields]) AND (anti-infective agents [MeSH Terms] OR periodontitis/drug therapy [MeSH Terms] OR antibiotic [All Fields] OR anti-bacterial agent [All Fields] OR antimicrobial agent [All Fields])

2. for EMBASE: ("periodontal guided tissue regeneration" OR (enamel AND derivative AND matrix) OR (bone AND graft) OR "bone morphogenetic protein") AND ("antibiotic agent" OR "antiinfective agent") AND ("periodontal disease" OR periodontitis OR intrabony OR infrabony OR furcation) AND ("controlled study"/de OR "human"/de)

3. for LILACS, Scopus, and Cochrane: (periodontal disease OR periodontitis OR intrabony OR furcation) AND (periodontal regeneration OR guided tissue regeneration OR bone substitute OR bone graft OR enamel derivative matrix OR Emdogain OR bone morphogenetic protein OR platelet derived growth factor in OR platelet rich fibrin) AND (systemic antibiotics OR antibiotics OR antimicrobial OR anti-infective).

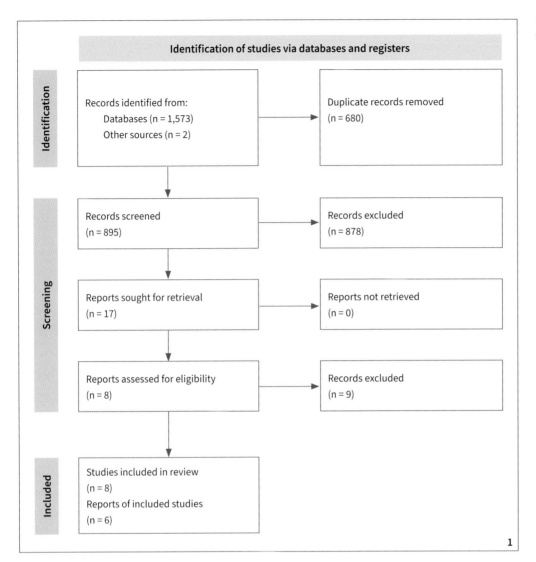

Fig 1 PRISMA flowchart of the selection process.

The search was limited to controlled studies and human subjects. Google Scholar was used for searching gray literature. Manual search was performed in Journal of Periodontology, Journal of Clinical Periodontology, Clinical Oral Investigation, International Journal of Periodontics and Restorative Dentistry, and Journal of Periodontal Research in the previous 15 years.

Study selection

Two independent reviewers (LC and BH) screened the eligibility with titles and abstracts. Full articles were obtained for possible inclusion for this review. Reasons of rejection were recorded. Discrepancies of inclusion or exclusion between two reviewers were solved via discussion with a third reviewer (YH).

Data extraction

Data were extracted and recorded in an Excel spreadsheet by one reviewer, followed by two reviewers cross-checking the data. The data collected included:

- first author and publication year
- study design and length of follow-up
- mean age of the subjects
- number and type of the periodontal defects
- type of systemic antibiotics and regimen
- type of regenerative procedures
- smoking status of the subjects
- clinical outcomes including PPD reduction and CAL gain.

Table 1 Summary of the excluded studies

Study	Reason for exclusion
Mabry et al[20]	Use of systemic plus local antimicrobials in the test group
Machtei et al[21]	Use of local antimicrobial agent
Dowell et al[22]	Use of local antimicrobial agent
Mombelli et al[23]	Systemic antibiotic therapy was given 2 weeks after the surgery
Zucchelli et al[24]	Use of local antimicrobial agent versus use of systemic antibiotics
Minabe et al[25]	3-month follow-up
Starvropoulos et al[26]	Use of local antimicrobial agent
Röllke et al[27]	Same subjects as the study by Eickholz et al[34]
Collins et al[28]	The periodontal surgery performed was not regenerative therapy

Risk of bias of individual studies

Using the revised Cochrane risk-of-bias tool for randomized trials (RoB 2),[19] quality assessment of the included studies was performed by two independent reviewers (LC and BH). Each study was assessed for the following risk of bias domains: randomization process, deviations from intended interventions, missing outcome data, measurement of the outcome, and selection of the reported result.

Statistical analysis

PPD and CAL of the defects at baseline were calculated as weighted mean differences (WMDs) and 95% confidence interval (CI). Studies with at least 6 months follow-up for postoperative PPD reduction and CAL gain were combined in the meta-analysis. A random-effects meta-analysis was performed to account for possible heterogeneity between studies. Results are presented as a weighted average of the treatment effect along with 95% CI.

Results

Study selection

The initial search from the electronic database yielded 895 papers (Fig 1). No additional studies were identified with manual search afterwards. Screening papers based on the title and abstract, a total of 17 studies was extracted for full-text analysis. Finally, eight studies met the inclusion criteria. The reasons for exclusion are listed in Table 1.

Study characteristics

Table 2 summarizes the characteristics of included studies. The studies included were all designed as prospective studies. Patients' age ranged from 18 to 88 years old. Six studies investigated the effects of systemic antibiotics on intrabony defects, whereas furcation defects were tested in two papers. The antibiotics regimen and materials used for regenerative procedures among studies varied. Test subjects in the study by Loos et al[30] initiated antibiotics 4 days prior to the surgery and continued for 4 days after the procedure. Patients in the test group were asked to take the medication 1 hour before the surgical intervention in addition to the use of postoperative antibiotics in two papers. Nonresorbable membrane was used in two trials,[29,36] whereas resorbable membrane alone or in combination with bone grafts were applied in four studies.[30,32,33,35] Enamel matrix derivative (EMD) was the material of choice in two publications.[31,34] The clinical outcomes reported were relatively short-term (6 to 24 months) in all studies. Two studies included only nonsmokers;[32,33] in contrast, current smokers were enrolled in four papers.[30,31,34,35]

Results of individual studies and meta-analyses

Intrabony defects

Of the six included studies, only one study revealed that the administration of systemic antibiotics led to statistically significant differences in CAL gain in favor of the test group.[29] This study used a nonresorbable membrane in the regenerative therapy. The membrane was removed 6 weeks after the GTR procedure,

Table 2 Summary of the included studies

Defect	Study	Study design	Subjects (no., age)	No. of defects	Antibiotics regimen	Treatment (materials)	Smoking habits	Clinical outcomes: PPD, CAL changes	
								CAL gain	PPD reduction
Intrabony defects	Nowzari et al[29]	Prospective	Test: 9 Pt (mean age 55 y; range 50–71 y); Control: 9 Pt (mean age 51 y; range 43–63 y)	Test: 9 defects; Control: 9 defects	500 mg augmentin 1 h prior to surgery, and 500 mg augmentin tid for 8 d	ePTFE membrane	Unknown	At 6 mo: Test: 3.3 mm; Control: 2.4 mm	At 6 mo: Test: 4.1 mm; Control: 2.7 mm
	Loos et al[30]	Prospective	Test: 13 Pt (mean age 39 ± 12 y; range 18–54 y); Control: 12 Pt (mean age 36 ± 11 y; range 16–58 y)	Test: 13 defects; Control: 12 defects	(Started 4 days before the surgery and to be continued 4 days after the surgery) Systemic amoxicillin (375 mg/tid/8 d) and metronidazole (250 mg/tid/8 d)	Bioresorbable polylactic acid membranes (Guidor)	Current smokers: 5 in test group; 7 in control group	At 6 mo: Test: 0.83 ± 0.34 mm; Control: 1.69 ± 0.34 mm. At 1 y: Test: 1.21 ± 0.38 mm Control: 1.60 ± 0.40 mm	At 6 mo: Test: 2.47 ± 0.49 mm; Control: 2.78 ± 0.49 mm. At 1 y: Test: 2.54 ± 0.38 mm; Control: 3.06 ± 0.40 mm
	Sculean et al[31]	Prospective	Test: 17 Pt; Control: 17 Pt (age: unknown)	Test: 13 defects; Control: 12 defects	Systemic amoxicillin 3 × 375 mg and metronidazole 3 × 250 mg daily for 7 d starting the day of surgery	EMD	Current smokers: 3 in test group; 4 in control group	At 1 y: Test: 3.5 mm; Control: 3.3 mm	At 1 y: Test: 4.6 mm; Control: 4.7 mm
	Abu-Ta'a[32]	Prospective	Test: 20 Pt (mean age 60 y); Control: 20 Pt (mean age 57 y; range 26–88 y)	Test: 20 defects; Control: 20 defects	Oral amoxicillin 1 g, 1 h preoperatively, and 2 g for 2 days postoperatively	EMD + DFDBA (modified papilla preservation technique)	Nonsmokers	At 1 y: Test: 4.3 ± 1.1 mm; Control: 4.1 ± 1.4 mm	At 1 y: Test: 4.7 mm; Control: 4.5 mm
	Pietruska et al[33]	Prospective	Test: 21 Pt (mean age 44.67 ± 9.76 y); Control: 20 Pt (mean age 38.75 ± 8.27 y)	Test: 21 defects; Control: 20 defects	Amoxicillin starting the day of the surgery and followed by 2 × 1 g/d for 7 d	DBBM + collagen membrane	Nonsmokers	At 1 y: Test: 3.6 ± 1.6 mm; Control: 2.7 ± 1.6 mm	At 1 y: Test: 3.8 ± 1.3 mm; Control: 2.7 ± 1.6 mm
	Eickholz et al[34]	Prospective	Test: 28 Pt (mean age 54.2 ± 10.3 y); Control: 29 Pt (mean age 49.8 ± 10.0 y)	Test: 28 defects; Control: 29 defects	200 mg doxycycline qd for 7 d postoperatively	EMD	Current smokers: 7 in test group; 6 in control group	At 1 y: Test: 2.78 ± 1.75 mm; Control: 2.76 ± 1.76 mm. At 2 y: Test: 2.74 ± 1.89 mm; Control: 2.95 ± 1.92 mm	At 1 y: Test: 3.48 ± 2.05 mm; Control: 3.29 ± 1.59 mm. At 2 y: Test: 3.69 ± 2.23 mm; Control: 3.4 ± 1.73 mm
Furcation defects	Vest et al[35]	Prospective	Test: 12 Pt; Control: 12 Pt (age: unknown)	Class II furcation defects (Md molar or buccal aspect of Mx molar). Test: 12 defects; Control: 12 defects	Systemic metronidazole 250 mg tid and ciprofloxacin 250 mg q12H for 1 wk starting the day of surgery followed by a 7-wk regimen of doxycycline hyclate 50 mg qd.	DFDBA + Bioresorbable polylactic acid membranes (Guidor)	Current smokers: 8 in test group; 5 in control group	At 9 mo: Test: 0.83 ± 1.75 mm; Control: 0.75 ± 1.22 mm	Vertical: Test: 1.58 ± 1.56 mm; Control: 1.08 ± 1.24 mm. Horizontal: Test: 1.75 ± 1.06 mm; Control: 2.08 ± 1.00 mm
	Demolon et al[36]	Prospective	Test: 5 Pt; Control: 8 Pt (All Pt: mean age 51 y)	Class II furcation defects (Md molar). Test: 10 defects; Control: 12 defects	Amoxicillin/clavulanate potassium during the first 10 postoperative days	ePTFE membrane	Unknown	At 1 y: Test: 1.0 mm; Control: 0.8 mm	Vertical: Test: 1.8 ± 1.1 mm; Control: 2.0 ± 1.2 mm. Horizontal: Test: 1.5 mm; Control: 1.4 mm

DFDBA, demineralized freeze-dried bone allograft; ePTFE, expanded polytetrafluoroethylene; Md, mandibular; Mx, maxillary; Pt, patient.

and the microbial samples were taken from the apical portion of the membrane. The quantity and composition of the microorganisms on the membrane were analyzed with anerobic culturing and DNA probes. It was demonstrated that the antibiotics group had significantly fewer microorganisms compared to the nonantibiotics group. The presence of periodontal pathogens on the nonresorbable membrane influenced the CAL gain recorded 6 months after the regenerative therapy.

Fig 2 Forest plot presenting the result of meta-analysis for intrabony defects in terms of PPD reduction.

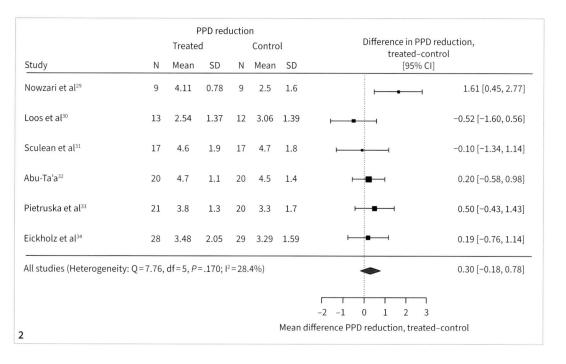

Fig 3 Forest plot presenting the result of meta-analysis for intrabony defects in terms of CAL gain.

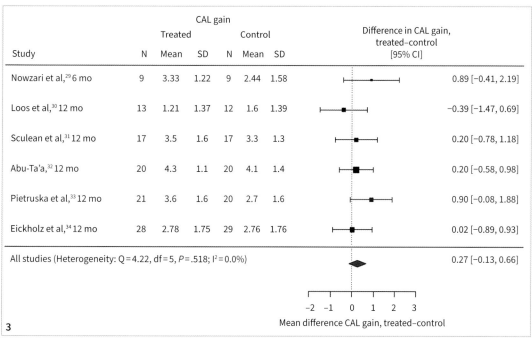

Five studies, in which resorbable materials or EMD were utilized, found significant improvement in clinical outcomes after the regenerative procedures; however, there were no statistically significant differences in PPD reduction and CAL gain between test and control groups in these studies.

Furcation defects

In the study by Vest et al,[35] a combination of bone grafts and resorbable membrane was applied on maxillary or mandibular buccal/lingual Class II furcation defects and no statistically significant differences were found in terms of changes in horizontal

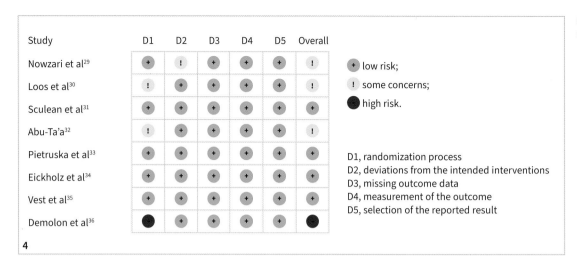

Fig 4 Risk of bias assessment.

Study	D1	D2	D3	D4	D5	Overall
Nowzari et al[29]	+	!	+	+	+	!
Loos et al[30]	!	+	+	+	+	!
Sculean et al[31]	+	+	+	+	+	+
Abu-Ta'a[32]	!	+	+	+	+	!
Pietruska et al[33]	+	+	+	+	+	+
Eickholz et al[34]	+	+	+	+	+	+
Vest et al[35]	+	+	+	+	+	+
Demolon et al[36]	●	+	+	+	+	●

+ low risk;

! some concerns;

● high risk.

D1, randomization process
D2, deviations from the intended interventions
D3, missing outcome data
D4, measurement of the outcome
D5, selection of the reported result

4

and vertical PPD and CAL 9 months after the surgery. The same study evaluated the effects of smoking and membrane exposure on the treatment outcomes. However, no correlation was reported although there was a trend of better healing outcomes in nonsmokers in both antibiotics and nonantibiotics groups compared to smokers, and the horizontal PPD reduction was the lowest in the control group when membrane was exposed.[35] Demolon et al[36] used a nonresorbable membrane for the treatment of mandibular Class II furcation defects. The test group received amoxicillin/clavulanate potassium for 10 days after the surgery. In their previous study,[37] clinical signs of inflammation were less pronounced in the antibiotics group during the observation period of 4 weeks. Nonetheless, the soft and hard tissue measurements between the two groups were not significantly different.

Meta-analysis

Meta-analysis was conducted for the six studies in which the intrabony defects were treated. The results of the meta-analysis are shown in Figs 2 and 3. As noted above, only one individual study showed any significant effect, for CAL gain. Heterogeneity measures (Q and I^2) indicate low heterogeneity across studies. Examination of funnel plots, although limited due to only six data points, did not show indications of asymmetry. For the combined results, differences for PPD reduction and CAL gain between test and control groups were 0.30 mm (95% CI −0.18 to 0.78) and 0.27 mm (95% CI −0.13 to 0.66), respectively, neither of which reached statistical significance (Figs 2 and 3). Due to the limited studies on furcation defects, meta-analysis was not performed.

Risk of bias assessment

Figure 4 demonstrates the results of the risk of bias assessment. While four publications were assessed as low risk of bias, three studies were considered in the category of some concerns. One study[36] was identified with high risk of bias mainly due to the unclear randomization process.

Discussion

The use of systemic antibiotics for regenerative periodontal surgery has been frequently applied, as preventing postsurgical infection is deemed essential for achieving optimal treatment outcomes.[38] However, the results from the present systematic review with meta-analysis revealed that the administration of systemic antibiotics might not affect the clinical outcomes of regenerative periodontal therapy based on the current evidence.

In the treatment of periodontitis, in addition to using conventional instruments for mechanical debridement, the adjunctive use of various chemotherapeutic agents and/or devices (eg, lasers) during nonsurgical or surgical therapies have been applied in clinical practice. Specifically, the combination of amoxicillin and metronidazole or metronidazole alone, administered systemically, have been shown to provide additional benefits to SRP in PPD reduction and CAL gain for patients with aggressive form of periodontitis.[39] Furthermore, a randomized clinical trial showed that patients diagnosed with generalized aggressive periodontitis, based on the 1999 classification, had greater PPD reduction and pocket closure when the adjunctive antibiotics

(500 mg amoxicillin and 500 mg metronidazole for 7 days) were prescribed during initial treatment compared to those who received antibiotics at retreatment.[40] It is unclear, however, whether the use of systemic antibiotics in regenerative procedures in these subjects would lead to different outcomes.

In the studies by Demolon et al,[36,37] it was concluded that administering systemic antibiotics might help controlling inflammation during the early healing phase. It should be noted that more than 50% of the treated sites in both groups had membrane exposure by week 4. Nevertheless, the treatment outcomes for the nonantibiotics group appeared to be comparable to the antibiotic group.[36,37] Conversely, Nowzari et al[29] revealed that patients receiving systemic augmentin had greater CAL gain 6 months after GTR treatment on intrabony defects than those not receiving antibiotics. Nevertheless, more treated sites in the control group had membrane exposure, and whether the differences resulted from the systemic antimicrobials or the negative effects of exposed membrane remains unknown. A case series study, in which intrabony defects were treated with GTR using a nonresorbable membrane, showed that minimal membrane exposure did not affect the obtained tissue gain before removing the membrane.[41] The authors stated that the stringent infection control protocol, involving systemic tetracycline for 7 days after the surgery, daily use of 0.2% chlorhexidine mouthwash and weekly professional cleaning, might contribute to the nonsignificant effects of membrane exposure. In contrast, after membrane removal, the coverage of regenerated tissues was an important factor in probing attachment level and bone gain at 1 year.[41]

Treatment outcomes after regenerative therapy on intrabony and furcation defects are affected by various factors. Froum et al[42] summarized four critical factors for regenerative therapy: thorough root debridement, space maintenance, stability of fibrin clot, and coverage of graft and/or barrier membrane. Patient-related, site-related, and technical factors should all be considered to interpret the clinical outcomes.[43,44] While the defect morphology dictates the selection of the materials, tension-free primary closure and patients' systemic factors are considered critical to the success of the treatment. Moreover, patients' ability to maintain optimal oral hygiene and compliance to periodontal maintenance visits play an important role in the long-term outcomes of regenerative periodontal therapy.

The various antibiotic regimen and materials used among studies is one of the limitations of this systematic review. Biomaterials may influence soft tissue wound healing since EMD has the potential to improve early wound healing,[45,46] whereas bacterial colonization of barrier membrane could exert negative effects.[47] It is possible that the influence of systemic antibiotics on treatment outcomes would be dependent on the materials used in the procedure. Aside from the limited studies included, the studies reported short-term clinical outcomes and subjects enrolled in these studies were relatively healthy. Hence, the results cannot be generalized to patients with systemic diseases. The correlation between smoking status and systemic antibiotics could not be assessed due to the small sample size in the studies.

Conclusion

Within the limitations of the present review, the use of adjunct systemic antibiotics in regenerative periodontal surgery did not appear to achieve more favorable clinical outcomes. Thus, the use of adjunct systemic antibiotics as part of the regenerative periodontal therapy might not be justifiable and should be reconsidered.

Acknowledgments

The authors acknowledge the effort of George Eckert, biostatistician at Indiana University School of Medicine, for performing statistical analyses. This study was funded by Department of Periodontology at the Indiana University School of Dentistry.

Disclosure

All authors declare that there are no conflicts of interest in regard to this manuscript. The authors do not have any financial interests in any of the products mentioned.

References

1. Papapanou PN, Sanz M, Buduneli N, et al. Periodontitis: Consensus report of workgroup 2 of the 2017 World Workshop on the Classification of Periodontal and Peri-Implant Diseases and Conditions. J Periodontol 2018;89(Suppl 1):S173–S182.

2. Eke PI, Borgnakke WS, Genco RJ. Recent epidemiologic trends in periodontitis in the USA. Periodontol 2000 2020;82:257–267.

3. Tonetti MS, Greenwell H, Kornman KS. Staging and grading of periodontitis: Framework and proposal of a new classification and case definition. J Periodontol 2018;89(Suppl 1): S159–S172.

4. Heitz-Mayfield LJ, Trombelli L, Heitz F, Needleman I, Moles D. A systematic review of the effect of surgical debridement vs non-surgical debridement for the treatment of chronic periodontitis. J Clin Periodontol 2002;29(Suppl 3):92–102.

5. Reynolds MA, Kao RT, Camargo PM, et al. Periodontal regeneration - intrabony defects: a consensus report from the AAP Regeneration Workshop. J Periodontol 2015;86:S105–S107.

6. Reddy MS, Aichelmann-Reidy ME, Avila-Ortiz G, et al. Periodontal regeneration – furcation defects: a consensus report from the AAP Regeneration Workshop. J Periodontol 2015;86:S131–S133.

7. Stavropoulos A, Bertl K, Spineli LM, Sculean A, Cortellini P, Tonetti M. Medium- and long-term clinical benefits of periodontal regenerative/reconstructive procedures in intrabony defects: Systematic review and network meta-analysis of randomized controlled clinical studies. J Clin Periodontol 2021;48:410–430.

8. Jepsen S, Gennai S, Hirschfeld J, Kalemaj Z, Buti J, Graziani F. Regenerative surgical treatment of furcation defects: A systematic review and Bayesian network meta-analysis of randomized clinical trials. J Clin Periodontol 2020;47(Suppl 22):352–374.

9. Position Paper: Systemic Antibiotics in Periodontics. J Periodontol 2004;75:1553–1565.

10. Drisko CH. Nonsurgical periodontal therapy. Periodontol 2000 2001;25:77–88.

11. Teughels W, Feres M, Oud V, Martin C, Matesanz P, Herrera D. Adjunctive effect of systemic antimicrobials in periodontitis therapy: A systematic review and meta-analysis. J Clin Periodontol 2020;47(Suppl 22):257–281.

12. Herrera D, Matesanz P, Martin C, Oud V, Feres M, Teughels W. Adjunctive effect of locally delivered antimicrobials in periodontitis therapy: A systematic review and meta-analysis. J Clin Periodontol 2020;47(Suppl 22):239–256.

13. Mombelli A, Almaghlouth A, Cionca N, Courvoisier DS, Giannopoulou C. Differential benefits of amoxicillin-metronidazole in different phases of periodontal therapy in a randomized controlled crossover clinical trial. J Periodontol 2015;86:367–375.

14. Mombelli A, Almaghlouth A, Cionca N, Cancela J, Courvoisier DS, Giannopoulou C. Microbiologic response to periodontal therapy and multivariable prediction of clinical outcome. J Periodontol 2017;88:1253–1262.

15. Hai JH, Lee C, Kapila YL, Chaffee BW, Armitage GC. Antibiotic prescribing practices in periodontal surgeries with and without bone grafting. J Periodontol 2020;91:508–515.

16. Powell CA, Mealey BL, Deas DE, McDonnell HT, Moritz AJ. Post-surgical infections: prevalence associated with various periodontal surgical procedures. J Periodontol 2005;76: 329–333.

17. Herrera D, Alonso B, Leon R, Roldan S, Sanz M. Antimicrobial therapy in periodontitis: the use of systemic antimicrobials against the subgingival biofilm. J Clin Periodontol 2008; 35:45–66.

18. Page MJ, McKenzie JE, Bossuyt PM, et al. The PRISMA 2020 statement: an updated guideline for reporting systematic reviews. BMJ 2021;372:n71.

19. Higgins JP, Savović J, Page MJ, Elbers RG, Sterne JA. Chapter 8: Assessing risk of bias in a randomized trial. In: Higgins J, Thomas J, Chandler J, et al (Eds). Cochrane Handbook for Systematic Reviews of Interventions: Cochrane, 2021. www.training.cochrane.org/handbook (Accessed 22 Nov 2022).

20. Mabry TW, Yukna RA, Sepe WW. Freeze-dried bone allografts combined with tetracycline in the treatment of juvenile periodontitis. J Periodontol 1985;56:74–81.

21. Machtei EE, Dunford RG, Norderyd OM, Zambon JJ, Genco RJ. Guided tissue regeneration and anti-infective therapy in the treatment of class II furcation defects. J Periodontol 1993;64:968–973.

22. Dowell P, al-Arrayed F, Adam S, Moran J. A comparative clinical study: the use of human type I collagen with and without the addition of metronidazole in the GTR method of treatment of periodontal disease. J Clin Periodontol 1995;22:543–549.

23. Mombelli A, Zappa U, Bragger U, Lang NP. Systemic antimicrobial treatment and guided tissue regeneration. Clinical and microbiological effects in furcation defects. J Clin Periodontol 1996;23:386–396.

24. Zucchelli G, Sforza NM, Clauser C, Cesari C, De Sanctis M. Topical and systemic antimicrobial therapy in guided tissue regeneration. J Periodontol 1999;70:239–247.

25. Minabe M, Kodama T, Kogou T, et al. Clinical significance of antibiotic therapy in guided tissue regeneration with a resorbable membrane. Periodontal Clin Investig 2001;23:20–30.

26. Stavropoulos A, Karring ES, Kostopoulos L, Karring T. Deproteinized bovine bone and gentamicin as an adjunct to GTR in the treatment of intrabony defects: a randomized controlled clinical study. J Clin Periodontol 2003; 30:486–495.

27. Rollke L, Schacher B, Wohlfeil M, et al. Regenerative therapy of infrabony defects with or without systemic doxycycline. A randomized placebo-controlled trial. J Clin Periodontol 2012;39:448–456.

28. Collins JR, Ogando G, Gonzalez R, et al. Adjunctive efficacy of systemic metronidazole in the surgical treatment of periodontitis: a double-blind parallel randomized clinical trial. Clin Oral Investig 2022;26:4195–4207.

29. Nowzari H, Matian F, Slots J. Periodontal pathogens on polytetrafluoroethylene membrane for guided tissue regeneration inhibit healing. J Clin Periodontol 1995;22:469–474.

30. Loos BG, Louwerse PH, Van Winkelhoff AJ, et al. Use of barrier membranes and systemic antibiotics in the treatment of intraosseous defects. J Clin Periodontol 2002;29:910–921.

31. Sculean A, Blaes A, Arweiler N, Reich E, Donos N, Brecx M. The effect of postsurgical antibiotics on the healing of intrabony defects following treatment with enamel matrix proteins. J Periodontol 2001;72:190–195.

32. Abu-Ta'a M. Adjunctive systemic antimicrobial therapy vs asepsis in conjunction with guided tissue regeneration: a randomized, controlled clinical trial. J Contemp Dent Pract 2016;17:3–6.

33. Pietruska M, Dolinska E, Milewski R, Sculean A. Effect of systemic antibiotics on the outcomes of regenerative periodontal surgery in intrabony defects: a randomized, controlled, clinical study. Clin Oral Investig 2021;25: 2959–2968.

34. Eickholz P, Rollke L, Schacher B, et al. Enamel matrix derivative in propylene glycol alginate for treatment of infrabony defects with or without systemic doxycycline: 12- and 24-month results. J Periodontol 2014;85: 669–675.

35. Vest TM, Greenwell H, Drisko C, et al. The effect of postsurgical antibiotics and a bioabsorbable membrane on regenerative healing in Class II furcation defects. J Periodontol 1999;70:878–887.

36. Demolon IA, Persson GR, Ammons WF, Johnson RH. Effects of antibiotic treatment on clinical conditions with guided tissue regeneration: one-year results. J Periodontol 1994;65: 713-717.

37. Demolon IA, Persson GR, Moncla BJ, Johnson RH, Ammons WF. Effects of antibiotic treatment on clinical conditions and bacterial growth with guided tissue regeneration. J Periodontol 1993;64:609–616.

38. Laurell L, Gottlow J. Guided tissue regeneration update. Int Dent J 1998;48:386–398.

39. Rabelo CC, Feres M, Goncalves C, et al. Systemic antibiotics in the treatment of aggressive periodontitis. A systematic review and a Bayesian Network meta-analysis. J Clin Periodontol 2015;42:647–657.

40. Griffiths GS, Ayob R, Guerrero A, et al. Amoxicillin and metronidazole as an adjunctive treatment in generalized aggressive periodontitis at initial therapy or re-treatment: a randomized controlled clinical trial. J Clin Periodontol 2011;38:43–49.

41. Tonetti MS, Pini-Prato G, Cortellini P. Periodontal regeneration of human intrabony defects. IV. Determinants of healing response. J Periodontol 1993;64:934–940.

42. Froum S, Lemler J, Horowitz R, Davidson B. The use of enamel matrix derivative in the treatment of periodontal osseous defects: a clinical decision tree based on biologic principles of regeneration. Int J Periodontics Restorative Dent 2001;21:437–449.

43. Reynolds MA, Kao RT, Nares S, et al. Periodontal regeneration - Intrabony defects: practical applications from the AAP Regeneration Workshop. Clin Adv Periodontics 2015;5: 21–29.

44. Aichelmann-Reidy ME, Avila-Ortiz G, Klokkevold PR, et al. Periodontal regeneration – Furcation defects: practical applications from the AAP Regeneration Workshop. Clin Adv Periodontics 2015;5:30–39.

45. Tonetti MS, Fourmousis I, Suvan J, et al. Healing, post-operative morbidity and patient perception of outcomes following regenerative therapy of deep intrabony defects. J Clin Periodontol 2004;31:1092–1098.

46. Sculean A, Schwarz F, Becker J, Brecx M. The application of an enamel matrix protein derivative (Emdogain) in regenerative periodontal therapy: a review. Med Princ Pract 2007;16:167–180.

47. Ling LJ, Hung SL, Lee CF, Chen YT, Wu KM. The influence of membrane exposure on the outcomes of guided tissue regeneration: clinical and microbiological aspects. J Periodontal Res 2003;38:57–63.

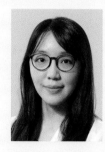

Lan-Lin Chiou

Lan-Lin Chiou   Assistant Professor, Division of Periodontology, School of Dental Medicine, University of Connecticut Health Center, Farmington, Connecticut, USA

Brandi Herron   Graduate student, Department of Periodontology, Indiana University School of Dentistry, Indianapolis, Indiana, USA

Glendale Lim   Private Practice, Chicago, Illinois, USA

Yusuke Hamada   Associate Professor, University of California, Los Angeles, Section of Periodontics, Los Angeles, California, USA

Correspondence: Yusuke Hamada, Director, Advanced Education in Periodontics, Clinical Instructor, Periodontics, UCLA School of Dentistry, 63-022A, 10833 Le Conte Ave., Los Angeles, CA 90095-1668, USA. Email: yusukehamada@dentistry.ucla.edu

First submission: 24 Sep 2022
Acceptance: 27 Nov 2022
Online publication: 6 Dec 2022

Five-year results following regenerative periodontal surgery with an enamel matrix derivative in patients with different smoking status

Siro Pietro De Ry, Med Dent*/Marco Pagnamenta, Med Dent*/Christoph Andreas Ramseier, PD, Dr Med Dent/
Andrea Roccuzzo, DDS/Giovanni Edoardo Salvi, Prof Dr Med Dent/Anton Sculean, Prof Dr Med Dent, MS, PhD, Dr hc mult

Objective: To evaluate the five-year results following regenerative periodontal surgery of intrabony defects using an enamel matrix derivative (EMD) in patients with different smoking status. **Method and materials:** The dental records of patients treated with regenerative periodontal surgery with EMD between 2001 and 2011 were screened. The clinical parameters at baseline (T0) and 6 months (T1) and 5 years (T2) after surgery were collected and analyzed in relation to patient's smoking status (smokers, former smokers, and nonsmokers). **Results:** A total of 71 sites were initially assessed in 38 patients. In total, 56 sites could be evaluated at T1, and 34 after 5 years (T2). At 6 months after surgery, a statistically significant mean probing pocket depth (PPD) reduction of 2.91 ± 1.60 mm and a mean clinical attachment level (CAL) gain of 1.89 ± 1.90 mm were measured. Nonsmokers revealed a greater, statistically not significant CAL gain compared to smokers (2.38 ± 2.12 mm vs 1.50 ± 1.71 mm). Although at 5 years the site-specific PPD values remained stable in nonsmokers, smokers showed an increase of 1.60 ± 2.41 mm. **Conclusions:** The present study provides evidence that regenerative periodontal surgery with EMD may lead to clinically relevant improvements even in smoking patients. However, the positive effect of EMD seems to be limited in time and can only partially compensate for the negative influence of smoking. (Quintessence Int 2022;53:832–838; doi: 10.3290/j.qi.b3418233)

Key words: enamel matrix derivative (EMD), intrabony defects, long-term results, periodontal regeneration, regenerative periodontal surgery, smoking

Periodontitis is a multifactorial inflammatory disease, initiated by periodontal pathogenic dental biofilm and subsequent inflammatory reaction which leads to progressive destruction of the tooth-supporting tissues.[1-4] It is now universally accepted that smoking is an important risk factor for the progression of periodontal disease.[5-7] It has been shown that smokers have an overall odds risk ratio of 2.82 for developing severe periodontal disease when compared with nonsmokers.[7] Furthermore, robust evidence is available indicating that together with poor oral hygiene, smoking is the strongest modifying risk factor for the development and progression of periodontal disease; the benefit of nonsurgical periodontal therapy is lower in smoking patients, and therefore additional surgery is frequently needed to stop further disease progression.[5-7]

Substantial evidence indicates that intrabony defects are associated with a greater risk of progressive loss of periodontal attachment and bone ultimately leading to tooth loss.[8] Thus, from a clinician's point of view, it is of utmost importance to treat intrabony defects to improve long-term tooth prognosis and prevent tooth loss. Regenerative periodontal surgery using an enamel matrix derivative (EMD) has been repeatedly demonstrated to be one of the most predictable treatment modalities to regenerate the tooth's supporting tissues (ie, root cementum, periodontal ligament, and alveolar bone), leading also to statistically and clinically significant improvements.[9]

Recent data indicate that about one third of the Swiss population smokes tobacco daily.[10] Despite the efforts made by dental practitioners and dental hygienists to get patients to stop tobacco consumption, smoking cessation is only successfully achieved in 4% to 30% of cases.[11] Since many periodontitis patients exhibiting intrabony defects are smokers, the question arises as to what extent regenerative periodontal surgery represents a realistic treatment in such scenarios. It has been repeatedly demonstrated that in smokers, regenerative periodontal surgery by means of guided tissue regeneration (GTR) yields statistically and clinically poorer outcomes compared with nonsmokers.[12,13] However, at present the evidence on the clinical outcomes following regenerative periodontal surgery in smokers is mainly limited to GTR, while studies evaluating the outcomes obtained with EMD are still sparse.[12-17]

Therefore, the aim of the present study was to evaluate in smokers the clinical outcomes following treatment of intrabony defects with open flap debridement (OFD) and EMD as compared to those in nonsmokers.

Method and materials

The study protocol was approved by the Ethical Committee of the Canton of Bern (KEK), Switzerland (Nr. 2018-01877). The study was performed according to the guidelines of the Helsinki Declaration (2013). Signed, informed consent was obtained from each patient.

Study population

This investigation was designed as a retrospective longitudinal cohort study evaluating data collected from patients treated at the Department of Periodontology, School of Dental Medicine, University of Bern, between 2001 and 2011. The list of all patients diagnosed with generalized chronic or aggressive periodontitis who underwent periodontal surgery with OFD and EMD (Emdogain, Straumann) was screened by two of the authors (SDR and MP).

The following inclusion criteria had to be fulfilled to qualify for the study:
- male and female patients aged ≥ 18 years
- patients with systemic health or controlled medical conditions
- conclusion of initial nonsurgical periodontal therapy
- presence of single or multiple intrabony defects treated with OFD and EMD without any additional use of bone grafts or GTR
- availability of pre- and postoperative patient's chart with anamnestic information, including smoking status and complete dental treatment records.

Patients were excluded from the study when:
- treatment performed with regenerative materials other than EMD alone (ie, bone grafts or GTR)
- the intrabony defect was associated with a furcation involvement
- the treated tooth was a fixed/removable partial denture abutment
- the tooth presented degree III mobility
- inadequate endodontic treatment and/or restoration
- the preoperative data were incomplete (ie, no periodontal chart)
- smoking status was unknown.

Patients with daily cigarette consumption of less than five were classified as smokers. People who quit smoking ≤ 5 years before surgery were considered to be former smokers. Patients with less than five cigarettes per day consumption or former smokers who underwent smoking cessation > 5 years before surgery were classified as a nonsmokers.

Initial nonsurgical periodontal therapy

In all patients, nonsurgical periodontal therapy was completed by postgraduate students or senior staff members of the Department of Periodontology and consisted of oral hygiene instructions, full-mouth scaling and root planing, and occlusal adjustment, if trauma from occlusion was diagnosed. Following reevaluation, patients were scheduled for periodontal surgery when persisting pockets of a depth of ≥ 5 mm associated with an intrabony defect detectable on intraoral radiographs were present.

Clinical parameters

At 3 months after nonsurgical periodontal therapy (T1), and at 6 months (T2) and 5 years after surgery (T3), the following clinical parameters were recorded:
- full-mouth Plaque Index scores (FMPI) (%)[18]
- full-mouth bleeding on probing (FMBOP) (%)[19]
- site-specific Plaque Index (PI)[18]
- site-specific bleeding on probing (BOP)[19]
- pocket probing depth (PPD, in mm) measured at the deepest site of the defect at baseline (T1).

All measurements were made at six sites per tooth: mesiobuccal (mb), midbuccal (b), distobuccal (db), mesiooral (mo), midoral (o), and distooral (do), using a Michigan periodontal probe (Deppeler).

Table 1 Full-mouth Plaque Index (FMPI) and full-mouth bleeding on probing (FMBOP) at baseline, and at 6 months and 5 years following regenerative periodontal surgery with EMD (patient-based analysis)

Parameter		All patients Mean ± SD/ P value	No. of sites	Smokers (A) Mean ± SD/ P value	No. of sites	Former smokers (B) Mean ± SD/ P value	No. of sites	Nonsmokers (C) Mean ± SD/ P value	No. of sites	P values between A & B & C[†]
FMPI (%)	Baseline (I)	17.15±12.67	61	16.75±7.99	28	14.67±11.17	9	18.54±17.20	24	.7245
	6 months (II)	13.05±11.95	44	11.52±5.47	21	7.33±4.08	6	16.94±17.59	17	.1735
	5 years (III)	26.00±21.19	5	21.25±21.17	4	NA	0	NA	1	NA
	P values between: I & II[#]	.0968	NA	.0092*	NA	.1511	NA	.7728	NA	NA
	II & III[#]	.2459		.0647*		NA		NA		
	I & II & III[†]	.0574		.0420*		NA		NA		
FMBOP (%)	Baseline (I)	23.24±14.73	67	26.24±15.80	29	25.44±19.85	9	19.55±11.14	29	.2012
	6 months (II)	10.95±8.06	55	13.17±8.98	23	6.83±5.81	6	9.92±7.27	26	.1547
	5 years (III)	7.16±5.38	38	7.56±4.89	16	7.00±4.65	6	6.81±6.32	16	.9261
	P values between: I & II[#]	<.0001*	NA	.0005*	NA	.0457	NA	.0004*	NA	NA
	II & III[#]	.0079*		.0168*		.9573		.1652		
	I & II & III[†]	<.0001*		<.0001*		NA		NA		

NA, not applicable; SD, standard deviation.
*Statistically significant, P<.05.
[#]Student t test (two-tailed).
[†]One-way ANOVA.

At 5 years after surgery (T3) the same parameters were recorded at four sites per tooth by an experienced dental hygienist.

Surgical procedure

Following local anesthesia, intrasulcular incisions were placed and mucoperiosteal flaps were raised vestibularly and orally. After complete granulation tissue removal, the roots were scaled and planed using hand and ultrasonic instruments and the defects were rinsed with a sterile saline solution (NaCl). The root surfaces were conditioned for 2 minutes with a 24% ethylenediaminetetraacetic acid (EDTA) gel (PrefGel, Straumann) to remove the smear layer. Following copious rinsing with sterile saline, EMD was applied onto the root surfaces and into the defect. Finally, the mucoperiosteal flaps were adapted to allow a tension-free closure and closed with vertical or horizontal mattress sutures.

Postsurgical care and maintenance

Patients were instructed to rinse twice daily with a 0.2% chlorhexidine solution for 60 seconds during the 2 weeks after the surgery and received a nonsteroidal anti-inflammatory drug (NSAID) against pain (3×500 mg mefenamic acid/day for 3 days).

After suture removal at 14 days postoperatively, the patients were then enrolled in an individually tailored maintenance program consisting of recall appointments every 3 to 6 months during the entire study period of 5 years.

Statistical analysis

All statistical analyses were performed using IBM SPSS Statistics for Windows, version 26.0.0.0 (IBM). Mean, percentage, and standard error values were calculated by means of descriptive statistics. Chi-square tests, Mann-Whitney-tests, Student t tests, and one-way analysis of variance (ANOVA) were used to test for statistical significance of differences between numerical variables within subgroups. Consecutive comparisons of follow-up data were adjusted using Bonferroni tests. P values<.05 were defined as statistically significant.

Results

Demographic data

A total of 38 patients (21 women and 17 men), with a mean age of 47.4±12.8 years (range 23 to 77) at baseline, were analyzed.

Table 2 Plaque Index and bleeding on probing (BOP) at baseline, and at 6 months and 5 years following regenerative periodontal surgery (patient-based analysis)

Parameter			All patients Mean ± SD/ P value	No. of sites	Smokers (A) Mean ± SD/ P value	No. of sites	Former smokers (B) Mean ± SD/ P value	No. of sites	Nonsmokers (C) Mean ± SD/ P value	No. of sites	P values between A & B & C[†]
PI (%)	Baseline (I)		0.15±0.36	61	0.14±0.36	28	0.33±0.50	9	0.08±0.28	24	.2032
	6 months (II)		0.14±0.35	44	0.10±0.30	21	0.00±0.00	6	0.24±0.44	17	.2783
	5 years (III)		0.00±0.00	5	0.00±0.00	4	NA	0	0.00±0.00	1	NA
	P values between:	I & II[#]	.8723	NA	.6184	NA	.1266	NA	.1804	NA	NA
		II & III[#]	.3830		.5284		NA		.5930		
		I & II & III[†]	.6590		.6761		NA		.3774		
BOP (%)	Baseline (I)		0.69±0.47	67	0.62±0.49	29	0.78±0.44	9	0.72±0.46	29	.5822
	6 months (II)		0.30±0.46	56	0.35±0.49	23	0.00±0.00	6	0.33±0.48	27	.2393
	5 years (III)		0.20±0.41	35	0.19±0.40	16	0.00±0.00	4	0.27±0.46	15	.5125
	P values between:	I & II[#]	<.0001	NA	.0529	NA	.0043*	NA	.0037*	NA	NA
		II & III[#]	.2780		.2800		1.0000		.6582		
		I & II & III[†]	<.0001*		.0111*		.0002*		.0019*		

NA, not applicable; SD, standard deviation.
*Statistically significant, $P<.05$.
[#]Mann–Whitney test.
[†]One-way ANOVA.

Patients contributed with one or more teeth with a total of 71 intrabony defects.

Thirteen patients (34.2%) were categorized as smokers and had a mean age of 44.7±12.4 years (range 23 to 71 years). The group of former smokers consisted of four patients (10.5%) with a mean age of 39.5±8.7 years (range 31 to 47 years), whereas the nonsmoker group included 21 patients (55.3%) with a mean age of 50.6±13.1 years (range 23 to 77 years).

Clinical data

Out of the 71 sites assessed initially, only 56 sites could be evaluated at T2 and 34 after 5 years (T3). At T1, mean FMPI and FM-BOP values were 17.15±12.67% and 23.24±14.73%, respectively, with no statistically significant difference between the three groups ($P=.7245$) (Table 1). At 6 months after surgery (T2), the FMPI percentages were slightly lower (13.05±11.95%), whereas the FMBOP showed a statistically significant reduction (10.95±8.06%, $P<.0001$) (Table 1).

The patient-based PI and BOP values are presented in Table 2. At T1, the site-specific PI value was 0.15±0.36 and the BOP was 0.69±0.47. No statistically significant difference was seen between the three groups in relation to site-specific PI

and BOP values ($P=.2032, .5822,$ and $.1716$, respectively). At 6 months after surgery (T2) the site-specific BOP values showed a statistically significant reduction from 0.69±0.47 at baseline (T1) to 0.30±0.46 ($P<.0001$).

No statistically significant differences in terms of PPD values were observed at baseline (T1) between the groups (Table 3). At T2, mean PPD measured 3.95±1.41 mm, with a statistically significant reduction of 2.91±1.60 mm ($P<.0001$), when comparing with baseline (T1).

When comparing the different groups, a statistically significant PPD reduction was measured compared to baseline. The mean PPD reduction measured 2.95±1.68 mm in smokers, 2.17±1.33 mm in former smokers, and 3.04±1.60 mm in nonsmokers, respectively. The difference in terms of PPD between the groups was not statistically significant when comparing smokers with nonsmokers ($P=.9039$ and $.1828$, respectively).

At 5 years after surgery (T3) data showed stable results in terms of PPD in former smokers (0.00±0.71 mm) with a slight additional reduction in nonsmokers (−0.36±1.74 mm). In smokers, there was an increase in site-specific PPD (1.60±2.41 mm) in the first five years. These differences in PPD at T3, between smokers and nonsmokers, were statistically significant ($P=.0248$) (Table 3) (Figs 1 to 3).

Table 3 Probing pocket depths (PPDs) at baseline, and at 6 months and 5 years following surgery

PPD parameter		All patients Mean ± SD/ P value	No. of sites	Smokers (A) Mean ± SD/ P value	No. of sites	Former smokers (B) Mean ± SD/ P value	No. of sites	Nonsmokers (C) Mean ± SD/ P value	No. of sites	P values between A & B & C[†]
Baseline (I)		6.73 ± 1.59	71	6.55 ± 1.64	19	6.23 ± 1.01	13	7.14 ± 1.71	29	.1716
6 months (II)		3.95 ± 1.41	56	3.73 ± 1.20	22	3.83 ± 2.14	6	4.14 ± 1.41	28	.5801
5 years (III)		3.88 ± 1.30	34	4.07 ± 1.53	15	3.80 ± 1.79	5	3.71 ± 0.83	14	.7677
P values between:	I & II[#]	<.0001*	NA	<.0001*	NA	.0036*	NA	<.0001*	NA	NA
	II & III[#]	.8265		.4561		.9785		.3004		

NA, not applicable; SD, standard deviation.
*Statistically significant, P<.05.
[#]Student t test (two-tailed).
[†]One-way ANOVA.

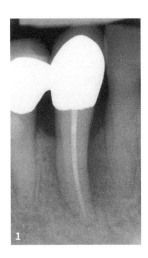 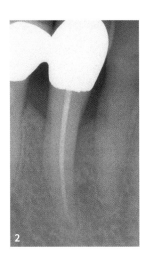 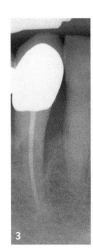

Fig 1 Preoperative radiograph prior to regenerative surgery with EMD depicting a deep intrabony defect located at the mandibular right canine (tooth 43) in a smoker patient.

Fig 2 At 6 months following regenerative surgery with EMD, a complete fill of the intrabony defect has occurred.

Fig 3 At 5 years following regenerative surgery with EMD, a bone defect is again visible at the mesial aspect of tooth 43.

Discussion

The present study has shown that in intrabony defects, regenerative periodontal surgery with EMD resulted in statistically significant clinical improvement evidenced by PPD reduction and CAL gain compared with baseline. At 6 months following surgery, mean CAL gain measured 1.89 mm, which is in line with the findings of previous reports.[9,14,15,20]

When comparing the clinical results 6 months after surgery between smokers and nonsmokers, there were no statistically significant differences in terms of PPD reduction and CAL gain. However, while for PPD reduction the results were similar, a tendency towards a greater CAL gain in nonsmoker patients was observed. This finding appears to suggest that even though nonsmoking patients had a tendency to yield better short-term results (ie, at 6 months after surgery) in terms of CAL gain, the use of EMD in conjunction with periodontal surgery seems also to be effective in smokers.

Another important finding of the present study was the differences in PPD stability between nonsmokers and smokers at T3 (ie, 5 years after surgery). Data analysis revealed that smokers had a statistically significant increase in PPD (ie, 1.60 mm) during the observation period of 5 years, while in nonsmoker patients these values were maintained stable. On one hand, these findings provide evidence for the beneficial effects of EMD to improve the clinical outcomes following regenerative surgery, while on the other hand, they provide additional evidence on the detrimental effects of smoking on the outcomes of regenerative periodontal surgery.

The finding that in intrabony defects, regenerative surgery with EMD may lead to statistically significant reductions in PPD and CAL gain is in agreement with a plethora of previously published data.[9,14,15,20] However, the mean CAL gain obtained in the present study measured 1.89 mm, which is in contrast with the other results that reported mean CAL gains between 2.1 and 4.6 mm.[9,14,15,20] These dissimilarities may be attributed to differences in baseline mean PPD values (ie, 6.73±1.59 mm) which, in the present study, were lower compared with those reported previously. It is well known that the magnitude of clinical improvements following regenerative periodontal surgery is directly related to the baseline probing depths (ie, the deeper the baseline pocket depths the greater the PPD reduction and CAL gain).[9,20] Another possible explanation for these discrepancies may be related to the operator-sensitivity of the regenerative surgical procedure (most patients included the present study were treated by postgraduate students during their specialty training and not by specialists with long experience in regenerative periodontal surgery). It has been clearly demonstrated that surgical-related variables, such as surgical skill, clinical experience, and knowledge have a significant impact on the clinical outcomes.[21]

When interpreting the present results, it should be kept in mind that most of the studies showing the negative effect of smoking on the results of regenerative surgery have used nonresorbable (ePTFE) or resorbable (polylactic acid) membranes and, until now, only a few studies have investigated the clinical outcomes obtained in intrabony defects treated with EMD in patients with different smoking status.[12,14,16,22]

In 1997, Heijl et al[14] published the results of a randomized controlled clinical trial using a split-mouth design in which intrabony defects were treated either with EMD alone (test) or placebo (control). Among the 33 patients included, 16 (48%) were smokers. When comparing the results in term of radiographic bone gain after 16 months, the authors reported that both test and control were more favorable in nonsmokers. Interestingly, the results of EMD treatment, calculated as a difference between test and control side in the same patient, was not dependent upon smoking habits.[14]

Later, Heden[23] reported better results in nonsmokers compared with smokers in term of radiographic bone gain 1 year after surgery in a case series study including 72 intrabony defects treated with EMD alone (3.3 and 2.6 mm, respectively). In contrast, in a case series study including 35 patients (11 smokers), Trombelli et al[16] found no statistically significant differences be-

tween smokers and nonsmokers in terms of CAL and PPD reduction at 11 months after regenerative surgery with EMD and a bone graft.

In the present study, a statistically significant difference in term of PPD change between nonsmokers and smokers was observed at 5 years. This finding is in agreement with several previous clinical studies analyzing the long-term stability after nonsurgical or conventional and regenerative periodontal surgery.[12,20,22,24,25]

When interpreting these findings, it should be kept in mind that this study has some limitations. Due to its retrospective design and the lack of controls, coupled with the questionable reliability of data reported by the patients on their smoking habits, the results need to be interpreted with caution. Moreover, the surgical access of the defects was made through intrasulcular incisions without papilla preservation approaches, which have been shown to additionally improve the clinical outcomes. As clearly demonstrated in a systematic review, surgical techniques have developed in the last two decades (and can significantly improve the clinical outcomes even without the use of any type of regenerative biomaterial).[26–29]

Conclusion

In conclusion, within its limits, the present study has shown that reconstructive periodontal surgery with EMD may lead to substantial clinical improvements even in smokers. However, the positive effect of EMD appears to be limited in time and can only partially compensate for the negative influence of smoking.

Disclosure

The authors declare not to have any potential conflict of interests related to the publication of this paper. To perform the present study, informed consent was not required. The study was self-funded and no external funding was received by any of the authors.

References

1. Darveau RP, Curtis MA. Oral biofilms revisited: A novel host tissue of bacteriological origin. Periodontol 2000 2021;86:8–13.
2. Hajishengallis G, Lamont RJ. Polymicrobial communities in periodontal disease: Their quasi-organismal nature and dialogue with the host. Periodontol 2000 2021;87:241–253.
3. Abusleme L, Hoare A, Hong BY, Diaz PI. Microbial signatures of health, gingivitis, and periodontitis. Periodontol 2000 2021;86:57–78.
4. Joseph S, Curtis MA. Microbial transitions from health to disease. Periodontol 2000 2021;86:201–209.
5. Buduneli N. Environmental factors and periodontal microbiome. Periodontol 2000 2021;85:112–125.
6. Chaffee BW, Couch ET, Vora MV, Holliday RS. Oral and periodontal implications of tobacco and nicotine products. Periodontol 2000 2021;87:241–253.

7. Johnson GGK, Guthmiller JMJ. The impact of cigarette smoking on periodontal disease and treatment. Periodontol 2000 2007;44:178–194.

8. Papapanou PN, Wennström JL. The angular bony defect as indicator of further alveolar bone loss. J Clin Periodontol 1991; 18:317–322.

9. Miron RJ, Sculean A, Cochran DL, et al. Twenty years of enamel matrix derivative: the past, the present and the future. J Clin Periodontol 2016;43:668–683.

10. Bundesamt für Statistik. Tabakkonsum in der Schweiz - Schweizerische Gesundheitsbefragung 2017. https://www.bfs.admin.ch/bfs/de/home/statistiken/gesundheit/determinanten/tabak.assetdetail.11827016.html. Accessed 30 Aug 2021.

11. Ramseier CA, Woelber JP, Kitzmann J, Detzen L, Carra MC, Bouchard P. Impact of risk factor control interventions for smoking cessation and promotion of healthy lifestyles in patients with periodontitis: A systematic review. J Clin Periodontol 2020;47(S22):90–106.

12. Tonetti MS, Pini-Prato G, Cortellini P. Effect of cigarette smoking on periodontal healing following GTR in infrabony defects. A preliminary retrospective study. J Clin Periodontol 1995;22:229–234.

13. Patel RA, Wilson RF, Palmer RM. The effect of smoking on periodontal bone regeneration: a systematic review and meta-analysis. J Periodontol 2012;83:143–155.

14. Heijl L, Heden G, Svärdström G, Ostgren A. Enamel matrix derivative (Emdogain) in the treatment of intrabony periodontal defects. J Clin Periodontol 1997;24(9 Pt 2): 705–714.

15. Heden G, Wennström J, Lindhe J. Periodontal tissue alterations following Emdogain treatment of periodontal sites with angular bone defects. A series of case reports. J Clin Periodontol 1999;26:855–860.

16. Trombelli L, Farina R, Minenna L, Toselli L, Simonelli A. Regenerative periodontal treatment with the single flap approach in smokers and nonsmokers. Int J Periodontics Restorative Dent 2018;38:e59–e67.

17. Estrin NE, Moraschini V, Zhang Y, Miron RJ. Use of enamel matrix derivative in minimally invasive/flapless approaches: a systematic review with meta-analysis. Oral Health Prev Dent 2022;20:233–242.

18. O'Leary TJ, Drake RB, Naylor JE. The plaque control record. J Periodontol 1972;43:38.

19. Lang NP, Joss A, Orsanic T, Gusberti FA, Siegrist BE. Bleeding on probing. A predictor for the progression of periodontal disease? J Clin Periodontol 1986;13:590–596.

20. Stavropoulos A, Bertl K, Spineli LM, Sculean A, Cortellini P, Tonetti M. Medium- and long-term clinical benefits of periodontal regenerative/reconstructive procedures in intrabony defects: Systematic review and network meta-analysis of randomized controlled clinical studies. J Clin Periodontol 2021;48:410–430.

21. Cortellini P, Tonetti MS. Clinical concepts for regenerative therapy in intrabony defects. Periodontol 2000 2015;68:282–307.

22. Stavropoulos A, Mardas N, Herrero F, Karring T. Smoking affects the outcome of guided tissue regeneration with bioresorbable membranes: A retrospective analysis of intrabony defects. J Clin Periodontol 2004;31:945–950.

23. Heden G. A case report study of 72 consecutive Emdogain-treated intrabony periodontal defects: clinical and radiographic findings after 1 year. Int J Periodontics Restorative Dent 2000;20:127–139.

24. Rosa EF, Corraini P, De Carvalho VF, et al. A prospective 12-month study of the effect of smoking cessation on periodontal clinical parameters. J Clin Periodontol 2011;38:562–571.

25. Rosa EF, Corraini P, Inoue G, et al. Effect of smoking cessation on non-surgical periodontal therapy: Results after 24 months. J Clin Periodontol 2014;41:1145–1153.

26. Graziani F, Gennai S, Cei S, Cairo F, Baggiani A, Miccoli M, Gabriele M, Tonetti M. Clinical performance of access flap surgery in the treatment of the intrabony defect. A systematic review and meta-analysis of randomized clinical trials. J Clin Periodontol 2012;39:145–156.

27. Calzavara D, Morante S, Sanz J, et al. The apically incised coronally advanced surgical technique (AICAST) for periodontal regeneration in isolated defects: a case series. Quintessence Int 2021;53:24–34.

28. Palkovics D, Molnar B, Pinter C, Gera I, Windisch P. Utilizing a novel radiographic image segmentation method for the assessment of periodontal healing following regenerative surgical treatment. Quintessence Int 2022;53:492–501.

29. Bartha V, Mohr J, Krumm B, Herz MM, Wolff D, Petsos H. Minimal periodontal basic care - no surgery, no antibiotics, low adherence. What can be expected? A retrospective data analysis. Quintessence Int 2022;53: 666–675.

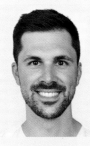

Siro Pietro De Ry

Siro Pietro De Ry* Postgraduate Student, Department of Periodontology, School of Dental Medicine, University of Bern, Bern, Switzerland

Marco Pagnamenta* Private practice, Melide (TI), Switzerland

Christoph Andreas Ramseier Assistant Professor, Department of Periodontology, School of Dental Medicine, University of Bern, Bern, Switzerland

Andrea Roccuzzo Postgraduate Student, Department of Periodontology, School of Dental Medicine, University of Bern, Bern, Switzerland

Giovanni Edoardo Salvi Associate Professor, Department of Periodontology, School of Dental Medicine, University of Bern, Bern, Switzerland

Anton Sculean Professor and Chairman, Department of Periodontology, School of Dental Medicine, University of Bern, Bern, Switzerland

*Both authors contributed equally to the manuscript.

Correspondence: Prof Anton Sculean, Department of Periodontology, School of Dental Medicine, University of Bern, Freiburgstrasse 7, 3010 Bern, Switzerland. Email: anton.sculean@unibe.ch

::: IMPLANTOLOGY

Prevalence and risk indicators of peri-implantitis: a university based cross-sectional study

Phoebus Tsaousoglou, DDS, MSc, Dr Med Dent/Georgios S. Chatzopoulos, DDS, MS/Lazaros Tsalikis, DDS, MSc, Dr Med Dent/Theodosia Lazaridou, DDS, MSc/Georgios Mikrogeorgis, DDS, MSc, PhD/Ioannis Vouros, DDS, MSc, Dr Med Dent

Objectives: To assess the prevalence of peri-implantitis and identify risk and protective indicators of peri-implantitis in a population that underwent implant therapy in a university dental clinic. **Method and materials:** Randomly selected patients from a postgraduate university dental clinic were invited to participate. Clinical and radiographic examinations were recorded. Peri-implantitis was defined as the presence of bleeding and/or suppuration on probing, probing depths of ≥6 mm, and bone loss ≥3 mm. Patient-, implant-, and bone- related factors were recorded and analyzed using a multivariate logistic regression analysis. **Results:** A total of 355 dental implants placed in 108 patients and exhibiting at least 1 year loading time were included. The prevalence of peri-implantitis was 21.3% at patient-level, while 10.7% at implant-level. Simultaneous guided bone regeneration (OR 2.76, 95% CI 1.07–7.12, P=.035), recurrent periodontitis (OR 3.11, 95% CI 1.02–9.45, P=.045) and significant medical history (OR 2.86, 95% CI 1.08–7.59, P=.034) were identified as risk indicators for peri-implantitis. The mean peri-implant bone loss was estimated to be 2.18±1.57 mm for the total number of implants, whereas implants diagnosed with peri-implantitis demonstrated 4.42±1.12 mm in a time period between 12 to 177 months. **Conclusion:** Within the limitations of the study, the prevalence of peri-implantitis in a cohort receiving dental implant therapy at a university dental clinic was 10.7% at implant level and 21.3% at patient level. Patient-reported systemic comorbidities and recurrent periodontitis as well as implants placed in ridge augmented sites were associated with greater risk of peri-implantitis.
(Quintessence Int 2023;54:558–568; doi: 10.3290/j.qi.b4069205)

Key words: cross-sectional studies, dental implants, peri-implantitis, periodontal diseases, risk factors

Dental implants are widely accepted as a well-established treatment of completely or partially edentulous patients due to their increased predictability that leads to improved functional and esthetic treatment outcome.[1] Oral rehabilitation with dental implants demonstrates high survival rates of 97.1% for fixed implant prostheses and 95% to 100% for removable prostheses.[2,3] Despite the high survival rate of implants, implant-supported restorations may encounter complications. The longevity and success of dental implants can be compromised by biologic and prosthetic complications due to various factors including surgical trauma, implant diameter, type of implant–abutment connection, abutment disconnection and mobility, presence of microgap, implant malpositioning, excess cement, as well as presence of inadequate width and thickness of attached mucosa.[4] These may lead to peri-implant infections that are diagnosed as peri-implant mucositis and peri-implantitis or even implant loss.[4]

According to the peri-implant diseases and conditions classification developed at the 2017 World Workshop of the American Academy of Periodontology and the European Federation of Periodontology, peri-implant health is considered when there is absence of peri-implant soft tissue inflammation (redness, swelling, and profuse bleeding on probing) and absence of additional bone loss following the initial healing.[5] Peri-implant mucositis is characterized by peri-implant signs of inflammation combined with no additional bone loss following the initial healing, whereas a diagnosis of peri-implantitis is established when the following criteria are fulfilled: signs of peri-implant inflammation, radiographic evidence of bone loss following the initial healing and increased probing depth measures.[5] Therefore, it is crucial to perform both clinical and radiographic assessment of an implant to establish a diagnosis. Peri-implant diseases are the primary reason for implant failure, and they are biofilm-mediated inflammatory conditions of the connective tissue that lead to progressive loss of the implant-supporting bone.[6,7]

The prevalence of peri-implant diseases varies widely due to the different case definitions used worldwide. A meta-analysis by Derks and Tomasi[8] estimated the weighted mean prevalence of peri-implant mucositis at 43% and peri-implantitis at 22%. Peri-implant mucositis is the precursor to peri-implantitis and the latter condition progresses in a non-linear, accelerating pattern.[9] In addition, due to the progressive nature of peri-implantitis, it may lead to implant loss if left untreated.[10] Peri-implantitis treatments can be either nonsurgical (mechanical, antiseptic, antibiotics, surface decontamination) and surgical (resective and regenerative), and these have displayed unpredictable results.[11] Therefore, it is imperative to efficiently implement strategies to prevent peri-implant mucositis and especially peri-implantitis and avoid recurrences. Implant complications jeopardize the treatment process and lead to a significant impact on patients and dental practitioners. Prosthetic complications are classified as technical or mechanical including fracture and chipping of the materials as well as implant fracture or abutment failures.[12] Technical complications may lead to implant treatment failure and therefore a comprehensive treatment planning is required prior to the initiation of the treatment.[13]

A number of factors have been found to play a pivotal role in the onset and progression of peri-implantitis. Inadequate oral hygiene, excess cement, history of periodontitis, smoking, inadequate periodontal maintenance, genetic factors, systemic diseases, medications, implant location, and bone grafting are among the critical factors associated with the success rate of implants and the incidence of peri-implantitis.[14-18] As peri-implantitis and periodontitis are biofilm-mediated inflammatory conditions, they exhibit similar risk factors and indicators that are associated with biofilm accumulation and host susceptibility. True risk factors of peri-implantitis have been identified in the literature including history of chronic periodontitis, poor plaque control, and no regular periodontal maintenance care.[7]

Studies have reported data on risk indicators of peri-implant diseases that include smoking, diabetes, presence of submucosal excess cement, lack of keratinized mucosa and positioning of implants, implant location, sex, diameter and surface, type of prosthesis, and access to interproximal hygiene.[7,19] Protective indicators have also been identified in the literature such as

interproximal flossing/brushing, proton pump inhibitors, the use of anticoagulants, as well as restoration type.[19,20]

In an effort to advance the field on the prevention of peri-implant diseases, identifying factors that may amplify or reduce the implant prognosis are of paramount importance. Data regarding potential risk factors and indicators of peri-implantitis may assist clinicians to treatment plan accordingly and facilitate a long-term treatment outcome.

The aims of the present cross-sectional university-based study were:
- to assess the prevalence of peri-implantitis in a population that underwent implant therapy in a university dental clinic
- to identify risk and protective indicators of peri-implantis
- to assess the peri-implant (marginal) bone loss.

Method and materials

The present observational cross-sectional study included patients who had osseointegrated dental implants placed in the post-graduate clinic of the Department of Periodontology and Implant Biology of the School of Dentistry at the Aristotle University of Thessaloniki, Greece, between 2005 and 2017. Patients' files were retrieved and evaluated for potential inclusion in the present investigation. Patients were considered eligible for the study when the following criteria were fulfilled:
- one or more two-piece bone level dental implants placed with a one or two stage surgical procedure
- healing period between implant placement and implant exposure ranged between 3 and 9 months
- implants in function for at least 1 year
- available records of clinical and radiographic parameters.

Patients diagnosed with metabolic syndrome were excluded from the study. Patients with incomplete records regarding their demographic characteristics, medical, dental, and periodontal status, as well as implant therapy were deemed ineligible for the present investigation. Following the initial screening phase, randomly selected eligible individuals by computer-generated randomization lists were contacted and invited to attend an implant recall visit. Individuals were excluded if they were not able to be reached, deceased, relocated, or refused to participate in the study. Among them, 108 accepted the invitation and were available for a clinical and radiographic examination. Informed consent was obtained from all subjects involved in the study. The study was performed in accordance with the principles stated in the Declaration of Helsinki (2002) as revised in 2013 concerning the patients and their data.

Clinical assessment

Full-mouth periodontal and peri-implant examination was performed using a manual periodontal probe (15 UNC probe, Hu-Friedy) at six sites per tooth/implant apart from third molars. Periodontal and peri-implant clinical status was assessed including plaque (presence/absence), bleeding on probing (presence/absence), periodontal and peri-implant probing depth (in millimeters), swelling, and suppuration on probing around implants. Implant failure and removal were also recorded, if applicable. With respect to plaque, bleeding, and probing depth, a mean value was calculated for each tooth/implant. Plaque and bleeding were recorded as percentages. All clinical measurements were performed by three calibrated examiners (PT, TL, and LT). A calibration procedure was carried out prior to the initiation of the study to assure reproducibility of the measurements using a sample of 10 nonparticipating subjects who were measured twice at a 7-day interval by each of the examiners. Clinical measurements ranged within ±1 mm for 94% of the recordings for intra-examiner and 89% for inter-examiner variability.

Radiographic assessment

A radiographic examination was performed using digital peri-apical radiographs and was carried out by an independent examiner (GMI), who was unaware of the clinical examination. All radiographs were taken following a standardized protocol with the parallel technique using the Visualix HDI direct digital intraoral radiography system (Gendex Dental System) and an Oralix AC Densomat X-ray machine (Gendex Dental System, 65 kV peak and 7.5 mA mean). Appropriate intraoral sensor alignment instruments (Rinn system: XCP Instruments, Rinn) were used for this purpose. Implant bone level was measured as the distance from the implant fixture shoulder to the first bone-to-implant contact on mesial and distal surfaces of each implant using a digital image processing and analysis software (VixWin Pro, Gendex Dental System).

Examined variables

The investigated variables were grouped into patient-, implant-, and bone-related characteristics.

The patient-related factors were as follows:
- Sex (male, female)
- Age (in years)
- Level of education (elementary, high school, secondary, university)
- Medical history (healthy, systemic diseases)

- Current medication intake (systematic medication intake including bisphosphonates, anticoagulants, antihypertensives, statins, thyroid medications, contraceptives, anticonvulsants, or no medication)
- Periodontal status (periodontal health, periodontal health with reduced periodontium due to history of periodontal disease, recurrent periodontal disease)
- Compliance with supportive periodontal treatment; patients' compliance to supportive periodontal treatment was considered based on the frequency of recall visits per year (two to three visits per year was accounted as compliant)
- Smoking habits (nonsmoker, former smoker, smoker)
- Oral hygiene habits including interdental brushing.

The implant-related factors were as follows:
- Implant surface (acid etched, acid etched and nanometer scale crystals of calcium phosphate, grit blasted and etched, grit blasted with TiO_2, coated surface with titanium plasma spray, airborne-particle abraded, and airborne-particle abraded and acid etched). All included implant systems were bone level implants and included the following implant systems: 3i Biomet, Astra, XiVe, Ankylos, IMZ, Southern, and Straumann
- Implant location (maxillary anteriors, maxillary posteriors, mandibular anteriors, mandibular posteriors)
- Type of prosthetic rehabilitation (single-unit implant crown, tooth-implant supported restoration, overdenture, implant-supported fixed dental prosthesis, implant-supported fixed dental prosthesis with cantilever)
- Immediate implant placement (yes, no)
- Time following implant placement (in months)
- Time of implant in function (in months)
- Peri-implant pocket depth (in millimeters)
- Bleeding on probing around implant(s) (presence, in percentage)
- Plaque accumulation around implant(s) (presence, in percentage)
- Diagnosis of peri-implantitis (presence/absence) based on the new classification of periodontal and peri-implant diseases: Bleeding and/or suppuration on gentle probing, probing depths of ≥6 mm, and bone levels ≥3 mm apical of the most coronal portion of the intra-osseous part of the implant.[21]

The bone-related factors were as follows:
- Guided bone regeneration (yes, no). Guided bone regeneration was performed prior to or simultaneously with the implant placement

Table 1 Demographic characteristics of the included patients and associations between patient-related parameters with the risk of peri-implantitis

Variables		Total population (N = 108 [100.0%])	Non-peri-implantitis (N = 85 [78.7%])	Peri-implantitis (N = 23 [21.3%])	P value
Sex	Male	44 (40.7%)	34 (40.0%)	10 (43.5%)	.763
	Female	64 (59.3%)	51 (60.0%)	13 (56.5%)	
Age (y)	20–39	13 (12.0%)	13 (15.3%)	0 (0.0%)	.078
	40–49	24 (22.2%)	20 (23.5%)	4 (17.4%)	
	≥50	71 (65.7%)	52 (61.2%)	19 (82.6%)	
Education	Elementary	8 (7.4%)	7 (8.2%)	1 (4.3%)	.861
	High school	16 (14.8%)	12 (14.1%)	4 (17.4%)	
	Secondary	37 (34.3%)	30 (35.3%)	7 (30.4%)	
	University	47 (43.5%)	36 (42.4%)	11 (47.8%)	
Medical history	Healthy	80 (74.1%)	67 (78.8%)	13 (56.5%)	.030*
	Systemic diseases (osteoporosis, hypertension, thyroid, thrombosis, osteoarthritis, Sjogren syndrome)	28 (25.9%)	18 (21.2%)	10 (43.5%)	
Administration of medication	No medication	74 (68.5%)	60 (70.6%)	14 (60.9%)	.474
	Medication intake (bisphosphonates, anticoagulants, antihypertensives, cholesterol drugs, thyroid drugs, contraceptives, digestive system drugs, anticonvulsants)	34 (31.5%)	25 (29.4%)	9 (39.1%)	
Smoking	Nonsmoker	41 (38.0%)	35 (41.2%)	6 (26.1%)	.247
	Former smoker	25 (23.1%)	17 (20.0%)	8 (34.8%)	
	Smoker	42 (38.9%)	33 (38.8%)	9 (39.1%)	
Periodontal status	Periodontal health	34 (31.5%)	28 (32.9%)	6 (26.1%)	.003*
	Periodontal health in reduced periodontium	39 (36.1%)	36 (42.4%)	3 (13.0%)	
	Recurrent periodontal disease	35 (32.4%)	21 (24.7%)	14 (60.9%)	
Compliance	No SPT	9 (8.3%)	8 (9.4%)	1 (4.3%)	.084
	1 SPTs/year	23 (21.3%)	14 (16.5%)	9 (39.2%)	
	2 SPTs/year	71 (65.7%)	58 (68.2%)	13 (56.5%)	
	3 SPTs/year	5 (4.6%)	5 (5.9%)	0 (0.0%)	
Interdental brushing	Yes	96 (88.9%)	77 (90.6%)	19 (82.6%)	.280
	No	12 (11.1%)	8 (9.4%)	4 (17.4%)	

*P < .05 (based on chi-square test comparing peri-implantitis and non-peri-implantitis patient groups).
SPT, supportive periodontal treatment.

- Sinus augmentation (yes, no). Sinus augmentation was performed prior to or simultaneously with the implant placement
- Peri-implant bone loss (in millimeters).

Statistical analysis

The statistical analysis was performed at both patient and implant level. Patient-level analysis included all patient-related factors whereas implant-level analysis included bone- and implant-related factors. The diagnosis of peri-implantitis is generally attributed to an implant, whereas in the current study this variable was also considered at the patient level. Patients having at least one implant with a diagnosis of peri-implantitis during the follow-up period were considered as peri-implantitis patients. For categorical variables (such as sex, periodontal status, smoking status, implant surface, implant location, prosthetic type, etc) the corresponding data were summarized by computing absolute (counts) and relative frequencies (percentages %). For scale variables (probing pocket depth, peri-implant bone loss, months following implant placement and loading, etc) measures of central tendency (mean values) and standard deviations (SDs) were computed. Univariate logistic regression was used to analyze the correlation between each indicator and the occurrence of peri-implantitis. Multivariate logistic regression was used to comprehensively analyze the influence of univariate factors with statistical significance (P values < .05). The odds ratio (OR) and its 95% confidence interval (95% CI) were used to represent the strength of association between risk

Table 2 Characteristics of the included implants and associations between implant- and bone-related parameters with the risk of peri-implantitis

Variables		Total implants (N = 355 [100.0%])	Non-peri-implantitis (N = 317 [89.3%])	Peri-implantitis (N = 38 [10.7%])	P value
Implant surface	Acid-etched	49 (13.8%)	45 (14.2%)	4 (10.5%)	.345
	Acid-etched and nanometer scale crystals of calcium phosphate	54 (15.2%)	49 (15.5%)	5 (13.2%)	
	Grit blasted and etched	71 (20.0%)	66 (20.8%)	5 (13.2%)	
	Grit blasted with TiO$_2$	113 (31.8%)	102 (32.2%)	11 (28.9%)	
	Coated with titanium plasma spray	25 (7.0%)	20 (6.3%)	5 (13.2%)	
	Sand blasted	25 (7.0%)	20 (6.3%)	5 (13.2%)	
	Sand blasted and acid-etched	18 (5.1%)	15 (4.7%)	3 (7.9%)	
Implant location	Maxillary anteriors	60 (16.9%)	52 (16.4%)	8 (21.2%)	.675
	Maxillary posteriors	134 (37.7%)	118 (37.2%)	16 (42.1%)	
	Mandibular anteriors	31 (8.7%)	29 (9.1%)	2 (5.3%)	
	Mandibular posteriors	130 (36.6%)	118 (37.2%)	12 (31.6%)	
Guided bone regeneration	Yes	38 (10.7%)	28 (8.8%)	10 (26.3%)	<.001*
	No	317 (89.3%)	289 (91.2%)	28 (73.7%)	
Sinus augmentation	Yes	28 (7.9%)	25 (7.9%)	3 (7.9%)	.999
	No	327 (92.1%)	292 (92.1%)	35 (92.1%)	
Immediate implant	Yes	1 (0.3%)	1 (0.3%)	0 (0.0%)	.729
	No	354 (99.7%)	316 (99.7%)	38 (100.0%)	
Prosthetic type	Single-unit implant crown	126 (35.5%)	114 (36.0%)	12 (31.6%)	.075
	Tooth-implant supported restoration	30 (8.5%)	26 (8.2%)	4 (10.5%)	
	Overdenture	123 (34.6%)	108 (34.1%)	15 (39.5%)	
	Implant-supported fixed dental prosthesis	61 (17.7%)	60 (18.9%)	3 (7.9%)	
	Implant-supported fixed dental prosthesis with cantilever	13 (3.7%)	9 (2.8%)	4 (10.5%)	
Healing mode	1 stage	6 (1.7%)	6 (1.9%)	0 (0.0%)	.392
	2 stages	349 (98.3%)	311 (98.1%)	38 (100.0%)	
Time following implant placement (mean ± SD value in months)		4.85 ± 2.04	4.88 ± 2.08	4.66 ± 1.67	.647
Time of implant in function (mean ± SD value in months)		63.04 ± 33.18	66.13 ± 32.32	82.71 ± 37.75	.075

*P < .05 (based on chi-square test comparing peri-implantitis and non-peri-implantitis implant groups).

factors and peri-implant disease. The significance level in all hypotheses testing procedures was predetermined at a = .05 (P < .05). All statistical analyses were performed with a statistical software program (SPSS v.22.0, IBM).

Results

A total of 355 dental implants placed in 108 patients and exhibited at least 1 year loading time were included in the present analysis. The demographic characteristics of the included patients and the associations between patient-related parameters with the risk of peri-implantitis are shown in Table 1. Most of the included patients were females (59.3%), aged ≥ 50 years (65.7%) and medically healthy (74.1%). The majority of the included

population exhibited a form of periodontal disease, either recurrent periodontal disease (32.4%) or periodontal health in reduced periodontium (36.1%). More than two thirds of this cohort received at least two supportive periodontal treatments per year and 88.9% of them reported regular interdental cleaning. At patient-level, the prevalence of peri-implantitis was 21.3%. In univariate analysis, peri-implantitis was associated with patients' medical history (P = .030) as well as periodontal status (P = .003).

The characteristics of the included implants and the associations between implant- and bone-related parameters with the risk of peri-implantitis are shown in Table 2. The total number of implants examined and included in the statistical analysis was 355. Amongst these implants, 31.8% were grit blasted with TiO$_2$, 74.3% were placed either in the maxillary (37.7%) or mandibu-

Table 3 Clinical and radiographic characteristics of the included implants

Variables		Total implants (N = 355 [100.0%])	Non-peri-implantitis (N = 317 [89.3%])	Peri-implantitis (N = 38 [10.7%])	P value
Probing pocket depth, mm (mean±SD)		4.94±1.71	4.61±1.33	7.66±2.07	<.001*
Peri-implant bone loss, mm (mean±SD)		2.18±1.57	1.91±1.39	4.42±1.12	<.001*
Bleeding on probing (implants)	Yes	225 (63.4%)	187 (59.0%)	38 (100.0%)	<.001*
	No	130 (36.6%)	130 (41.0%)	0 (0.0%)	
Plaque (implants)	Yes	63 (17.7%)	58 (18.3%)	5 (13.2%)	.433
	No	292 (82.3%)	259 (81.7%)	33 (86.8%)	

*P<.05.

lar (36.6%) posterior regions, and approximately one tenth of them received guided bone regeneration (10.7%) or sinus augmentation (7.9%) procedures. Single-unit implant crowns (35.5%) and overdentures (34.6%) were the most common prosthetic rehabilitations used. The vast majority of the included implants healed following a two-stage protocol (98.3%) with the mean time between implant placement and restoration being 4.85± 2.04 months. The mean time of implant in function was 63.04± 33.18 months. At implant-level, the prevalence of peri-implantitis was 10.7%. In univariate analysis, guided bone regeneration (P=.003) was associated with peri-implantitis.

The clinical and radiographic characteristics of the included implants are demonstrated in Table 3. The mean probing pocket depth in the 38 implants presenting with peri-implantitis was 7.66±2.07 mm and the mean peri-implant bone loss was 4.42± 1.12 mm. All implants diagnosed with peri-implantitis exhibited bleeding on probing and only 13.2% of them had plaque accumulation. All clinical and radiographic variables were significantly different between peri-implantitis and non-peri-implantitis dental implants (P<.001) apart from plaque (P=.433). Regarding radiographic peri-implant bone level, the peri-implant bone level alterations were found to be ≤2 mm in almost half (49.3%) of the installed implants. Approximately 50% of the implants were examined in a time period from 60 to 183 months after implant installation, and 51% from 56 months to 177 months following prostheses loading, respectively.

Multivariate logistic regression analyses were performed at patient- and implant-level to identify associations between independent factors and peri-implantitis. Results of the multivariate analyses are presented in Table 4. A statistically significant association between guided bone regeneration (P=.035) with the occurrence of peri-implantitis was determined at the implant level. Particularly, implants placed in guided bone regenerated sites presented significantly (P=.035) higher ORs for

developing peri-implantitis (OR 2.76, 95% CI 1.07–7.12). At the patient-level, the periodontal (P=.045) and systemic medical (P=.034) status of the patients were significantly associated with peri-implantitis. For individuals diagnosed with recurrent periodontitis, the ORs were estimated to be 3.11 (95% CI 1.02–9.45) and similarly medically compromised patients showed 2.86 higher odds to have peri-implantitis (OR 2.86, 95% CI 1.08–7.59) than systemically healthy subjects.

Discussion

The objectives of this study focused on assessing the prevalence of peri-implantitis as well as identifying risk indicators for the occurrence of peri-implantitis in a population who received implant treatment at a university postgraduate clinic. In addition, the peri-implant bone loss was analyzed in the same population. This cross-sectional investigation included patients treated at the Aristotle University of Thessaloniki and has shown that peri-implantitis affected 10.7% of implants and 21.3% of patients. Simultaneous guided bone regeneration, recurrent periodontitis, and patient-reported systemic comorbidities were identified as risk indicators for peri-implantitis. The mean peri-implant bone loss was estimated to be 2.18± 1.57 mm for the total number of implants, while implants diagnosed with peri-implantitis demonstrated 4.42±1.12 mm between 12 to 177 months. Almost half of the included implants (49.3%) displayed bone loss of ≤2 mm.

When comparing the present results with the available literature, the prevalence of peri-implantitis is in agreement with recent systematic reviews that have estimated the overall prevalence of peri-implantitis in various populations.[9,22] A limiting factor that influences the ability to compare different studies is the use of various definitions of disease. In a study by Koldsland et al,[23] the prevalence of peri-implant disease ranged be-

Table 4   Multivariate logistic regression analyses at patient- and implant-level to identify associations between independent factors and peri-implantitis

Level	Variable		OR (95% CI)	P value
Implant level	Guided bone regeneration	Yes	2.76 (1.07–7.12)	.035*
		No	1.00 (reference)	
Patient level	Periodontal status	Periodontal health	1.00 (reference)	
		Periodontal health in reduced periodontium	0.39 (0.09–1.69)	.208
		Recurrent periodontal disease	3.11 (1.02–9.45)	.045*
	Medical history	Healthy	1.00 (reference)	
		Systemic diseases (osteoporosis, hypertension, thyroid, thrombosis, osteoarthritis, Sjogren syndrome)	2.86 (1.08–7.59)	.034*

*P<.05.
CI, confidence interval; OR, odds ratio.

tween 11.3% and 47.1% based on the different definitions of disease severity. Other reasons for the variability in the reported prevalence between studies may be associated with differences in the study designs. A number of studies have included in their analysis only one implant system, whereas in the current study different implant brands were utilized. In the present investigation, the criteria for peri-implantitis diagnosis were based on the consensus of the 2017 World Workshop on the Classification of Periodontal and Peri-Implant Diseases and Conditions.[21] In addition, the present results are applicable to clinical practice due to the diversity of the included population, treated with different implant systems as well as different surgeons and restorative dental practitioners. Moreover, the included cohort received implant treatment with various prosthetic types including single-unit implant crowns, tooth-implant supported restorations, implant-supported overdentures, implant-supported fixed dental prostheses, and implant-supported fixed dental prostheses with cantilever.

In an effort to identify risk indicators, a number of different patient-, implant-, and bone-related parameters were evaluated. The initial medical, periodontal, and dental records of the included patients were assessed in combination with data that were acquired during the recall visit. Guided bone regeneration demonstrated a significant association with peri-implantitis (P=.035). Marginal bone loss around implants placed simultaneously with bone graft may be significantly higher than implants inserted following a delayed implant placement protocol.[24] Moreover, bone augmentation has been associated with an increased risk of implant failure and therefore implants placed in augmented sites are at risk of failure.[25] Hence, alveolar bone augmentation should be performed, when needed, prior to implant placement to ensure adequate bone formation

and healing.[26] In contrast, a systematic review and meta-analysis that assessed the implant treatment outcomes in grafted and non-grafted sites revealed that implants inserted into previously grafted areas display high survival rates and lower marginal bone loss than implants placed in non-grafted sites.[27]

In the present investigation, patients with recurrent periodontal disease demonstrated 3.11 higher odds to exhibit peri-implantitis (P=.045). This is in agreement with previous research which concluded that periodontitis patients experience greater risk of implant failure as well as peri-implantitis long-term (5 years after implant loading).[28] According to the 6th European Association for Osseointegration consensus report in 2021, history of periodontitis may influence the occurrence of peri-implantitis to a much higher degree.[29] In addition, implants placed in sites with prior tooth loss due to periodontal disease have 0.5 mm more marginal bone loss after 5 years.[30] The association between periodontitis and peri-implantitis may be due to the similar etiologies of the diseases that are believed to be microbially mediated.[31] Peri-implantitis patients may harbor an increased number of pathogenic bacterial species, a higher bacterial load, or an impaired immune response.[32] Periodontitis patients exhibiting residual periodontal probing depths of at least 5 mm display a significant higher risk for peri-implantitis and implant loss or in general a higher risk of biologic complications.[33] The significance of compliance with supportive periodontal therapy for the long-term success of implants has also been confirmed, reinforcing the need for periodontally compromised patients to be more compliant.[34] The appropriate maintenance program can lead to similar success rates between periodontally compromised and healthy patients.[34] The majority of the included individuals received at least two supportive periodontal treatments per year, and 88.9% of them reported regular interdental cleaning.

Patients with systemic diseases including osteoporosis, hypertension, thyroid, thrombosis, osteoarthritis, and Sjogren syndrome exhibited an increased risk for peri-implantitis (OR 2.86, 95% CI 1.08–7.59, $P = .034$) compared with those who were systemically healthy. Underlying systemic diseases may influence implant failure and the risk of peri-implantitis.[35] In regards to the potential influence of common systemic diseases on implant survival, the level of evidence is currently low and there is a limited number of randomized control trials.[36] Moreover, it has been demonstrated that hyperglycemia is associated with a higher risk for peri-implantitis development, and this effect is dose-dependent, leading to greater risk for peri-implantitis and greater severity of peri-implantitis as hyperglycemia is more severe.[37] Greater values for peri-implant measures have also been detected in individuals with cardiovascular disease.[38] These associations may be attributed to the increased or decreased inflammatory responses of the systemic diseases in peri-implant tissues, the medications and/or life-style factors which therefore may influence the implant outcome.

In the present investigation, the mean peri-implant bone loss after 12 to 177 months of loading was estimated to be 2.18 ± 1.57 mm. The mean time of implant in function was 63.04 ± 33.18 months. Moreover, peri-implant bone loss of ≤2 mm was recorded in almost half (49.3%) of the installed implants. In a recent systematic review and meta-analysis that assessed the marginal bone loss in rough threaded and machined smooth neck implants, the estimated bone loss was 0.39 mm (95% CI 0.61–0.18 mm) after 3 to 6 months of loading and 0.43 mm (95% CI 0.65–0.22 mm) after 1 year or longer.[39] However, the present study evaluated implants during a longer follow-up time. Only implants in function for at least 1 year were eligible for inclusion in the analysis. In a retrospective clinical study that included different implant systems with a follow-up of 1 to 11 years, the mean marginal bone loss 1.37 ± 1.5 mm.[40] The difference between these findings and the results of the present investigation may be attributed to the increased peri-implant bone loss identified in the peri-implantitis implants. Bone remodeling is normally expected following implant placement. Other authors have reported that a marginal bone loss of 1.5 to 2.0 mm during the first year represents a good treatment outcome.[41-43] Implant surface was not associated with the incidence of peri-implantitis in the present cross-sectional study. This is in agreement with recent systematic reviews and consensus reports when clinical data were taken into consideration.[29,44]

When it comes to protective factors for peri-implantitis, interproximal flossing/brushing, proton pump inhibitors, use of anticoagulants, as well as restoration type have been reported in the literature.[19,20] Interproximal flossing/brushing is expected to be protective for disease onset when biofilm-mediated inflammatory conditions are considered. Similarly, the association of the restoration type (fixed dental prostheses vs single crowns) with the development of peri-implantitis may also be explained by the more difficult access to oral hygiene instructions. None of these parameters were found to be significant in the present investigation. This might be due to the inclusion of compliant patients who regularly attended the clinic for periodontal maintenance. Moreover, none of the included individuals reported intake of proton pump inhibitors which may explain the insignificant findings regarding medication intake. The reported protective role of anticoagulants in the literature may be explained by their secondary anti-inflammatory effects.[45] However, in the present cross-sectional study, fewer than five individuals reported use of anticoagulants.

The results of the present study showed that smoking is not associated with peri-implantitis. Although smoking has been greatly associated with periodontitis, attachment loss, and tooth loss, the majority of investigations failed to clearly identify smoking as a risk factor/indicator for peri-implantitis as reported in the proceedings of the 2017 Word Workshop on the Classification of Periodontal and Peri-implant Diseases and Conditions.[7,46,47] This might be attributed to the various confounding factors that may be present or may be related to the differences in categorization of smoking habits. All studies include patient-reported information regarding smoking status, and this was the case in the present study.[7] Patient's age and sex as well as implant location were not associated with the onset of peri-implantitis in the current investigation. This is in agreement with a systematic review and meta-analysis of the literature.[48] The association between compliance to preventive periodontal maintenance therapy and peri-implantitis has been established. In a 5-year clinical study, the prevalence of peri-implantitis in individuals adhering to maintenance protocols was 18%, while for non-compliers this was significantly increased to 43.9%.[49] In the present study, no significant association was reported between compliance and peri-implantitis incidence. This might be due to the inclusion of patients who attended the clinic for periodontal maintenance regularly (at least two appointments per year). Monje et al[50] demonstrated that compliance to at least two peri-implant maintenance therapies per year is crucial to prevent peri-implantitis.

No standardized radiographic assessment of the bone levels was possible due to the nature of the study. Hence, this limits the ability to make interpretation about the causality of the identified risk/protective indicators. However, the aim of the present study was to assess a number of patient-, implant-, and bone-related factors using multivariate analysis in order to identify risk/protective indicators of peri-implantitis. Prospective longitudinal studies are required for the identification of true risk factors. All information regarding patients' medical status and medications were self-reported and no medical examination was performed to assess the patients systemically. In addition, all systemic conditions were analyzed together as a group due to the presence of many different systemic diseases among the individuals in the cohort that could not be statistically compared individually. The inclusion of patients receiving dental implant therapy of different systems that were treated by different surgeons and restorative dental practitioners at a university dental clinic should also be considered when interpreting the results. The prevalence of peri-implantitis in the present study was in agreement with the literature.[22,51]

Conclusions

Within the limitations of the study, the prevalence of peri-implantitis in a cohort receiving dental implant therapy at a university dental clinic was 10.7% at the implant level and 21.3% at the patient level. Simultaneous guided bone regeneration, periodontal disease, and patient-reported systemic comorbidities were the most significant risk indicators that were associated with the development of peri-implantitis. The mean peri-implant bone loss was estimated to be 2.18 ± 1.57 for the evaluated implants. Randomized clinical trials or prospective longitudinal cohort studies are required to demonstrate true causality.

Acknowledgment

The authors report there are no conflicts of interest.

References

1. Hjalmarsson L, Gheisarifar M, Jemt T. A systematic review of survival of single implants as presented in longitudinal studies with a follow-up of at least 10 years. Eur J Oral Implantol 2016;9(Supp 1):S155–S162.

2. Pjetursson BE, Asgeirsson AG, Zwahlen M, Sailer I. Improvements in implant dentistry over the last decade: comparison of survival and complication rates in older and newer publications. Int J Oral Maxillofac Implants 2014;29(Suppl):308–324.

3. Di Francesco F, De Marco G, Gironi Carnevale UA, Lanza M, Lanza A. The number of implants required to support a maxillary overdenture: a systematic review and meta-analysis. J Prosthodont Res 2019;63:15–24.

4. Romanos GE, Delgado-Ruiz R, Sculean A. Concepts for prevention of complications in implant therapy. Periodontol 2000 2019;81:7–17.

5. Renvert S, Persson GR, Pirih FQ, Camargo PM. Peri-implant health, peri-implant mucositis, and peri-implantitis: Case definitions and diagnostic considerations. J Periodontol 2018;89(Suppl 1):S304–S312.

6. Gargallo-Albiol J, Tavelli L, Barootchi S, Monje A, Wang HL. Clinical sequelae and patients' perception of dental implant removal: a cross-sectional study. J Periodontol 2021; 92:823–832.

7. Schwarz F, Derks J, Monje A, Wang HL. Peri-implantitis. J Periodontol 2018;89 (Suppl 1):S267–S290.

8. Derks J, Tomasi C. Peri-implant health and disease. A systematic review of current epidemiology. J Clin Periodontol 2015;42 (Suppl 16):S158–S171.

9. Derks J, Schaller D, Håkansson J, Wennström JL, Tomasi C, Berglundh T. Peri-implantitis - onset and pattern of progression. J Clin Periodontol 2016;43:383–388.

10. Karlsson K, Derks J, Håkansson J, Wennström JL, Petzold M, Berglundh T. Interventions for peri-implantitis and their effects on further bone loss: A retrospective analysis of a registry-based cohort. J Clin Periodontol 2019;46:872–879.

11. Polyzois I. Treatment planning for periimplant mucositis and periimplantitis. Implant Dent 2019;28:150–154.

12. Salvi GE, Bragger U. Mechanical and technical risks in implant therapy. Int J Oral Maxillofac Implants 2009;24(Suppl):69–85.

13. Sailer I, Karasan D, Todorovic A, Ligoutsikou M, Pjetursson BE. Prosthetic failures in dental implant therapy. Periodontol 2000 2022;88:130–144.

14. Klinge B, Flemming T, Cosyn J, et al. The patient undergoing implant therapy. Summary and consensus statements. The 4th EAO Consensus Conference 2015. Clin Oral Implants Res 2015;26(Suppl 11):64–67.

15. Fretwurst T, Nelson K. Influence of medical and geriatric factors on implant success: an overview of systematic reviews. Int J Prosthodont 2021;34:s21–s26.

16. Song X, Li L, Gou H, Xu Y. Impact of implant location on the prevalence of peri-implantitis: A systematic review and meta- analysis. J Dent 2020;103:103490.

17. Carra MC, Rangé H, Swerts PJ, Tuand K, Vandamme K, Bouchard P. Effectiveness of implant-supported fixed partial denture in patients with history of periodontitis: A systematic review and meta-analysis. J Clin Periodontol 2022;49:208–223.

18. Stacchi C, Troiano G, Rapani A, et al. Factors influencing the prevalence of peri-implantitis in implants inserted in augmented maxillary sinuses: A multicenter cross-sectional study. J Periodontol 2021;92:1117–1125.

19. Rodrigo D, Sanz-Sánchez I, Figuero E, et al. Prevalence and risk indicators of peri-implant diseases in Spain. J Clin Periodontol. 2018;45:1510–1520.

20. Romandini M, Lima C, Pedrinaci I, Araoz A, Soldini MC, Sanz M. Prevalence and risk/protective indicators of peri-implant diseases: A university-representative cross-sectional study. Clin Oral Implants Res 2021;32: 112–122.

21. Berglundh T, Armitage G, Araujo MG, et al. Peri-implant diseases and conditions: Consensus report of workgroup 4 of the 2017 World Workshop on the Classification of Periodontal and Peri-Implant Diseases and Conditions. J Clin Periodontol 2018;45 (Suppl 20):S286–S291.

22. Diaz P, Gonzalo E, Villagra LJG, Miegimolle B, Suarez MJ. What is the prevalence of peri-implantitis? A systematic review and meta-analysis. BMC Oral Health 2022;22:449.

23. Koldsland OC, Scheie AA, Aass AM. Prevalence of peri-implantitis related to severity of the disease with different degrees of bone loss. J Periodontol 2010;81:231–238.

24. Grunau O, Terheyden H. Lateral augmentation of the sinus floor followed by regular implants versus short implants in the vertically deficient posterior maxilla: a systematic review and timewise meta-analysis of randomized studies. Int J Oral Maxillofac Surg 2022;16:S0901-5027(22)00466-0.

25. Lin G, Ye S, Liu F, He F. A retrospective study of 30,959 implants: Risk factors associated with early and late implant loss. J Clin Periodontol 2018;45:733–743.

26. Yang Y, Hu H, Zeng M, et al. The survival rates and risk factors of implants in the early stage: a retrospective study. BMC Oral Health 2021;21:293.

27. Ramanauskaite A, Borges T, Almeida BL, Correia A. Dental implant outcomes in grafted sockets: a systematic review and meta-analysis. J Oral Maxillofac Res 2019; 10:e8.

28. Derks J, Håkansson J, Wennström JL, Tomasi C, Larsson M, Berglundh T. Effectiveness of implant therapy analyzed in a Swedish population: early and late implant loss. J Dent Res 2015;94:44S–51S.

29. Schwarz F, Alcoforado G, Guerrero A, et al. Peri-implantitis: Summary and consensus statements of group 3. The 6th EAO Consensus Conference 2021. Clin Oral Implants Res 2021;32(Suppl 21):245–253.

30. Ferreira SD, Martins CC, Amaral SA, et al. Periodontitis as a risk factor for peri-implantitis: systematic review and meta-analysis of observational studies. J Dent 2018;79:1–10.

31. Lafaurie GI, Sabogal MA, Castillo DM, et al. Microbiome and microbial biofilm profiles of peri-implantitis: a systematic review. J Periodontol 2017;88:1066–1089.

32. Kornman KS. Mapping the pathogenesis of periodontitis: a new look. J Periodontol 2008;79:1560–1568.

33. Pjetursson BE, Helbling C, Weber HP, et al. Peri-implantitis susceptibility as it relates to periodontal therapy and supportive care. Clin Oral Implants Res 2012;23:888–894.

34. Cortellini S, Favril C, De Nutte M, Teughels W, Quirynen M. Patient compliance as a risk factor for the outcome of implant treatment. Periodontol 2000 2019;81:209–225.

35. Seki K, Hasuike A, Hagiwara Y. Clinical evaluation of the relationship between systemic disease and the time of onset of peri-implantitis: a retrospective cohort study. J Oral Implantol 2023;49:55–61.

36. Diz P, Scully C, Sanz M. Dental implants in the medically compromised patient. J Dent 2013;41:195–206.

37. Al-Sowygh ZH, Ghani SMA, Sergis K, Vohra F, Akram Z. Peri-implant conditions and levels of advanced glycation end products among patients with different glycemic control. Clin Implant Dent Relat Res 2018;20:345–351.

38. Wang IC, Ou A, Johnston J, et al. Association between periimplantitis and cardiovascular diseases: a case-control study. J Periodontol 2022;93:633–643.

39. Zhang Q, Yue X. Marginal bone loss around machined smooth neck implants compared to rough threaded neck implants: a systematic review and meta-analysis. J Prosthodont 2021;30:401–411.

40. Rokn A, Aslroosta H, Akbari S, Najafi H, Zayeri F, Hashemi K. Prevalence of peri-implantitis in patients not participating in well-designed supportive periodontal treatments: a cross-sectional study. Clin Oral Implants Res 2017;28:314–319.

41. Papaspyridakos P, Chen CJ, Singh M, Weber HP, Gallucci GO. Success criteria in implant dentistry: a systematic review. J Dent Res 2012;91:242–248.

42. Roos-Jansåker AM, Lindahl C, Renvert H, Renvert S. Nine- to fourteen-year follow-up of implant treatment. Part II: presence of peri-implant lesions. J Clin Periodontol 2006;33:290–295.

43. Tarnow DP, Cho SC, Wallace SS. The effect of inter-implant distance on the height of inter-implant bone crest. J Periodontol 2000;71:546–549.

44. Stavropoulos A, Bertl K, Winning L, Polyzois I. What is the influence of implant surface characteristics and/or implant material on the incidence and progression of peri-implantitis? A systematic literature review. Clin Oral Implants Res 2021;32 (Suppl 21):203–229.

45. Müller KA, Chatterjee M, Rath D, Geisler T. Platelets, inflammation and anti-inflammatory effects of antiplatelet drugs in ACS and CAD. Thromb Haemost 2015;114:498–518.

46. Axelsson P, Paulander J, Lindhe J. Relationship between smoking and dental status in 35, 50-, 65-, and 75-year-old individuals. J Clin Periodontol 1998;25:297–305.

47. Tomar SL, Asma S. Smoking-attributable periodontitis in the United States: findings from NHANES III. National Health and Nutrition Examination Survey. J Periodontol 2000; 71:743–751.

48. Dreyer H, Grischke J, Tiede C, et al. Epidemiology and risk factors of peri-implantitis: a systematic review. J Periodontal Res 2018;53:657–681.

49. Costa FO, Takenaka-Martinez S, Cota LO, Ferreira SD, Silva GL, Costa JE. Peri-implant disease in subjects with and without preventive maintenance: a 5-year follow-up. J Clin Periodontol 2012;39:173–181.

50. Monje A, Wang HL, Nart J. Association of preventive maintenance therapy compliance and peri-implant diseases: a cross-sectional study. J Periodontol 2017;88:1030–1041.

51. Rakic M, Galindo-Moreno P, Monje A, et al. How frequent does peri-implantitis occur? A systematic review and meta-analysis. Clin Oral Investig 2018;22:1805–1816.

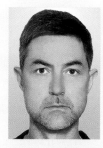

Phoebus Tsaousoglou

Phoebus Tsaousoglou Periodontist, Department of Preventive Dentistry, Periodontology and Implant Biology, Faculty of Dentistry, School of Health Sciences, Aristotle University of Thessaloniki, Greece

Georgios S. Chatzopoulos Periodontist, Department of Preventive Dentistry, Periodontology and Implant Biology, Faculty of Dentistry, School of Health Sciences, Aristotle University of Thessaloniki, Greece; and Adjunct Assistant Professor, Division of Periodontology, Department of Developmental and Surgical Sciences, Minneapolis, MN, USA

Lazaros Tsalikis Professor, Department of Preventive Dentistry, Periodontology and Implant Biology, Faculty of Dentistry, School of Health Sciences, Aristotle University of Thessaloniki, Greece

Theodosia Lazaridou Periodontist, Private practice

Georgios Mikrogeorgis Associate Professor, Department of Endodontology, Faculty of Dentistry, School of Health Sciences, Aristotle University of Thessaloniki, Greece

Ioannis Vouros Professor, Department of Preventive Dentistry, Periodontology and Implant Biology, Faculty of Dentistry, School of Health Sciences, Aristotle University of Thessaloniki, Greece

Correspondence: Georgios S. Chatzopoulos, Department of Preventive Dentistry, Periodontology and Implant Biology, School of Dentistry, Faculty of Health Sciences, Aristotle University of Thessaloniki, University, Campus, 54124 Thessaloniki, Greece. Email: gschatzo@dent.auth.gr

First submission: 6 Feb 2023
Acceptance: 15 Apr 2023
Online publication: 4 May 2023

Effects of ozone therapy on periodontal and peri-implant surgical wound healing: a systematic review

Luiz Felipe Palma, MSc, PhD/Cristiano Joia, MSc/Leandro Chambrone, MSc, PhD

Objective: To evaluate the effectiveness of the use of adjuvant ozone therapy in the healing process of wounds resulting from periodontal and peri-implant surgical procedures by answering the following focused question: "Can adjuvant ozone therapy improve wound healing outcomes related to periodontal and peri-implant surgical procedures?". **Method and materials:** MEDLINE (via PubMed), EMBASE, and Cochrane Central Register of Controlled Trials (CENTRAL) databases were searched, without language restriction, for peer-reviewed articles published until 23 March 2022, in addition to manual search. Only controlled clinical trials (randomized or not) were considered. The risk of bias was evaluated by the Cochrane risk-of-bias tool for RCTs – version 1 (RoB1). Data were pooled into evidence tables and a descriptive summary was presented. **Results:** Of the 107 potentially eligible records, only seven studies were included. Four addressed free/deepithelialized gingival grafts with a palatal donor area, two evaluated implant sites, and one comprised gingivectomy and gingivoplasty. A total of 225 patients were evaluated in the included studies, considering control and test groups (ozone and other adjuvant therapies for comparison). Ozone therapy had a positive effect on outcomes directly or indirectly related to periodontal/peri-implant surgical wound healing. Furthermore, it could also increase the stability of immediately loaded single implants installed in the posterior mandible. **Conclusion:** In general, ozone therapy seems to both accelerate the healing processes of periodontal/peri-implant wounds and increase the secondary stability of dental implants; however, considering the limited evidence available and the risk of bias in the included studies (none classified as low risk), a definitive conclusion cannot be drawn. *(Quintessence Int 2023;54: 100–110; doi: 10.3290/j.qi.b3512007)*

Key words: dental implants, ozone, ozone therapy, periodontal surgery, wound healing/surgery

Many periodontal and peri-implant surgical procedures have been proposed in recent decades to improve patients' oral health-related quality of life.[1-5] These procedures are generally associated with the resolution of functional or esthetic alterations, discomfort, pain, or even psychosocial issues.[6,7] Peri-implant surgical procedures aim mainly to offer access for proper removal of biofilm and calculus from the implant surface, allowing for healing and reducing the risk of peri-implantitis progression. Augmentative techniques may be performed concomitantly, in order to achieve new osseointegration and bone defect regeneration.[8,9] Likewise, the main goal of surgical periodontal procedures is to gain access for performing adequate debridement of the root surfaces and to establish optimal gingival contours.[10]

Healing is defined as the whole physiologic process responsible for repairing the integrity of injured tissues.[1,11-18] This process depends not only on adequate technical performance but also on comprehensive knowledge of the biologic principles involved.[1] The healing of oral tissues occurs as a result of a complex cascade of molecular and cellular events that may be grouped into:
- hemostatic phase (or hemostasis)
- inflammatory phase
- proliferative phase
- maturation and remodeling phase.[1,8-15]

Normally, these phases overlap to some extent and vary in duration according to the type of tissue and local and systemic conditions such as smoking, microbial infections, and the shape and extent of the surgical wound.[1,11,12] Other relevant aspects of the postoperative phase of the periodontal/peri-implant treatment are the occurrence and prevention of adverse effects (eg, pain, discomfort, and bleeding) and the quality of tissue healing processes.[1,11-18]

Some adjuvant therapies have been proposed for microbial control in the surgical area, reducing postsurgical morbidity and/or accelerating (improving) tissue healing processes.[19-22] In this sense, the topical use of ozone (in the forms of ozonated water, ozonated oil, or ozone gas) has been suggested in periodontology and implantology for antimicrobial control[23-25] or as an adjuvant for tissue repair and regeneration.[19-21,26,27] The antimicrobial activity, its most known propriety, is based on oxidative processes that lead to detrimental effects on both constitution and metabolism of bacteria, fungi, viruses, and protozoa, without inducing resistance.[28]

Recently other therapeutic effects of ozone have gained attention, such as its influence on cellular and humoral immune systems, stimulating immunocompetent cells proliferation and immunoglobulins and biologically active substances synthesis (interleukins, leukotrienes, and prostaglandins).[29] Moreover, ozone is capable of activating macrophage function and increasing the sensitivity of microorganisms to phagocytosis, besides favoring better interactions between dental implant surfaces and biologic tissues (proliferation and differentiation of mesenchymal cells and reduction of pro-inflammatory cytokine).[29] Finally, the effects on blood cells and circulatory system elements would lead to benefits on oxygen metabolism, cellular energy, antioxidant defense system, and microcirculation.[30]

The effects of ozone therapy on the healing of periodontal and peri-implant surgical wounds, however, have not been systematically compiled and evaluated so far. Thus, this systematic review aims to evaluate the effectiveness of adjuvant ozone therapy in the healing of wounds resulting from periodontal and peri-implant surgical procedures.

Method and materials

General information

This systematic review was developed in accordance with the PRISMA guidelines[31] and the Cochrane Handbook for Systematic Reviews of Interventions.[32]

PICO strategy, focused question, types of studies, and inclusion/exclusion criteria

Only interventional studies characterized as randomized clinical trials (RCTs) or controlled (nonrandomized) clinical trials were considered eligible for inclusion. Case reports, case series, and observational studies were excluded from this systematic review. Interventional studies reporting outcomes from nonsurgical periodontal or peri-implant treatment were also not considered.

The focused question "Can adjuvant ozone therapy improve wound healing outcomes related to periodontal and peri-implant surgical procedures?" was formulated according to the following PICO strategy:[33]

- Population: Adult patients (≥18 years) undergoing periodontal or peri-implant surgical procedures
- Intervention: use of ozone compounds (ie, ozonized water, ozonized oil, or ozone gas) as adjunctive/complementary strategy to surgical procedures in periodontal or peri-implant treatment
- Comparison: surgical procedures in periodontal or peri-implant treatment
- Outcomes of interest: assessment of any clinical, radiographic, laboratory, or patient-reported outcomes related to surgical wound healing.

Outcome variables

Three major types of outcome variables were considered for this systematic review:

- Clinical outcome variables: defined as structural and biologic assessments performed by researchers during a clinical examination (eg, probing depth, clinical attachment level, depth of gingival recessions, changes in keratinized tissue width, or other clinical scores/outcomes relevant to the surgical approaches of interest)
- Variables from patient-reported outcomes (PROMs): defined as assessments of the quality of life or other outcomes reported by patients on different aspects of the therapy such as general satisfaction, preferences, perceived pain/discomfort, the occurrence of adverse events, and esthetics and function alterations, using standardized assessment methods (eg, visual analog scale [VAS] or questionnaires).
- Variables from images, imaging exams, histology, cytology, or laboratory tests: any analysis that characterizes tissue healing processes.

Table 1 The search strategy for MEDLINE

No.	Search terms
#1	periodontal surgery OR gingivectomy OR gingival recession/surgery OR palatal tissue harvesting OR dental implants OR implant placement
#2	ozone OR ozone therapy OR ozonated water OR ozonated oil OR gaseous ozone therapy
#3	#1 AND #2

Search strategy

Comprehensive search strategies were established to identify peer-reviewed studies for inclusion in this systematic review. The MEDLINE (via PubMed), EMBASE, and CENTRAL databases were searched without language and publication date restrictions for papers published up to and including 23 March 2022.

MeSH terms, keywords, and other free terms were used for searching and Boolean operators (OR, AND) were applied to combine searches. Detailed search strategies were developed for each database based on that used in MEDLINE (Table 1). Moreover, the reference list of any potential article was examined (manual search).

Assessment of validity and data extraction

Two independent reviewers (CJ and LC) screened the titles, abstracts, and full texts of the articles identified by searching. Any disagreement was resolved via discussion between the reviewers. When necessary, a third reviewer was consulted (LFP). Studies meeting the inclusion criteria underwent validity assessment and data extraction. Data on the following issues were extracted and recorded in duplicate (CJ and LC) using custom-designed data extraction forms:

- citation, publication status, and year of publication
- location of the trial
- study design
- characteristics of the participants
- outcome measures
- methodologic quality
- conclusions
- source of funding and conflict of interest.

Quality assessment and assessment of the risk of bias

The risk of bias of each included randomized clinical trial was assessed in duplicate using the Cochrane risk-of-bias tool for RCTs - version 1 (RoB1).[34] Each domain was ranked as low (+), high (-), or unclear (?). The criteria included the assessment of:

- randomization sequence generation
- allocation concealment
- blinding of participants and personnel
- blinding of outcome assessment
- incomplete outcome data
- selective reporting
- other bias.

Moreover, the studies were categorized into a low, high, or unclear risk of bias, according to the following criteria:

- low risk of bias (plausible bias unlikely to seriously alter the results) if all domains were at low risk of bias
- high risk of bias (plausible bias that seriously weakens confidence in the results) if one or more domains were at high risk of bias
- unclear risk of bias (plausible bias that raises some doubt about the results) if one or more domains were at unclear risk of bias.

In addition, nonrandomized studies were automatically considered to be at a high risk of bias.[35,36]

Data synthesis and statistical analyses

Data were pooled into evidence tables, and a descriptive summary was performed to determine the quantity of data, checking further for study variations in terms of the characteristics and results.

Results

General results

A total of 107 records were identified by both electronic and manual searches (Fig 1). After removing the duplicates, 64 publications were screened for eligibility and then 56 were excluded

Fig 1 PRISMA 2020 search flow diagram.

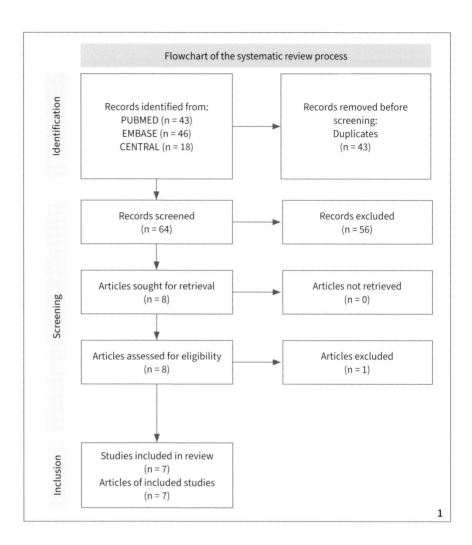

based on their title and/or abstract. Subsequently, the full-text version of eight articles[19,21,37-42] was evaluated. Seven articles were then considered eligible for inclusion in this systematic review[19,37-42] and one was excluded as it does not present a control group.[21]

Included studies

A total of 225 patients were evaluated in the included studies and no adverse effect from the ozone compounds was reported.[19,37-42] Four studies addressed clinical conditions related to free/deepithelialized gingival grafts with palatal donor areas,[37,39,40,42] totaling 104 patients (47 controls, 45 treated with ozone therapy, and 12 treated with photobiomodulation therapy). Two studies evaluated dental implant sites, one with immediately loaded implants and 25 patients (25 control sites, 25 sites sub-

mitted to photobiomodulation therapy, and 50 sites submitted to ozone therapy under two protocols)[38] and another one with conventionally loaded implants and 60 patients (30 controls and 30 submitted to ozone therapy).[41] Furthermore, one study evaluated 36 patients requiring gingivectomy and gingivoplasty (12 controls, 12 submitted to photobiomodulation therapy, and 12 submitted to ozone therapy).[19]

Four studies (57%) were conducted in Turkey[19,37,38,42] and three (43%) in India.[39-41] Moreover, all of them were university-based studies, except for one which did not present such information.[19] Although all studies reported no conflicts of interest,[19,37-42] one declared funding (material donation) from a private company[39] and the others either declared funding from the authors/universities or did not report such information. Table 2 presents a summary of the included studies and some general characteristics.

Table 2 Characteristics of the included studies

Study	Participants	Interventions	Outcome measures	Adverse effects	Authors' conclusions	Others
Isler et al[37]	36 healthy patients with gingival recessions requiring FGG with a palatal donor area. Nonsmokers.	The laser group (n=12) received 4 sessions of PBM therapy on the donor site (0, 3, and 7 days). The ozone group (n=12) received 4 sessions of ozone therapy on the donor site (0, 3, and 7 days). The control group (n=12) received no therapy.	Remaining wound area on the palate: a technique with H_2O_2 and digital photographs at 1, 3, 7, and 14 days. Pain, discomfort, changes in eating habits, burning sensation, amount of analgesics consumed: VAS at 1, 2, 3, 7, 14, and 30 days.	None.	Adjunctive ozone therapy could have a significantly beneficial effect on the acceleration of palatal wound healing following FGG procedures. Both PBM and ozone treatment modalities reduced postoperative discomfort as compared with spontaneous healing.	Location: Turkey. University-based study. Funding: authors/university. Conflict of interest: no.
Karaca et al[38]	25 healthy patients requiring immediately loaded mandibular single implants, bilaterally (slightly out of occlusion). Nonsmokers.	Group 1 received 25 implants and PBM therapy sessions on the site (0, 2, 4, 6, 8, 10, 12, and 14 days). Group 2 received 25 implants and ozone therapy sessions (3 minutes) on the site (3 times a week for 2 weeks). Group 3 received 25 implants and ozone therapy sessions (6 min) on the site (3 times a week for 2 weeks). The control group received 25 implants and no additional therapy.	Pain: VAS at 0, 1, 3, 5, and 7 days. Implant resonance frequency: implant stability quotient after surgery and at 6 months.	None.	Within the limitations of this study, it is concluded that both laser therapy and ozone therapy with prolonged application time increase implant stability in the immediate slightly functional loading of single implants in the posterior mandible. However, the standard application of ozone did not seem to have any effect on implant stability.	Location: Turkey. University-based study. Funding: university. Conflict of interest: no.
Patel et al[40]	20 healthy patients with gingival recessions requiring FGG with a palatal donor area. Nonsmokers.	The ozone group (n=10) received ozone therapy sessions on surgical wounds (donor and graft sites) once a day for 1 week. The control group (n=10) received a placebo in the palatal wounds, in the same way as the other group.	Cytological evaluation by scraping the sites: indices of keratinization and superficial cells evaluated at the beginning of the study, after 24 h, on the 3rd, 7th, 14th, and 21st days and 2, 3, 8, and 18 months after surgery.	None.	The results of this study indicate that the application of ozonated oil to the grafted and palatal donor sites of FGGs is of significant benefit in achieving early epithelial healing when compared to nonozonated oil. The topical application of ozonated oil provided a positive influence on the healing of FGG surgical sites (grafted site and palatal donor site). The regenerative changes observed after topical application of ozonated oil in the epithelial cells of healing tissue were significant, ultimately resulting in rapid keratinization and better healing of the gingival tissue.	Location: India. University-based study. Funding: authors. Conflict of interest: no.
Patel et al[39]	18 healthy patients with gingival recessions requiring FGG with a palatal donor area. Nonsmokers.	The ozone group (n=8) received ozone therapy sessions on surgical wounds once a day for 1 week. The control group (n=10) received a placebo in the same way as the other group.	Planimetric parameters: wound size and shape factor at baseline, 24 h, 5, 7, 14, 21, and 28 postoperative days. Cytological evaluation by scraping the sites: keratinization indices and superficial cells evaluated at baseline, 24 h, 3, 7, 14, and 21 days, and 2 and 3 months postoperatively.	None.	The results showed significant improvement in wound size and epithelial healing after topical ozonated oil application compared to control oil on palatal wounds.	Location: India. University-based study. Funding: Gnosis Wellness Center Inc, British Colombia, Canada (material donation). Conflict of interest: no.
Shekhar et al[41]	60 healthy patients requiring single, conventionally loaded dental implants. Nonsmokers.	The control group (n=30) received osteotomies with conventional saline irrigation. The ozone group (n=30) received osteotomies with ozonized water as the irrigant and topical application of ozone gas before implant insertion.	Inflammation: C-reactive protein biomarker one day before implant placement and 48 h after. Pain: VAS at 24 and 48 h and 7 days. Healing: Landry, Turnbull, and Howley index at 7 and 14 days.	None.	The present study showed the beneficial effect of ozone among patients undergoing dental implantation in terms of reduced pain and inflammation and faster tissue healing.	Location: India. University-based study. Funding: authors. Conflict of interest: no.

Table 2 Characteristics of the included studies (contd.)

Study	Participants	Interventions	Outcome measures	Adverse effects	Authors' conclusions	Others
Tasdemir et al[42]	30 patients with gingival recessions requiring deepithelialized gingival graft with a palatal donor area. Nonsmokers.	The ozone group (n = 15) received ozone therapy shortly after surgery and on days 1 and 3. The control group (n = 15) did not receive any additional therapy.	Surgery parameters: length of operation, graft waiting time from collection to suturing on the recipient site, graft height, thickness and width, and the number of analgesic tablets needed daily. Blood perfusion in the recipient sites: laser doppler flowmetry on the day of surgery (1 h after recovery from local anesthesia), on day 1 (before ozone therapy, shortly after, and a further 2 h after), on day 2, on day 3 (before ozone therapy, immediately after, and 2 h after) and days 6, 8, 10, and 13. Pain: VAS at 1, 2, 3, 6, 8, 10, and 13 days. Surgery-related quality of life: OHIP-14 questionnaire at 6 and 13 days.	None.	Within the limits of the present study, it was concluded that ozone therapy enhanced blood perfusion units in the first postoperative week. The increase in blood perfusion may be interpreted as improvement in wound healing. This outcome is also consistent with the increase in quality of life and decrease in postoperative pain in the ozone-treated group.	Location: Turkey. University-based study. Funding: university. Conflict of interest: no.
Uslu and Akgül[19]	36 healthy patients requiring gingivectomy and gingivoplasty. Nonsmokers.	The control group (n = 12) received only gingivectomy and gingivoplasty. The ozone group (n = 12) received gingivectomy and gingivoplasty and ozone application soon after surgery and at 3 and 7 days. The laser group (n = 12) received gingivectomy and gingivoplasty and application of PBM therapy soon after surgery and at 3 and 7 days.	Pain: VAS at 3, 7, 14, and 28 days and analgesic consumption. Quality of life: OHIP-14 questionnaire before surgery and at 7 and 14 days. Wound healing: method using H_2O_2 at 3, 7, 14, and 28 days after surgery.	None.	Within the limitations of the present study, PBM and ozone applications after gingivectomy improve the quality of life of the patients	Location: Turkey. Context: not reported. Funding: authors. Conflict of interest: no.

FGG, free gingival graft; OHIP, Oral Health Impact Profile; PBM, photobiomodulation; VAS, visual analog scale.

Quality and risk of bias of the included studies

The assessment of the methodologic quality of the included studies is reported in Fig 2. Overall, no RCT[19,37,39-42] was considered to be at low risk of bias, as well as the nonrandomized clinical trial.[38]

Three RCTs presented an unclear risk of bias[39,40,42] and the others a high risk of bias.[19,37,41] Lack of information or inadequacy of randomization,[19,39-41] allocation concealment,[39-41] and blinding of patients[19,37,41,42] or examiners[41,42] were the domains most commonly associated with a higher risk of bias among the RCTs included in this systematic review.

Individual outcomes from each study

In the study conducted by Isler et al,[37] which used a clinical method based on the application of H_2O_2, there was no difference between the groups (laser, ozone, and control) in any evaluation period considering the repair of palatal donor sites for free gingival graft. Using a digital image analysis method, in 14 days, the ozone group (36.04 ± 9.66 mm²) had smaller areas of remaining wounds in relation to the control group (48.21 ± 13.22 mm², P = .034). With regards to pain scores, no differences were obtained between the groups at any time, likewise for analgesic taking in the first week, changes in eating habits, and burning sensation. However, the control group showed greater discomfort compared to the laser (values not reported objectively, P = .002) and ozone groups on the seventh day (values not reported objectively, P < .001).

When pain at implant sites was evaluated by Karaca et al,[38] no difference was observed between the groups treated with laser therapy, ozone therapy (regardless of protocol), and the controls. However, after 6 months, higher implant stability indexes were obtained (P = .008) in the groups that received spectively, there was a decrease both in the mean size of the wound in the ozone group (39.58±3.240 mm²; 11.80±2.550 mm²; 5.51±1.470 mm²; 3.10±0.440 mm²; 0.00±0.000 mm²) compared with the other group (53.93±5.820 mm²; 30.01±4.210 mm²; 13.49±3.370 mm²; 8.98±1.690 mm²; 2.05±0.618 mm²), as well as in the shape factor (0.93±0.031% and 0.80±0.038%, P=.000; 1.07±0.208% and 0.87±0.066%, P=.011; 0.81±0.068% and 0.94±0.105%, P=.008; 1.19±0.303% and 0.92±0.127%, P=.020; 0.00±0.000% and 0.75±0.105%, P=.000). Evaluating cytologically the sites, the authors also observed that the keratinization and superficial cell indices of the ozone group showed an early decrease, similar to the control group, from the beginning to 24 hours. On day 3, however, the ozone group showed a greater decrease in keratinization (2.45±0.330 and 0.94±0.170, P=.000) and superficial cells indices (2.38±0.43 and 1.87±0.15, P=.003). On days 7, 14 and 21, respectively, the ozone group showed a faster increase in keratinization (5.71±0.340 and 2.00±0.290, P=.000; 21.65±1.920 and 11.39±2.750, P=.000; 38.81±2.490 and 25.02±2.620, P=.000) and superficial cell indices (16.82±1.82 and 7.47±2.40, P=.000; 62.85±4.04 and 41.89±1.66, P=.000; 92.57±1.51 and 72.34±1.30, P=.000) and, finally, in the second and third months, respectively, the keratinization index was higher in the ozone group (52.35±1.850 and 42.49±1.720, P=.000; 65.70±2.220 and 51.61±1.05, P=.000).

Another study carried out by Patel et al[40] evaluated histologically wound healing in ozone and control groups, both at the recipient and palatal donor sites of free gingival graft. On the third day, the ozone group showed a decrease in keratinization (16.61±1.75 and 24.83±2.67, P=.000) and superficial cell indices (63.06±2.57 and 70.73±2.06, P=.000) at the grafted sites; however, in the palatal donor area, there were higher values in both indices in the ozone group (2.46±0.350 and 0.94±0.170, P=.000; and 2.41±0.39 and 1.87±0.15, P=.000). On days 7, 14, and 21, respectively, the ozone group showed a faster increase in the keratinization index compared with the other group regarding both the donor (5.65±0.40 and 2.00±0.29, P=.000; 22.13±1.42 and 14.08±1.78, P=.000; 39.75±3.03 and 25.02±2.62, P=.000) and recipient areas (23.56±1.33 and 12.31±0.69, P=.000; 40.84±2.00 and 21.21±1.90, P=.000; 53.01±2.69 and 35.08±2.57, P=.000). The same was observed in relation to the index of superficial cells in donor (16.98±1.75 and 7.47±2.40, P=.000; 63.57±2.27 and 43.05±1.82, P=.000; 92.70±1.36 and 72.34±1.30, P=.000) and recipient areas (43.81±3.33 and 23.30±2.30, P=.000; 72.75±2.12 and 52.69±1.36, P=.000; 96.88±0.98 and 83.06±1.96, P=.000). After 2, 3, and 8 months, respectively, the keratinization index was also higher in the ozone group at both wound sites (donors: 52.55±1.73 and 42.49±1.72, P=.000; 65.92±2.02 and

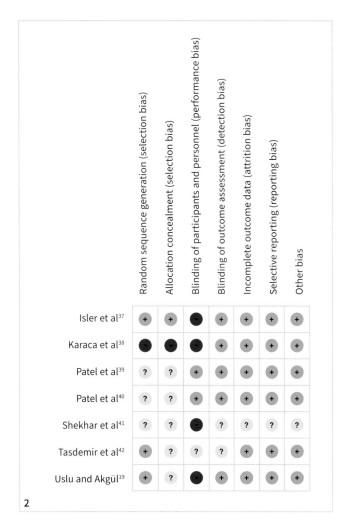

Fig 2 Risk of bias in each included study. Note: the study of Karaca et al[35] is a nonrandomized clinical trial.

photobiomodulation therapy (79±2.51 implant stability quotient [ISQ]) and ozone therapy for 6 minutes (80±3.01 ISQ) compared with the control group (77±2.14 ISQ) and the group that received ozone therapy for 3 minutes (77±4.29 ISQ).

Patel et al,[39] by planimetric analysis of wounds at palatal donor sites for free gingival graft, did not report any difference in the mean size of wounds after 24 hours between the ozone and control groups. On days 5, 7, 14, 21, and 28 (P=.000), re-

51.61±1.05, *P*=.000; 92.18±2.69 and 91.26±2.31, *P*=.000) (receptors: 70.80±1.13 and 62.55±1.76, *P*=.000; 86.64±3.17 and 74.47±2.35, *P*=.000; 96.80±1.53 and 91.03±1.61, *P*=.000), while the superficial cell index after 2, 3, 8, and 18 months was the same (index 100±0, without statistical analysis) and remained constant at both sites.

By quantification of C-reactive protein, Shekhar et al[41] evaluated inflammation on dental implant sites treated or not with ozonated compounds during the surgery and found that ozone therapy could reduce the biomarker within 48 hours (0.36±0.03 mg/dL and 0.88±0.05 mg/dL, *P*<.001). Regarding pain, within 24 and 48 hours and 7 days, the ozone group had lower scores compared with the control group (58.03±2.95 and 78.93±4.06, *P*<.001; 36.53±3.33 and 64.57±4.29, *P*<.001; 3.50±0.63 and 37.70±4.17, *P*<.001). Concerning the healing index, the ozone group was responsible for the highest values at 7 and 14 days (4.23±0.43 and 3.07±0.45, *P*<.001; 4.97±0.18 and 4.03±0.18, *P*<.001).

Tasdemir et al[42] addressed the effect of ozone therapy both on the recipient areas of deepithelialized gingival graft and their palatal donor areas. There were no differences between the control and ozone groups regarding several clinical and surgery-related variables. However, blood perfusion in the recipient sites (assessed by laser Doppler flowmetry) showed higher units in the ozone group in almost all study periods (on the day of surgery [1 hour after recovery from local anesthesia], on day 1 [before ozone therapy, right after, and 2 hours after], on day 2, on day 3 [before ozone therapy, right after, and 2 more hours after], and on days 6, 8, 10, and 13): 97.6±5.19 and 97.7±7.12, *P*=.98; 110.9±5.53 and 129.5±5.2, *P*<.001; 110.9±6.7 and 129.4±5.5, *P*<.001; 111.3±5.8 and 132.2±5.1, *P*<.001; 134.9±4.8 and 154.8±6.7, *P*<.001; 150±2.6 and 177.9±6.3, *P*<.001; 149.7±3.3 and 178±6.0, *P*<.001; 149.8±3.2 and 179.4±6.9, *P*<.001; 175.8±9.6 and 206.4±7.9, *P*<.001; 200.7±7.1 and 210.7±7.7, *P*<.001; 212.4±6.0 and 198.6±4.8, *P*<.001; 204.7±4.9 and 191.1±3.9, *P*<.001. Furthermore, the ozone group also showed higher scores of quality of life on the sixth day (24.5 and 22.6, standard deviations [SDs] not reported, *P*=.006) but no longer from the thirteenth day. At 1, 2, 3, 6, and 8 days, respectively, the ozone group had the lower averages of pain from receptor (4.7 and 3.0; 3.2 and 1.8; 2.0 and 0.8; 1.8 and 0.6; 0.2 and 0.0; unreported SDs, *P*<.05) and donor sites (6.4 and 3.7; 4.8 and 2.4; 2.8 and 1.2; 2.2 and 0.13; 1.0 and 0.0; SDs not reported, *P*<.05). Finally, the patients in the ozone group required fewer analgesic tablets (8.08±1.0 and 5.1±0.9, *P*<.001).

Uslu and Akgül[19] submitted patients to gingivectomy and gingivoplasty and evaluated the effects of ozone and low-level laser therapies on pain, quality of life, and wound healing. The pain scores were higher in the control group than in the laser group on day 3 (29.5±5.13 and 19.75±4.37, *P*=.002) and higher in the control group than in the ozone and laser groups on day 7 (10.25±5.29 and 4.75±3.84 and 1.5±3.21, *P*=.000); on the other hand, the scores of the ozone group were higher than those of the laser group on day 3 (23±6.99 and 19.75±4.37, *P*=.002) and day 7 (4.75±3.84 and 1.5±3.21, *P*=.001). At 14 and 28 days, there was no difference in pain between either group. The total score obtained from the Oral Health Impact Profile-14 questionnaire in the control group was higher than that in the laser group only on day 7 (18.67±3.39 and 14.25±3.33, *P*=.022). The score obtained from the third question at 7 and 14 days, however, was lower in the laser group than in the control and ozone groups (data not objectively reported, *P*<.05). There were no differences concerning epithelialization at any time between the groups, but the use of analgesics was more frequent in the control group (data not reported, *P*<.05).

Discussion

Summary of the main results

Ozone therapy, in different forms of application, seemed to have a positive effect on the outcomes directly or indirectly related to periodontal/peri-implant wound healing (palatal donor sites of free/deepithelialized gingival graft or recipient sites, areas submitted to gingivectomy/gingivoplasty).[19,37,39-42] Data from the included studies indicated a faster healing response when sites treated with ozone were compared with control ones but only early in the clinical course.

In contrast, the results from both laser therapy and ozone therapy with prolonged application time suggested increasing the stability of immediately loaded single implants installed in the posterior mandible. However, the standard application of ozone did not appear to have any effect on implant stability.[38]

Quality of evidence

No included study showed a low risk of bias because of lack of information or inadequacy of randomization,[19,39-41] allocation concealment,[39-41] blinding of patients[19,37,41,42] or examiners,[41,42] or even due to the study design itself (controlled clinical trial).[38] These conditions may not essentially affect the results achieved by the studies but reporting them clearly is of paramount importance to the audience.

Limitations and potential biases in the review process

As the outcomes (factors directly or indirectly related to peri-implant/periodontal tissue repair[19,37,39-42] or stability of dental implants[38]), study periods, methods, and samples addressed in the studies were quite heterogenous, it was not possible to combine the extracted data to generate pooled estimates (ie, pairwise meta-analyses would include potential biases and lead to doubted results) (Table 2). This fact is easily noticed in studies that have a photobiomodulation therapy group or in those that compare more than one protocol of ozone therapy.[19,37,38]

The authors believe that these controversial questions emerged mainly from the limited number of studies available in the literature about ozone therapy in periodontal and peri-implant surgical wound healing. A systematic review without meta-analyses is also representative but it may be less precise to answer the formulated focused question(s).[32,33] These aspects may be considered the main limitations of the present study.

Agreements and disagreements with other studies or systematic reviews

To the best of the present authors' knowledge, there is no systematic review about the effect of ozone therapy on periodontal and peri-implant surgical wound healing, even without considering the type of surgical procedure or the ozone compound. This fact makes it difficult to discuss properly the present findings based on the most current literature.

The benefits of ozone therapy in the repair of human wounds/ulcers from other etiologies, however, have already been addressed by some systematic reviews. Wen et al[43] reported that ozone may accelerate the improvement of wound areas and reduce the rate of amputation in chronically refractory wounds and ulcers. Fitzpatrick et al,[44] likewise, suggested that chronic wounds seem to heal in a shorter period when ozone is used. Bomfim et al[45] concluded that the use of ozone as an adjuvant treatment for ulcers of the lower limbs (especially diabetic foot) could be advantageous for tissue repair; on the other hand, the results of a meta-analysis by Liu et al[46] indicated that there is no evidence concerning the superiority of ozone therapy over conventional therapy regarding the reduction of ulcer areas, the number of ulcers healed, adverse events, and amputation rate in diabetic patients. For Di Fede et al,[47] conservative surgery combined with several adjuvant, noninvasive procedures such as ozone may promote partial or total healing of medication-related osteonecrosis of the jaw in any stage, with better results in variables of different natures.

Although nonsurgical periodontal and peri-implant therapies are out of the scope of this paper, another systematic review reported quite similar results. Moraschini et al[48] indicated that ozone presents antimicrobial activity and good biocompatibility with periodontal cells and tissues; however, due to the heterogeneity across the available studies, besides confounding factors and short follow-up periods, there is no reliable evidence that ozone therapy is beneficial as an adjunct to scaling and root planing. On the other hand, a meta-analysis conducted by Deepthi and Bilichodmath[25] on the effects of ozone as an adjunct to mechanical therapy in patients with periodontitis showed that local ozone application may be a potential atraumatic, and promising antimicrobial agent (ie, a suitable tool during supportive periodontal therapy). For them, this clinical benefit probably arises from the ability of ozone to inactivate microorganisms. :::

Conclusion

In general, ozone therapy seems to present a positive effect on both the healing of periodontal/peri-implant wounds and secondary stability of dental implants; however, taking into account that the available evidence is quite limited and no study included in this systematic review had a low risk of bias, a definitive conclusion cannot be drawn.

Implications for practice and future research

Ozone therapy is undoubtedly an important and promising adjuvant therapeutic modality for periodontal and peri-implant surgical procedures; however, the decision-making process for selecting the best compound, concentration, and technique remains unclear. Likewise, the methods and evaluation periods of clinical outcomes, as well as those reported by patients, require standardization in future studies.

Disclosure

The authors have not declared any conflicts of interest.

References

1. Chambrone L, Avila-Ortiz G. Tissues: Critical Issues in Periodontal and Implant-Related Plastic and Reconstructive Surgery. 1st ed. Chicago: Quintessence Publishing, 2022.

2. Avila-Ortiz G, Bartold PM, Giannobile W, et al. Biologics and cell therapy tissue engineering approaches for the management of the edentulous maxilla: a systematic review. Int J Oral Maxillofac Implants 2016;31(Suppl): s121–s164.

3. Li G, Zhou T, Lin S, Shi S, Lin Y. Nanomaterials for craniofacial and dental tissue engineering. J Dent Res 2017;96:725–732.

4. Obregon F, Vaquette C, Ivanovski S, Hutmacher DW, Bertassoni LE. Three-dimensional bioprinting for regenerative dentistry and craniofacial tissue engineering. J Dent Res 2015;94(9 Suppl):143S–152S.

5. Larsson L, Decker AM, Nibali L, Pilipchuk SP, Berglundh T, Giannobile WV. Regenerative medicine for periodontal and peri-implant diseases. J Dent Res 2016;95:255–266.

6. Sischo L, Broder HL. Oral health-related quality of life: what, why, how, and future implications. J Dent Res 2011;90:1264–1270.

7. Inglehart MR, Bagramian RA. Oral Health-Related Quality of Life. 1st ed. Chicago: Quintessence Publishing, 2002.

8. Montero E, Roccuzzo A, Molina A, Monje A, Herrera D, Roccuzzo M. Minimal invasiveness in the reconstructive treatment of peri-implantitis defects (Epub ahead of print, 28 Jul 2022). Periodontol 2000 doi: 10.1111/prd.12460.

9. Schwarz F, Jepsen S, Obreja K, Galarraga-Vinueza ME, Ramanauskaite A. Surgical therapy of peri-implantitis. Periodontol 2000 2022;88:145–181.

10. Heitz-Mayfield LJ, Lang NP. Surgical and nonsurgical periodontal therapy. Learned and unlearned concepts. Periodontol 2000 2013;62:218–231.

11. Polimeni G, Xiropaidis AV, Wikesjo UM. Biology and principles of periodontal wound healing/regeneration. Periodontol 2000 2006;41:30–47.

12. Susin C, Fiorini T, Lee J, De Stefano JA, Dickinson DP, Wikesjo UM. Wound healing following surgical and regenerative periodontal therapy. Periodontol 2000 2015; 68:83–98.

13. Cardaropoli G, Araujo M, Lindhe J. Dynamics of bone tissue formation in tooth extraction sites. An experimental study in dogs. J Clin Periodontol 2003;30:809–818.

14. Trombelli L, Farina R, Marzola A, Bozzi L, Liljenberg B, Lindhe J. Modeling and remodeling of human extraction sockets. J Clin Periodontol 2008;35:630–639.

15. Nyman S, Lindhe J, Karring T, Rylander H. New attachment following surgical treatment of human periodontal disease. J Clin Periodontol 1982;9:290–296.

16. Caton J, Nyman S, Zander H. Histometric evaluation of periodontal surgery. II. Connective tissue attachment levels after four regenerative procedures. J Clin Periodontol 1980;7:224–231.

17. Polson AM, Caton J. Factors influencing periodontal repair and regeneration. J Periodontol 1982;53:617–625.

18. Sculean A, Gruber R, Bosshardt DD. Soft tissue wound healing around teeth and dental implants. J Clin Periodontol 2014; 41(Suppl 15):S6–S22.

19. Uslu MÖ, Akgül S. Evaluation of the effects of photobiomodulation therapy and ozone applications after gingivectomy and gingivoplasty on postoperative pain and patients' oral health-related quality of life. Lasers Med Sci 2020;35:1637–1647.

20. Acikan I, Sayeste E, Bozoglan A, et al. Evaluation of the effects of topical application of chlorhexidine, ozone, and metronidazole on palatal wound healing: a histopathological study. J Craniofac Surg 2022;33:1929–1933.

21. Tualzik T, Chopra R, Gupta SJ, Sharma N, Khare M, Gulati L. Effects of ozonated olive oil and photobiomodulation using diode laser on gingival depigmented wound: A randomized clinical study. J Indian Soc Periodontol 2021;25:422–426.

22. Chaudhry K, Rustagi N, Bali R, et al. Efficacy of adjuvant ozone therapy in reducing postsurgical complications following impacted mandibular third-molar surgery: A systematic review and meta-analysis. J Am Dent Assoc 2021;152:842–854.e1.

23. Rapone B, Ferrara E, Santacroce L, et al. The gaseous ozone therapy as a promising antiseptic adjuvant of periodontal treatment: a randomized controlled clinical trial. Int J Environ Res Public Health 2022;16;19:985.

24. Moreo G, Mucchi D, Carinci F. Efficacy ozone therapy in reducing oral infection of periodontal disease: a randomized clinical trial. J Biol Regul Homeost Agents 2020;34 (4 Suppl 1):31–36.

25. Deepthi R, Bilichodmath S. Ozone therapy in periodontics: a meta-analysis. Contemp Clin Dent 2020;11:108–115.

26. Laçin N, İzol BS, Gökalp Özkorkmaz E, Deveci B, Deveci E. Effects of alloplastic graft material combined with a topical ozone application on calvarial bone defects in rats. Folia Morphol (Warsz) 2020;79:528–547.

27. Eroglu ZT, Kurtis B, Altug HA, Sahin S, Tuter G, Baris E. Effect of topical ozone therapy on gingival wound healing in pigs: histological and immuno-histochemical analysis. J Appl Oral Sci 2018;10;27:e20180015.

28. Silva EJNL, Prado MC, Soares DN, Hecksher F, Martins JNR, Fidalgo TKS. The effect of ozone therapy in root canal disinfection: a systematic review. Int Endod J 2020;53:317–332.

29. Isler SC, Soysal F, Akca G, Bakirarar B, Ozcan G, Unsal B. The effects of decontamination methods of dental implant surface on cytokine expression analysis in the reconstructive surgical treatment of peri-implantitis. Odontology 2021;109:103–113.

30. Azarpazhooh A, Limeback H. The application of ozone in dentistry: a systematic review of literature. J Dent 2008;36: 104–116.

31. Page MJ, McKenzie JE, Bossuyt PM, et al. The PRISMA 2020 statement: An updated guideline for reporting systematic reviews. J Clin Epidemiol 2021;134:178–189.

32. Higgins JPT, Thomas J, Chandler J, et al (eds). Cochrane Handbook for Systematic Reviews of Interventions version 6.2 (updated February 2021). Cochrane, 2021. www.training.cochrane.org/handbook. Accessed 25 Sept 2022.

33. Schardt C, Adams MB, Owens T, Keitz S, Fontelo P. Utilization of the PICO framework to improve searching PubMed for clinical questions. BMC Med Inform Decis Mak 2007; 7:16.

34. Higgins JPT, Green S (eds). Cochrane Handbook for Systematic Reviews of Interventions Version 5.1.0 (updated March 2011). The Cochrane Collaboration, 2011. www.handbook.cochrane.org. Accessed 25 Sept 2022.

35. Chambrone L, Rincón-Castro MV, Poveda-Marín AE, et al. Histological healing outcomes at the bone-titanium interface of loaded and unloaded dental implants placed in humans: A systematic review of controlled clinical trials. Int J Oral Implantol (Berl) 2020;13:321–342.

36. Chambrone L, Chambrone LA, Lima LA. Effects of occlusal overload on peri-implant tissue health: a systematic review of animal-model studies. J Periodontol. 2010;81: 1367–1378.

37. Isler SC, Uraz A, Guler B, Ozdemir Y, Cula S, Cetiner D. Effects of laser photobiomodulation and ozone therapy on palatal epithelial wound healing and patient morbidity. Photomed Laser Surg 2018;36: 571–580.

38. Karaca IR, Ergun G, Ozturk DN. Is low-level laser therapy and gaseous ozone application effective on osseointegration of immediately loaded implants? Niger J Clin Pract 2018;21:703–710.

39. Patel PV, Kumar V, Kumar S, Gd V, Patel A. Therapeutic effect of topical ozonated oil on the epithelial healing of palatal wound sites: a planimetrical and cytological study. J Investig Clin Dent 2011;2:248–258.

40. Patel PV, Kumar S, Vidya GD, Patel A, Holmes JC, Kumar V. Cytological assessment of healing palatal donor site wounds and grafted gingival wounds after application of ozonated oil: an eighteen-month randomized controlled clinical trial. Acta Cytol 2012; 56:277–284.

41. Shekhar A, Srivastava S, Kumar Bhati L, et al. An evaluation of the effect of ozone therapy on tissues surrounding dental implants. Int Immunopharmacol 2021;96: 107588.

42. Taşdemir Z, Alkan BA, Albayrak H. Effects of ozone therapy on the early healing period of deepithelialized gingival grafts: a randomized placebo-controlled clinical trial. J Periodontol 2016;87:663–671.

43. Wen Q, Liu D, Wang X, et al. A systematic review of ozone therapy for treating chronically refractory wounds and ulcers. Int Wound J 2022;19:853–870.

44. Fitzpatrick E, Holland OJ, Vanderlelie JJ. Ozone therapy for the treatment of chronic wounds: A systematic review. Int Wound J 2018;15:633–644.

45. Bomfim TL, Gomes IA, Meneses DVC, Araujo AAS. Effectiveness of ozone therapy as an adjunct treatment for lower-limb ulcers: a systematic review. Adv Skin Wound Care 2021;34:1–9.

46. Liu J, Zhang P, Tian J, et al. Ozone therapy for treating foot ulcers in people with diabetes. Cochrane Database Syst Rev 2015;2015: CD008474.

47. Di Fede O, Canepa F, Panzarella V, et al. The treatment of medication-related osteonecrosis of the jaw (MRONJ): A systematic review with a pooled analysis of only surgery versus combined protocols. Int J Environ Res Public Health 2021;18:8432.

48. Moraschini V, Kischinhevsky ICC, Calasans-Maia MD, et al. Ineffectiveness of ozone therapy in nonsurgical periodontal treatment: a systematic review and meta-analysis of randomized clinical trials. Clin Oral Investig 2020;24:1877–1888.

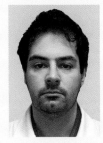

Luiz Felipe Palma

Luiz Felipe Palma Graduate Dentistry Program, Ibirapuera University, São Paulo, Brazil; and Department of Pathology, Federal University of São Paulo, São Paulo, Brazil

Cristiano Joia Graduate Dentistry Program, Ibirapuera University, São Paulo, Brazil

Leandro Chambrone Graduate Dentistry Program, Ibirapuera University, São Paulo, Brazil; Evidence-Based Hub – CiiEM, Egas Moniz - Cooperativa de Ensino Superior, Caparica, Almada, Portugal; and Unit of Basic Oral Investigation (UIBO), Faculty of Dentistry, Universidade El Bosque, Bogota, Colombia

Correspondence: Luiz Felipe Palma, Ibirapuera University, Av. Interlagos, 1329 - Chácara Flora, São Paulo, SP – Brazil, 04661-100. Email: luizfelipep@hotmail.com

First submission: 16 May 2022
Acceptance: 18 Sep 2022
Online publication: 28 Nov 2022

Impact of the COVID-19 pandemic on head and neck cancer patients: systematic review and meta-analysis

Mayara Santos de Castro, DDS, MSc/Bárbara Maria de Souza Moreira Machado, DDS, MSc/
Mariane Carolina Faria Barbosa, DDS, MSc/Lélio Fernando Ferreira Soares, DDS, MSc/
Felipe Fornias Sperandio, DDS, MSc, PhD, FRCD(C)/Marina Lara de Carli, DDS, PhD/
Suzane Cristina Pigossi, DDS, MSc, PhD/Daniela Coelho de Lima, DDS, MSc, PhD

Objectives: This manuscript presents a systematic review of the impact of the COVID-19 pandemic on head and neck cancer (HNC) patients. A meta-analysis was made to compare the number of treated/operated HNC patients in the pre-COVID-19 era versus the COVID-19 era. This investigation was based on previous reports showing a delay in the diagnosis and treatment of new cases of cancer during the pandemic. Worsening in cancer prognosis would be expected as a result of the delayed treatments. **Method and materials:** An electronic search was conducted using the PubMed/MEDLINE, Embase, Web of Science, Scopus, and The Cochrane Library databases. Relevant articles were selected based on specific inclusion criteria. **Results:** A total of 8,942 HNC patients were included. A higher prevalence in male (1,873) in comparison to female (1,695) was observed considering 3,568 patients. Regarding staging, the majority of cases were stage III to IV. The treatment type more frequently described was surgery. Positive diagnosis for COVID-19 in the pre-oncologic treatment was reported for 242 patients, and for post-oncologic treatment in 119 patients. Mortality by COVID-19 was reported for 27 HNC patients. The meta-analysis revealed a significantly smaller number of surgeries/oncologic treatments of HNC patients performed (2,666) in the COVID-19 era when compared to the pre-COVID-19 era (3,163) (Mantel–Haenszel odds ratio=0.81, 95% CI=0.65 to 1.00, P=.05). **Conclusion:** The impact of the COVID-19 pandemic on HNC patients occurred mainly in the number of surgeries/oncologic treatments, showing a significantly smaller number of surgeries/oncologic treatments performed in the COVID-19 era rather than the pre-COVID-19 era. (Quintessence Int 2023;54:320–327; doi: 10.3290/j.qi.b3908931)

Key words: COVID-19, head and neck cancer, meta-analysis, pandemic, SARS-CoV-2, systematic review

The early phase of the Coronavirus disease-2019 (COVID-19) pandemic was characterized by health care systems undergoing massive reprioritization and reorganization in order to control the outbreak of the disease given an overload of hospitalizations, which resulted in cancer patients receiving potentially suboptimal or delayed treatments.[1] Additionally, the literature suggests that the "lockdown" carried out in several cities around the world and the fear of contracting COVID-19 in hospital environments may have delayed the diagnosis of new cases of cancer as well as the initiation of oncologic treatment.[2] As a result, a worsening in the prognosis of cancer patients would be expected.[1-3]

Specifically, head and neck cancer (HNC) includes tumors located in the lips, oral cavity, oropharynx, hypopharynx, larynx, nasopharynx, maxillary sinus, salivary gland, and thyroid.[4-6] In 2018, HNC was the seventh most frequent type of cancer in the world (890,000 new cases and 450,000 deaths).[7] HNC increasing tumor size and potential complications such as airway compromise and risk of severe bleeding would result in undesired disease progression and distant metastases as treatment is postponed.[1]

Tevetoğlu et al[1] showed that the tumor size (T3–T4) for HNC patients and the number of regional metastases for tumors located in the oral cavity increased significantly in 2020, which points to locoregionally advanced disease during the COVID-19 pandemic. It is important to emphasize that the delay in HNC treatment (surgery and/or radiotherapy [RT] and/or chemotherapy [CT]) has a significant impact on the overall survival and quality of patients life.[8] Increased HNC T sizes due to a delay in diagnosis/treatment would require more mutilating surgical resections and more complex surgical reconstructions. Moreover, HNC patients are considered risk patients for COVID-19 given higher risk of infection, especially due to immunosuppressive CT.[9]

Preliminary studies appear to indicate that cancer patients diagnosed with COVID-19 are more vulnerable and with poorer outcomes and mortality.[10,11] Based on that, the real impact of the COVID-19 pandemic on HNC patients needs to be addressed. In this way, this manuscript aims to present a systematic review of the impact of the COVID-19 pandemic on HNC patients. A meta-analysis was conducted to compare the number of treated/operated HNC patients in the pre-COVID-19 era (PCE) versus the COVID-19 era (CE).

Method and materials

Protocol

This systematic review was performed and reported according to Preferred Reporting Items for Systematic Reviews and Meta-Analyses (PRISMA) guidelines[12] and a protocol was registered in the International Prospective Register of Systematic Reviews (PROSPERO, No. CRD42021297555). This article does not contain any studies with human participants or animals performed by any of the authors. For this type of study, formal consent was not required.

Focused question

The focused question of this study was "Did the COVID-19 pandemic affect the diagnosis, treatment, and prognosis of HNC patients?" This question was established according to the Population, Exposure, Comparison, and Outcome (PECO) strategy, as described below:
- Population: HNC patients
- Exposure: COVID-19 pandemic
- Comparison: PCE and CE
- Outcome: diagnosis, treatment, prognosis, and SARS-CoV-2 infection.

Literature search

An extensive electronic search was conducted covering all articles published until 22 May 2021, using the PubMed/MEDLINE, Embase, Web of Science, Scopus, and The Cochrane Library databases. The keywords selected according to Medical Subject Heading (MeSH) terms and PECO strategy are described in Appendix 1.

Eligibility criteria

The original research articles were selected according to the following inclusion criteria:
- case reports, case series, and observational and clinical studies with data on HNC patients obtained during the COVID-19 pandemic
- articles comparing HNC data obtained in PCE and CE
- only articles with a publication date corresponding to the decreed period of the COVID-19 pandemic were included
- HNC with primary locations in lips, oral cavity (including tongue), oropharynx, hypopharynx, larynx, nasopharynx, maxillary sinus, salivary gland, and thyroid according to Mowery et al.[5]

The exclusion criteria adopted were as follows:
- cancer localized in the head and neck skin
- laboratory studies (in vitro and in vivo), review articles, conference proceedings, protocol articles, letters to the editor, duplicate publications
- impossibility of obtaining data only about HNC
- articles published in a language other than English.

Study selection

The studies were selected by two independent researchers (MSC and BMSMM) in an unblinded standardized manner. Titles and abstracts were screened for eligibility, considering the inclusion/exclusion criteria described above. Full texts of the studies that met the eligibility criteria were selected and were accessed by both authors for inclusion. Disagreements between the investigators were resolved by consensus or were referred to a third review author (SCP) for the final decision. Studies that met the eligibility criteria were processed for data extraction.

Data extraction process

Two independent authors (MSC and BMSMM) extracted the following data from included articles: authors, year of publication,

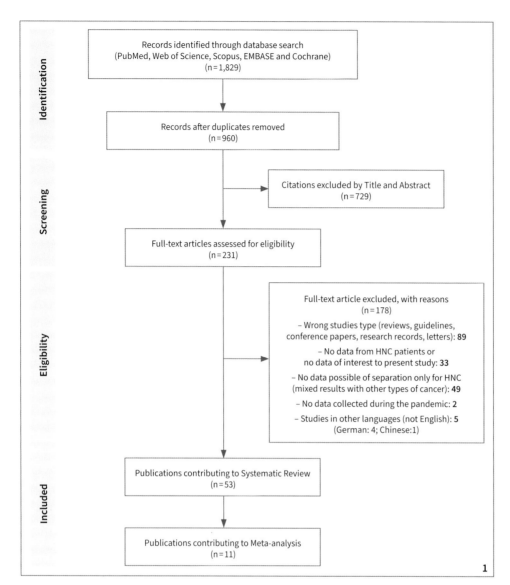

Fig 1 PRISMA flowchart outlining the selection process for the inclusion of studies in the systematic review.

Within the figure:

Identification

Records identified through database search
(PubMed, Web of Science, Scopus, EMBASE and Cochrane)
(n = 1,829)

Records after duplicates removed
(n = 960)

Screening

Citations excluded by Title and Abstract
(n = 729)

Full-text articles assessed for eligibility
(n = 231)

Eligibility

Full-text article excluded, with reasons
(n = 178)

– Wrong studies type (reviews, guidelines, conference papers, research records, letters): 89

– No data from HNC patients or no data of interest to present study: 33

– No data possible of separation only for HNC (mixed results with other types of cancer): 49

– No data collected during the pandemic: 2

– Studies in other languages (not English): 5 (German: 4; Chinese:1)

Included

Publications contributing to Systematic Review
(n = 53)

Publications contributing to Meta-analysis
(n = 11)

1

nationality of patients, number of patients, mean age of patients, sex (male/female), primary location of HNC, TNM, staging, metastasis, oncologic treatment type (surgery and/or RT and/or CT), mortality by HNC, COVID-19 diagnosis (made before and after oncologic treatment), and mortality by COVID-19. The qualitative data were organized and presented in Appendix 2. At this stage, the quantitative data from studies were also accessed for later realization to the meta-analysis.

Quality assessment

Two authors (MSC and BMSMM) assessed the quality of the included studies separately. Any disagreement was discussed with a third reviewer (SCP). The methodologic quality of case reports and case series was evaluated using the framework for appraisal suggested by Murad et al.[13] For prospective cohort studies, the Newcastle-Ottawa methodologic quality assessment was carried out.[14] The cross-sectional studies were submitted to the Joanna Briggs Institute (JBI) Critical Appraisal tool for systematic reviews of cross-sectional studies.[15]

Statistical analysis

A meta-analysis was performed to compare the number of surgeries/oncologic treatments performed for HNC patients during the PCE and CE. Studies with different periods of data collection between the PCE and CE were excluded from the meta-analysis. Moreover, subgroup analyses were made considering the period of analysis (March to May 2019 vs March to May 2020 and April to September 2019 vs April to September 2020) and data on resection surgeries. Data were extracted from each study with subsequent determination of the odds ratios (ORs) with 95% confidence intervals (CIs) by the Mantel–Haenszel method. A considerable heterogeneity would indicate a random-effects model analysis. I^2 statistics and Cochran test Q (χ^2) were used to assess the heterogeneity between the studies included. Values of I^2 can be interpreted as low (25% to 50%), moderate (50% to 75%), and high (75% and higher) levels of heterogeneity.[14] In this way, a dichotomous meta-analysis of the number of treated/operated HNC patients in the reported studies comparing PCE and CE was obtained. Meta-analyses, generation of forest plots, assessment of heterogeneity, and publication bias were performed using the statistical software Review Manager.[16] Statistical significance was set at alpha 5% ($P \le .05$) for all meta-analysis results.

Results

Literature search

The initial search from databases provided a total of 1,829 potential articles (PubMed/MEDLINE=499; Embase=475; Web of Science=341; Scopus=198; and The Cochrane Library=316). After removal of duplicates, 960 remained. Of these, 729 articles were not included after their corresponding titles and abstracts were reviewed and did not meet the inclusion criteria. The full texts of the remaining 231 articles were evaluated. A total of 53 articles (case reports=10; case series=11; retrospective studies=8; prospective studies=3; cohort studies=6; and cross-sectional studies=15) were included in the systematic review (qualitative analysis); from these, 11 studies were included in the meta-analysis (quantitative analysis) (Fig 1).

Qualitative data synthesis

A total of 8,942 HNC patients were reported on all included studies (Appendix 2). The age of the patients varied from 15 to 88 years with a mean of 54.5 years (only 26 of included articles described this information totalizing 2,717 patients). Sex data (male/female) were reported only for 3,568 patients (male=1,873; and female=1,695) in 32 included studies. HNC mortality was reported for 242/2,067 patients (data from seven studies), leading to an approximate mortality rate of 11.7%.

Regarding HNC characteristics, squamous cell carcinoma (SCC) was the most cited prevalent HNC type. The primary location of HNC was described in 3,928 cases included (data from 31 articles) and the most common primary location of HNC was the thyroid (2,799 cases), followed by oral cavity (325), nasopharynx (216), larynx (205), tongue (163), lip (130), oropharynx (48), salivary gland (23), parotid (6), hypopharynx (6), neck (5), vocal cord (1), and maxillary sinus (1). HNC with no primary location specification was assigned to 5,014 cases (data from 22 articles).

Size of tumor (T) was reported only in 420 cases from 8,942 (T1–T2=202 cases; and T3–T4=218) (data from 11 articles). Regarding cancer spread data, 835 cases showed metastases to nearby lymph nodes (N0=253 cases; N1=523; N2=36; N3=22; and "N+"=1) (data from 12 articles) and 37 cases reported distant metastases (spread of cancer to other parts of the body) (Mx=1 case; M0=7; and M1=29) (data from nine articles). In total, 729 cases reported staging (191 cases were stage I to II and 538 cases were stage III to IV [data from eight articles]).

The oncologic treatment type performed was mentioned for 6,293 patients (surgery=4,622; RT=487; CT=471; chemoradiotherapy [CRT]=33; radioactive iodine ablation therapy [RIA]=25; immunotherapy=5; and palliative=650) (data from 43 articles). HNC mortality was reported for 242 patients (data from seven articles, with a total of 2,067 patients).

COVID-19 diagnosis was described in 16 studies. The diagnosis was made by RT-PCR in all studies. A positive COVID-19 diagnosis was reported for 242 patients that were pre-oncologic treatment (data from seven articles). As for post oncologic treatment data, 119 patients were diagnosed with COVID-19 (data from 11 articles). Mortality by COVID-19 was reported in 27 HNC patients (data from four articles).

Fourteen articles described data comparing HNC patients in the PCE and CE and the main outcomes are shown in Appendix 3.

Quality assessment

With regards to the quality of the included articles, only one case series manuscript was included in this meta-analysis and showed moderate quality (Appendix 4). Two cohort studies were included and presented high quality (Appendix 5). For cross-sectional studies, a total of eight articles were added to this meta-analysis (Appendix 6), being five studies classified under moderate risk of bias and three studies classified under low risk of bias.

Quantitative data synthesis

Eleven studies were included in the present meta-analysis (case series=1; cohort studies=2; and cross-sectional studies=8).[1,17-26] The following demographics pooled data were

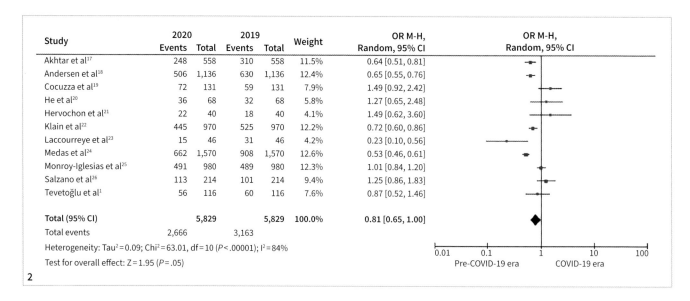

Study	2020 Events	Total	2019 Events	Total	Weight	OR M-H, Random, 95% CI
Akhtar et al[17]	248	558	310	558	11.5%	0.64 [0.51, 0.81]
Andersen et al[18]	506	1,136	630	1,136	12.4%	0.65 [0.55, 0.76]
Cocuzza et al[19]	72	131	59	131	7.9%	1.49 [0.92, 2.42]
He et al[20]	36	68	32	68	5.8%	1.27 [0.65, 2.48]
Hervochon et al[21]	22	40	18	40	4.1%	1.49 [0.62, 3.60]
Klain et al[22]	445	970	525	970	12.2%	0.72 [0.60, 0.86]
Laccourreye et al[23]	15	46	31	46	4.2%	0.23 [0.10, 0.56]
Medas et al[24]	662	1,570	908	1,570	12.6%	0.53 [0.46, 0.61]
Monroy-Iglesias et al[25]	491	980	489	980	12.3%	1.01 [0.84, 1.20]
Salzano et al[26]	113	214	101	214	9.4%	1.25 [0.86, 1.83]
Tevetoğlu et al[1]	56	116	60	116	7.6%	0.87 [0.52, 1.46]
Total (95% CI)		5,829		5,829	100.0%	0.81 [0.65, 1.00]
Total events	2,666		3,163			

Heterogeneity: Tau^2=0.09; Chi^2=63.01, df=10 (P<.00001); I^2=84%
Test for overall effect: Z=1.95 (P=.05)

Fig 2 Forest plot comparing the number of surgeries/oncologic treatments of HNC patients performed in the pre-COVID-19 era vs the COVID-19 era.

found for HNC patients: mean age±SD (PCE=51.6±7.2 years, and CE=52.0±6.0), and sex (PCE=male 68.4%±11.2%, and female 32.1%±11.7%; and CE=male 63.8%±3.2%, and female 34.9%±2.0%).

In Fig 2, the number of surgeries/oncologic treatments of HNC patients was compared between the PCE and CE. The period of data collection was divergent between studies and a considerable heterogeneity was observed among these studies (χ^2=63.01; P<.00001; I^2=84%). In the CE, there was a significantly smaller number of surgeries/oncologic treatments that were performed for HNC patients (2,666) compared to the PCE (3,163). The pooled OR was 0.81 (95% CI=0.65 to 1.00). Therefore, these results indicate a smaller number of treatments for HNC patients during the COVID-19 pandemic (P=.05).

In Appendix 7, a total of two studies[22,24] with the same data collection period (March to May 2019 vs March to May 2020) were included. A considerable heterogeneity was also observed among these studies (χ^2=17.51; P<.0001; I^2=94%). Here again, significantly smaller surgeries/oncologic treatments were performed in CE (651) than in PCE (861) (P=.05). The pooled OR was 0.52 (95% CI=0.28 to 0.99).

Similarly, Appendix 8 depicts a total of two studies[17,19] that compared the period of April to September 2019 to April to September 2020 and reveals a greater number of surgeries/oncologic treatments reported in the PCE (369) compared with the the CE (320); however, this result was not significant (P=0.90).

The pooled OR was 0.95 (95% CI=0.42 to 2.17). A considerable heterogeneity was also observed among these studies (χ^2=9.36; P<.002; I^2=89%).

Six studies[1,16,20,23-25] compared the resection surgeries performed in HNC patients in the PCE vs CE (Appendix 9). A considerable heterogeneity was observed among these studies (χ^2= 43.75; P<.00001; I^2=89%). In accordance, a smaller amount of resection surgeries were reported in the CE (1,592) when compared to the PCE (1,886); however, this result was not significant (P=.33). The pooled OR was 0.85 (95% CI=0.61 to 1.18).

Discussion

Similar to the present review, a higher prevalence of HNC was described in patients in the fifth decade of life and male.[27-31] Moreover, HNC arising from the mucosal epithelium of the oral cavity, pharynx, and larynx, namely squamous cell carcinoma (SCC), is among the most common head and neck malignancies,[27] consistent with the current review. In addition, tobacco consumption, alcohol abuse, or both have long been acknowledged as major risk factors for the development of SCC in the head and neck. Human papillomavirus (HPV) and Epstein–Barr virus (EBV) have also been associated with oropharyngeal and nasopharyngeal carcinoma, respectively; other HNC risk factors include environmental factors, toxic exposures, and diet.[27]

HNC staging comprises disease classification according to the tumor-node-metastasis (TNM) system.[32] The literature showed that HNC that presented with more advanced stages at diagnosis (stage III to IV) have a worse prognosis when compared to earlier stages of the disease (stage I to II).[1,27,32] In the current review, most HNC patients whose TNM data were reported presented with larger tumor sizes (T3 or T4) at time of diagnosis. Regarding the comparison between PCE and CE, a higher proportion of T3 or T4 tumors was reported in CE rather than in PCE.[1,33] Moreover, a lower number of HNC cases was diagnosed in CE in comparison to PCE.[1,17,22-24,33,34] Tevetoğlu et al[1] showed that the tumor size (T3–T4) for HNC patients and the number of regional metastases for tumors located in the oral cavity increased significantly in 2020, which points to locoregionally advanced disease during the COVID-19 pandemic. These results together may suggest that the COVID-19 pandemic has caused a delay in HNC diagnosis.

Regarding HNC treatment (surgery and/or RT and/or CT), surgery was the most commonly reported treatment in the present review, followed by RT and CT, respectively. Surgery is often chosen for oral cavity cancers, whereas RT might be more often employed for pharyngeal and laryngeal cancers.[27] For a small primary HNC with no clinical nodal involvement, or only a single node involvement, cure rates of over 80% can be achieved with single modality intervention (surgery or RT).[35] For more advanced HNC or positive nodal/metastasis, postoperative RT and/or CT reduces the risk of recurrence and improves survival.[36] RT and/or CT may also be chosen for inoperable HNC cases, in order to reduce tumor size.[27,37]

The present meta-analysis showed a significantly smaller number of surgeries/oncologic treatments for HNC patients in the CE rather than the PCE. A delay in HNC treatment may result in an increase in tumor size (requiring more complex and more mutilating surgeries), the spread of the disease (nodal or distant metastasis), in addition to worse prognosis and survival rates.[38] Overall, the reduced number of patients referred for HNC treatment in CE suggests a reduction in cancer treatments in order to prioritize COVID-19-related treatment.[26] Moreover, difficulties in patient transportation, fear of acquiring COVID-19 infection, efforts to arrange for budget and meals during travels, and lack of social support, among others, were challenges faced by patients that also complicated the access for HNC treatment.[17]

Regarding hospitalization of HNC patients, Batra et al[34] reported a median hospital stay that was significantly longer in CE (10 days: range 1 to 19 days) when compared to PCE (7 days: range 2 to 37 days). The authors suggest that this occurred due to the waiting period for the COVID-19 RT-PCR test result and the increased postponements that were seen during the pan-

demic.[34] There were also a few occasions where the swabs were repeated when the results were inconclusive, which also increased the time of hospital stay.[34]

In addition to HNC diagnosis/treatment, screening for other types of cancer such as colorectal, breast, prostate, cervical, and melanoma was postponed in many countries as COVID-19 hospitalization rates overwhelmed hospitals; surgeries and chemotherapy treatments were also delayed.[39,40] Jazieh et al[41] assessed the impact of the COVID-19 pandemic on cancer care worldwide and concluded that such detrimental impact was widely spread and varied in magnitude among the medical centers worldwide. In addition, it is also important to point out that advances in cancer research and therapeutic developments were also hampered during the early stages of the pandemic.[39]

Regarding other life-saving non-COVID-19 treatments, the pandemic has hindered human papillomavirus (HPV) vaccinations, which is essential for reducing the risk of cervical and oropharyngeal cancers.[42] Furthermore, repercussions around the COVID-19 pandemic have indirectly affected the prevention and treatment of myriad diseases.[39] Finally, regarding patients in need for hemodialysis, Guidotti et al[43] reported that COVID-19 challenged the dialysis centers with a much higher incidence rate of infections and a very high mortality rate compared to the general population during the first and second wave of the pandemic. Collectively, these observations showed that not only HNC diagnosis/treatment was affected by the COVID-19 pandemic, but other life-saving non-COVID-19 treatments also faced difficulties and may have been overlooked during that period.

This systematic review and meta-analysis has some study limitations. For instance, the included studies showed considerable heterogeneity between them, lack of data for qualitative and quantitative analysis, and discrepant periods of comparison between CE and PCE. A meta-analysis to assess the impact of the COVID-19 pandemic on HNC diagnosis in a more precise manner was not performed due to the lack and variability of data in the included studies. As expected, the long-term effects of the COVID-19 pandemic on HNC recurrence and mortality rates cannot be yet evaluated given the currently limited follow-up period. Concerning the diagnosis of COVID-19 in the pre- and post-oncologic treatment phases, the total number of HNC patients tested for COVID-19 could not be calculated due to the lack of information in the included studies. The absence of these data made it impossible to determine the number of patients contaminated with SARS-CoV-2 during their respective cancer treatment. Thus, such limiting factors may have influenced the results, and future studies will be necessary to further investigate the real dimension of the COVID-19 pandemic on HNC.

Conclusion

The impact of the COVID-19 pandemic on HNC patients occurred mainly on the number of surgical/oncologic treatments. There were significantly fewer surgeries and oncologic treatments performed in the CE when compared to the PCE.

Acknowledgments

The present study was financially supported by the Conselho Nacional de Desenvolvimento Científico e Tecnológico (CNPq), Grant/Award Number: MCTIC Universal Nr: 408884/2018–5, and Coordenação de Aperfeiçoamento de Pessoal de Nível Superior (CAPES), Grant/Award Nr: Finance Code 001. The authors declare that they have no conflict of interest.

References

1. Tevetoğlu F, Kara S, Aliyeva C, Yıldırım R, Yener HM. Delayed presentation of head and neck cancer patients during COVID-19 pandemic. Eur Arch Otorhinolaryngol 2021;278: 5081–5085.

2. Ianculovici C, Kaplan I, Kleinman S, Zadik Y. Guest Editorial: COVID-19 and the risk of delayed diagnosis of oral cancer. Quintessence Int 2020;51:785–786.

3. Eliav E. Editorial: Oral cancer: Can we do better? Quintessence Int 2017;48:91.

4. Mehanna HJCO. Head and neck cancer part 1: epidemiology, presentation, and preservation. Clin Otolaryngol 2011;36:65–68.

5. Mowery AJ, Conlin MJ, Clayburgh DR. Elevated incidence of head and neck cancer in solid organ transplant recipients. Head Neck 2019;41:4009–4017.

6. Patterson RH, Fischman VG, Wasserman I, et al. Global burden of head and neck cancer: economic consequences, health, and the role of surgery. Otolaryngol Head Neck Surg 2020;162:296–303.

7. Bray F, Ferlay J, Soerjomataram I, Siegel RL, Torre LA, Jemal A. Global cancer statistics 2018: GLOBOCAN estimates of incidence and mortality worldwide for 36 cancers in 185 countries. CA Cancer J Clin 2018;68:394–424.

8. Schutte HW, Heutink F, Wellenstein DJ, et al. Impact of time to diagnosis and treatment in head and neck cancer: a systematic review. Otolaryngol Head Neck Surg 2020; 162:446–457.

9. Elkrief A, Wu JT, Jani C, et al. Learning through a pandemic: the current state of knowledge on COVID-19 and Cancer. Cancer Discov 2022;12:303–330.

10. Dai M, Liu D, Liu M, et al. Patients with cancer appear more vulnerable to SARS-CoV-2: A multicenter study during the COVID-19 outbreak. Cancer Discov 2020;10:783–791.

11. Onder G, Rezza G, Brusaferro S. Case-fatality rate and characteristics of patients dying in relation to COVID-19 in Italy. JAMA 2020;323:1775–1776.

12. Page MJ, McKenzie JE, Bossuyt PM, et al. The PRISMA 2020 statement: an updated guideline for reporting systematic reviews. BMJ 2021;372:n71.

13. Murad MH, Sultan S, Haffar S, Bazerbachi F. Methodological quality and synthesis of case series and case reports. BMJ Evid Based Med 2018;23:60–63.

14. Higgins JP, Thompson SG, Deeks JJ, Altman DG. Measuring inconsistency in meta-analyses. BMJ 2003;327:557–560.

15. Saletta JM, Garcia JJ, Caramês JMM, Schliephake H, da Silva Marques DN. Quality assessment of systematic reviews on vertical bone regeneration. Int J Oral Maxillofac Surg 2019;48:364–372.

16. RevMan, version 5.4, Copenhagen: The Nordic Cochrane Center, The Cochrane Collaboration, 2020.

17. Akhtar N, Rajan S, Chakrabarti D, et al. Continuing cancer surgery through the first six months of the COVID-19 pandemic at an academic university hospital in India: A lower-middle-income country experience. J Surg Oncol 2021;123:1177–1187.

18. Andersen PA, Rasmussen KMB, Channir HI, et al. The impact and prevalence of SARS-CoV-2 in patients with head and neck cancer and acute upper airway infection in a tertiary otorhinolaryngology referral center in Denmark. Eur Arch Otorhinolaryngol 2021;278: 3409–3415.

19. Cocuzza S, Maniaci A, Pavone P, et al. Head and neck cancer: the new scenario in the pandemic covid-19 period. WCRJ 2021;8:e1917.

20. He J, Yang L, Tao Z, et al. Impact of the 2019 novel Coronavirus disease (COVID-19) epidemic on radiotherapy-treated patients with cancer: a single-center descriptive study. Cancer Manag Res 2021;13:37–43.

21. Hervochon R, Atallah S, Levivien S, Teissier N, Baujat B, Tankere F. Impact of the COVID-19 epidemic on ENT surgical volume. Eur Ann Otorhinolaryngol Head Neck Dis 2020;137:269–271.

22. Klain M, Nappi C, Maurea S, et al. Management of differentiated thyroid cancer through nuclear medicine facilities during Covid-19 emergency: the telemedicine challenge. Eur J Nucl Med Mol Imaging 2021; 48:831–836.

23. Laccourreye O, Mirghani H, Evrard D, et al. Impact of the first month of Covid-19 lockdown on oncologic surgical activity in the Ile de France region university hospital otorhinolaryngology departments. Eur Ann Otorhinolaryngol Head Neck Dis 2020;137: 273–276.

24. Medas F, Ansaldo GL, Avenia N, et al. The THYCOVIT (Thyroid Surgery during COVID-19 pandemic in Italy) study: results from a nationwide, multicentric, case-controlled study. Updates Surg 2021;73:1467–1475.

25. Monroy-Iglesias MJ, Tagliabue M, Dickinson H, et al. Continuity of Cancer Care: The surgical experience of two large cancer hubs in London and Milan. Cancers (Basel) 2021;13:1597.

26. Salzano G, Maglitto F, Guide A, et al. Surgical oncology of the head and neck district during COVID-19 pandemic. Eur Arch Otorhinolaryngol 2021;278:3107–3111.

27. Johnson DE, Burtness B, Leemans CR, Lui VWY, Bauman JE, Grandis JR. Head and neck squamous cell carcinoma. Nat Rev Dis Primers 2020;6:92.

28. Pulte D, Brenner H. Changes in survival in head and neck cancers in the late 20th and early 21st century: a period analysis. Oncologist 2010;15:994–1001.

29. Bhattacharjee A, Vishwakarma GK, Banerjee S, Shukla S. Disease progression of cancer patients during COVID-19 pandemic: a comprehensive analytical strategy by time-dependent modelling. BMC Med Res Methodol 2020;20:209.

30. Lou SC, Xu DJ, Li XD, Huan Y, Li J. Study of psychological state of cancer patients undergoing radiation therapy during novel coronavirus outbreak and effects of nursing intervention. Precision Med Sci 2020;9:83–89.

31. Yang Y, Shen C, Hu C. Effect of COVID-19 epidemic on delay of diagnosis and treatment path for patients with nasopharyngeal carcinoma. Cancer Manag Res 2020;12:3859–3864.

32. Amin MB, Greene FL, Edge SB, et al. The eighth edition AJCC cancer staging manual: continuing to build a bridge from a population-based to a more "personalized" approach to cancer staging. CA Cancer J Clin 2017;67:93–99.

33. Riju J, Tirkey AJ, Mathew M, et al. Analysis of early impact of COVID-19 on presentation and management of oral cancers – an experience from a tertiary care hospital in South India. Indian J Surg Oncol 2021;12:242–249.

34. Batra TK, Tilak MR, Pai E, et al. Increased tracheostomy rates in head and neck cancer surgery during the COVID-19 pandemic. Int J Oral Maxillofac Surg 2021;50:989–993.

35. Lee NCJ, Kelly JR, Park HS, et al. Patterns of failure in high-metastatic node number human papillomavirus-positive oropharyngeal carcinoma. Oral Oncol 2018;85:35–39.

36. Bernier J, Domenge C, Ozsahin M, et al. Postoperative irradiation with or without concomitant chemotherapy for locally advanced head and neck cancer. N Engl J Med 2004;350:1945–1952.

37. Bresadola V, Biddau C, Puggioni A, et al. General surgery and COVID-19: review of practical recommendations in the first pandemic phase. Surg Today 2020;50:1159–1167.

38. Olsen SH, Friborg J, Ellefsen B, at al. Incidence and survival of head and neck cancer in the Faroe Islands. Int J Circumpolar Health 2021;80:1894697.

39. Wells CR, Galvani AP. Impact of the COVID-19 pandemic on cancer incidence and mortality. Lancet Public Health 2022;7:e490–e491.

40. Ospina AV, Bruges R, Mantilla W, et al. Impact of COVID-19 infection on patients with cancer: experience in a Latin American country: The ACHOCC-19 study. Oncologist 2021;26:e1761–e1773.

41. Jazieh AR, Akbulut H, Curigliano G, et al. Impact of the COVID-19 pandemic on cancer care: a global collaborative study. JCO Glob Oncol 2020;6:1428–1438.

42. Damgacioglu H, Sonawane K, Chhatwal J, et al. Long-term impact of HPV vaccination and COVID-19 pandemic on oropharyngeal cancer incidence and burden among men in the USA: A modeling study. Lancet Reg Health Am 2022;8:100143.

43. Guidotti R, Pruijm M, Ambühl PM. COVID-19 pandemic in dialysis patients: the Swiss experience. Front Public Health 2022;10:795701.

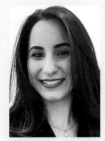

Mayara Santos de Castro

Mayara Santos de Castro   Postgraduate Student, School of Dentistry, Federal University of Alfenas, Alfenas, Brazil

Bárbara Maria de Souza Moreira Machado   Postgraduate Student, School of Dentistry, Federal University of Alfenas, Alfenas, Brazil

Mariane Carolina Faria Barbosa   Postgraduate Student, Department of Pediatric Dentistry, Federal University of Minas Gerais, Belo Horizonte, Brazil

Lélio Fernando Ferreira Soares   Postgraduate Student, School of Dentistry, Federal University of Alfenas, Alfenas, Brazil

Felipe Fornias Sperandio   Assistant Professor, Oral Pathologist, Oral Medicine Specialist, College of Dentistry, University of Saskatchewan, Saskatoon, SK, Canada

Marina Lara de Carli   Adjunct Professor, School of Dentistry, Federal University of Alfenas, Alfenas, Brazil

Suzane Cristina Pigossi   Professor, Department of Periodontology, School of Dentistry, Federal University of Uberlândia, Uberlândia, MG, Brazil

Daniela Coelho de Lima   Associate Professor, School of Dentistry, Federal University of Alfenas, Alfenas, Brazil

Correspondence: Mayara Santos de Castro, School of Dentistry, Federal University of Alfenas, 700 Gabriel Monteiro da Silva Street, Alfenas, MG 37130-001, Brazil. Email: maya.castro@outlook.com

First submission: 16 Nov 2022
Acceptance: 4 Feb 2023
Online publication: 17 Feb 2023

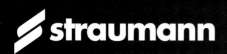
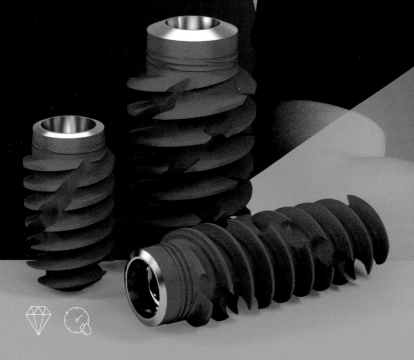

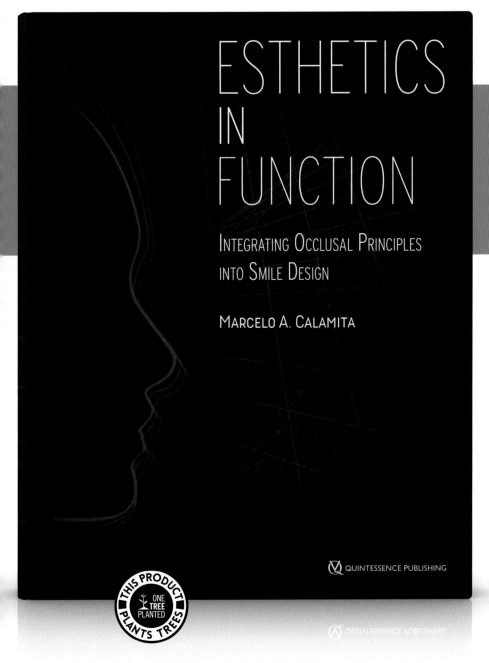

ESTHETICS
IN
FUNCTION

INTEGRATING OCCLUSAL PRINCIPLES
INTO SMILE DESIGN

MARCELO A. CALAMITA

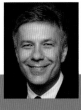

Marcelo A. Calamita

Esthetics in Function

Integrating Occlusal Principles
into Smile Design

648 pages, 1,490 illus.
ISBN 978-1-78698-134-9, €248

This comprehensive book, written by
a top expert in the field, is about the
preservation and enhancement of smile
esthetics. The richly illustrated content
aims to enhance the understanding
of the static and dynamic principles
acting on the stomatognathic system.
The book's main themes – treatment
planning and occlusion – are
inseparable factors for the success
of every restorative treatment. The
clearly presented protocols contain all
the relevant aspects related to these
themes for the achievement of excellent,
consistent, and predictable results.
The content is based on an extensive
literature review and the best-quality
scientific evidence available at the time
of publication, accompanied by the
author's valuable commentary and notes.

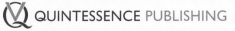

www.quint.link/esthetic-function   books@quintessenz.de   +49 (0)30 761 80 667

A blind randomized controlled pilot trial on recombinant human bone morphogenetic protein-2 in combination with a bioresorbable membrane on periodontal regeneration in mandibular molar furcation defects

Ankita A. Agrawal, MDS/Prasad V. Dhadse, MDS, Fellow HPE/Bhairavi V. Kale, MDS/
Komal R. Bhombe, MDS/Kiran K. Ganji, MDS/Andrej M. Kielbassa, Prof Dr med dent Dr h c

Objectives: In preparation of a definitive randomized clinical trial (RCT), the current parallel-grouped triple-blind pilot RCT assessed the efficacy of recombinant human bone morphogenetic protein-2 (rhBMP-2) with polylactic acid/polyglycolic acid (PLA/PGA) membrane for improvement of periodontal tissue regeneration in Class II furcation type defects. **Method and materials:** With the present single-center investigation, 24 patients/24 mandibular molars revealing Class II furcation lesions with involved buccal surfaces were randomly allocated and treated surgically, using either a PLA/PGA membrane alone (control, n = 12) or in combination with rhBMP-2 (n = 12). Assessors, participants, and the statistician were blinded to the treatment groups. Clinical parameters including Plaque Index (PI), Papillary Bleeding Index (PBI), clinical attachment level, vertical probing depth, horizontal probing depth, and gingival recession were assessed at baseline and 6 months postsurgery. **Results:** Baseline values concerning the investigated parameters were comparable between both groups (P > .05). After 6 months, clinical attachment level gain was similar (P = .76), while greater reductions in vertical probing depth (P = .01) and horizontal probing depth (P = .05), along with less gingival recession (P = .03) were observed in the PLA/PGA + rhBMP-2 group (compared to the controls). An increased number of completely closed furcation type defects was observed in the PLA/PGA + rhBMP-2 group (with no adverse effects). **Conclusions:** When treating Class II furcation lesions, the use of rhBMP-2 (combined with PLA/PGA membranes) seems advantageous. The presented set-up seems feasible with regards to recruitment, randomization, acceptance, retention, and adherence to the study protocol.
(Quintessence Int 2023;54:104–124; doi: 10.3290/j.qi.b3631815)

Key words: furcation defects, Class II furcation, periodontal therapy, pilot study, polylactic acid/polyglycolic acid (PLA/PGA) membrane, randomized clinical trial, recombinant bone morphogenetic proteins, regeneration

Treatment of furcation-involved teeth is a challenge for every clinician; anatomical predisposition limits the accessibility to the area, impeding the respective treatment efforts, thus often rendering the latter unpredictable.[1,2] Improving the prognosis of the teeth with involved furcation areas by attaining a complete defect closure is considered a desirable goal of furcation therapy.[3,4] Both the type of tooth involved and the degree of furcation involvement have been regarded as influencing factors for choosing the most promising treatment mode.[5]

The advent of recently developed techniques and the availability of biomaterials such as the use of enamel matrix protein derivatives (EMD), recombinant human platelet derived growth factor (rhPDGF), and hyaluronic acid (HA) have provided both clinicians and researchers with sophisticated therapeutic options for the management of Class II furcation type defects.[6] The use of these biomaterials in combination with either bone graft substitutes or membranes aiming at guided tissue regeneration (GTR) has been considered an effective modality when treating infrabony defects and Class II furcation type lesions, thus exhibiting improvement in clinical parameters and bone fill.[7] However, lack of novel therapies that might provide improved prospects impel the clinician to seek predictable periodontal regeneration, which is still considered an elusive goal.[8]

Demonstration of the formation of cartilage and bone in ectopic sites using demineralized bone matrix has attracted attention to the ability of bone morphogenetic proteins (BMP)[9] to induce differentiation of perivascular mesenchymal cells into osteoprogenitor cells. The use of recombinant human bone morphogenetic proteins (rhBMP) has resulted in clinically relevant bone formation in the reconstruction of periodontal defects,[10] oral/maxillofacial defects,[11] and dental implant fixation in animal models.[12] The clinical efficacy of rhBMP-2 has been established in feasibility and safety studies involving alveolar ridge augmentation for dental implant placement.[13,14]

The rapid release kinetics of rhBMP-2[15] necessitates the need for a carrier in order to keep the BMP in situ, and to ensure space maintenance. Absorbable collagen sponge (ACS) material is one of the most commonly used carriers.[15,16] However, lack of space maintenance with the use of ACS has been shown to result in limited bone formation in the treated defects.[17,18] Moreover, degradable polymers have been developed as a carrier for BMP.[19,20] The controlled release of rhBMP-2 was demonstrated when incorporated in poly(lactic acid-co-glycolic acid).[21]

The successful use of biodegradable membranes with low toxicity to promote periodontal regeneration has been reported.[22] The properties of the biodegradable membrane should permit selective repopulation of periodontal ligament (PDL) cells onto the root surfaces, followed by degradation to non-toxic by-products (lactic acid, glycolic acid, carbon dioxide, and water) only when this process is complete. Polylactic acid/polyglycolic acid (PLA/PGA) is a synthetic bioabsorbable membrane made from a copolymer of lactide and glycolide. The time of degradation of PLA/PGA membranes (polyglactin-910) was found to be 30 to 50 days, and has been reported to facilitate periodontal regeneration.[23] With this background in mind, the current study protocol was designed both to provide preliminary evidence on the clinical efficacy of the intervention when using rhBMP-2 along with a PLA/PGA membrane in periodontal tissue regeneration of Class II furcation type defects, and to assess the feasibility of the chosen setup. The null hypotheses stated that *(1)* rhBMP-2, along with a PLA/PGA membrane, does not contribute to gain in clinical attachment levels (CALs) for Class II furcation type defects (if compared to the sole use of a PLA/PGA membrane), and that *(2)* it does not lead to differing results regarding the vertical and horizontal defect depths, or the extent of gingival recessions.

Method and materials

Study population

As yet, no data from previous studies having evaluated PLA/PGA + rhBMP-2 with Class II furcation type defects are available, thus suggesting a triple-blinded pilot investigation. The present research design was a randomized, parallel designed, controlled clinical pilot trial, and the investigation was carried forward in the Department of Periodontics and Implantology, Sharad Pawar Dental College, Datta Meghe Institute of Medical Sciences, Wardha, Maharashtra, India. The research protocol was initially approved (2 September 2016) by the Institutional Ethics Committee at Datta Meghe Institute of Medical Sciences (Sawangi [M], Wardha, Maharashtra, India; vote number DMIMS (DU)/IEC/2016-17/6239). G*Power (Ver 3.1.9.7, Heinrich-Heine-Universität Düsseldorf) suggested that 24 participants would be needed in a paired samples t test to detect Cohen d = 0.43 with 80% power (α = .05, two-tailed); the effect size of 0.43 was set as the smallest effect size to be considered. This calculated sample size was equivalent to the minimum proposal of 12 patients per study leg with a randomized clinical pilot trial.[24]

The present pilot study was conducted from December 2018 to September 2019. A total of 76 patients were examined, and participants meeting the following selection criteria were included. A total of 24 Class II furcation defects (according to Lindhe) were selected in 24 patients on first mandibular molars involving buccal surfaces, after initial dental and periodontal therapy (see Fig 1).[25] The test group was treated using bioabsorbable PLA/PGA membranes (BioMesh-s, Samyang Biopharma) plus rhBMP-2 (BMP-2, Life Technologies), whereas the controls were treated using the PLA/PGA membranes only. Patients were provided with detailed information about the research and the basic similarity between the treatment approaches, including risks, foreseeable discomforts, and anticipated benefits; participation was voluntary, and no incentives were given to the patients. Differences between the research question and the care they might otherwise receive were elucidated, and written informed consent was obtained. All participants agreed to be blinded for treatment allocation and/or to groups.

Only participants diagnosed with chronic periodontitis (1999 classification) were selected, and patients suffering from aggressive periodontitis were excluded. Patients with presence of Class II furcation type defects involving buccal surfaces of the mandibular molars with horizontal and vertical furcation probing depth of ≤ 3 mm after initial therapy were enrolled for the study. Inclusion criteria were proximal bone heights of the experimental

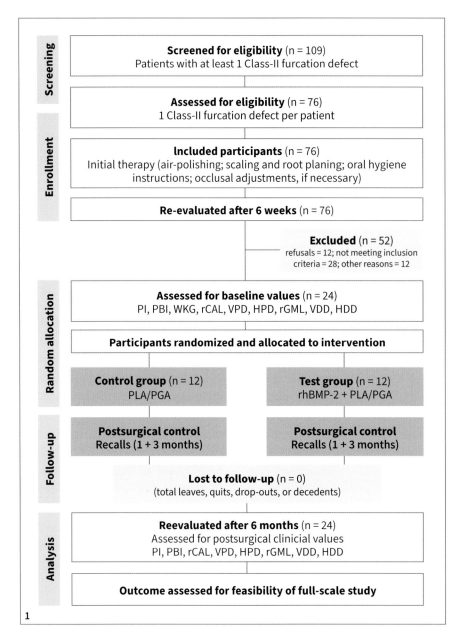

Fig 1 Flow diagram, adapted with reference to CONSORT extension to pilot trials[26] (HDD, horizontal defect depth; HPD, horizontal probing depth; PBI, Papillary Bleeding Index; PI, Plaque Index; rCAL, relative clinical attachment level; rGML, relative gingival marginal level; VDD, vertical defect depth; VPD, vertical probing depth; WKG, width of keratinized gingiva).

tooth to be located coronal to the interradicular bone levels, presence of adequate width of keratinized gingiva (≥3 mm), gingival margins coronal to the furcation fornix, no tooth mobility, and intact tooth surfaces with a normal pulp response on electric pulp testing (Waldent, Waldent Innovations). Systemically compromised subjects, pregnant or lactating mothers, smokers or users of other tobacco products, patients with previous history of periodontal surgical therapy at the selected site, confirmed allergy to the graft material, exhibiting tooth mobility of the selected tooth, or patients being noncompliant to a periodontal maintenance program were excluded. This study was conducted by following the guidelines for reporting parallel group randomized trials with reference to the CONSORT extension to pilot trials,[26,27] with regard to the respective flowchart (Fig 1).

Presurgical therapy

Air polishing procedures were done according to manufacturer's instructions using an air polishing system (Cavitron Prophy Jet, Dentsply Sirona), along with mildly abrasive sodium carbonate powdered particles (Cavitron Prophy-Jet Prophy Powder, Dentsply Sirona). Initial therapy such as scaling and root planing using scalers and curettes (Hu-Friedy) was performed following examination and diagnosis. Oral hygiene instructions were reinforced until patients attained 80% to 85% of plaque control. A reassessment was carried out 6 weeks after the initial therapy (presurgical phase), in order to determine how the patient responded to the ongoing treatment, and to specify the requirements for periodontal regenerative surgery. A computer-generated blocked randomization list (Randlist, DatInf) was used to generate a random sequence for the selected patients. This included the generation of random allocation sequential numbers on opaque envelopes. After the patient had drawn the number in sequence, patient's baseline data and details were printed on the envelope before opening, to disclose treatment allocation. The principal investigator monitored the complete process of random allocation concealment. Investigators were not unblinded with the follow-ups.

Clinical measurements

Prior to administering local lidocaine anesthesia (Lignox 2% A, Indoco Remedies) and before starting the surgical procedures, baseline measurements were taken, and Plaque Index (PI) as well as Papillary Bleeding Index (PBI) were recorded. Other clinical variables, including width of keratinized gingiva (WKG; a minimum of 3 mm was necessary as inclusion criterion, and this was determined prior to finishing the recruitment), relative clinical attachment level (rCAL; probing depth and gingival margin level measurements were added), vertical probing depth (VPD), and relative gingival marginal level (R-GML; measured as the distance between the gingival margin and the cementoenamel junction) were assessed using customized acrylic stents (DPI RR Cold Cure, DPI), with grooves to allow for reproducible periodontal probe positioning.[28] Horizontal probing depth (HPD) was measured with the help of a Nabers probe (2N, Hu-Friedy).[29] Only the deepest measurement per defect was taken into consideration for calculation of the results. A reevaluation of furcation defects was performed 6 months after therapy to assess the results. All pre- and postsurgical measurements were taken by the same assessors (BVK and KRB; both periodontists with clinical experience of several years); the latter were blinded to the respective treatment legs.

Surgical procedure

Just prior to the surgery, a presurgical rinse with chlorhexidine gluconate solution (Orahex, Nicholas Piramal) was employed for 1 minute. Extraoral asepsis was performed with povidine iodine solution (Betadine, Win-Medicare). After achieving adequate anesthesia (Lignox 2% A, Indoco Remedies), intracrevicular incisions were carried out on the buccal surfaces of teeth, in each case including one tooth adjacent (mesial and distal) to the treatment site. The incisions were made as interproximally as possible, for preservation of the interdental papilla, and to obtain primary closure of the wound. The releasing incisions were given when needed with the aim to achieve adequate accessibility, and to ensure coronal displacement of the periodontal flap. A mucoperiosteal flap was then reflected using a periosteal elevator (P9X, Hu-Friedy). The pocket epithelium was curetted out (Hu-Friedy) carefully. The furcation defect was debrided, the roof of the defect and the exposed surfaces of the root were scaled and planed using hand instruments such as furcation curettes (Hu-Friedy). Intrasurgical measurements including horizontal and vertical defect depths were recorded after obtaining hemostasis and irrigation with physiologic saline solution (Sodium Chloride 0.9% IV Infusion, Baxter). With respect to the horizontal defect depths (HDD), the furcation defects were measured at the deepest location using two periodontal probes (UNC 15 probe, Hu-Friedy),[28] being put across the prominent root surface in order to bridge the first probe (see Fig 2b). The furcation's vertical defect depth (VDD) was determined vertically at its deepest point, utilizing the fornix as a fixed reference point (see Fig 2c). The final patient's eligibility for the trial was confirmed if the furcation defect depth was less than 3 mm (measured vertically and horizontally). Again, blinding of patients was ensured for the entire duration of the study.

In the test group, the flap was presutured without placing a knot in order to allow for rapid wound closure following the placement of the PLA/PGA membrane with rhBMP-2. A bioabsorbable PLA/PGA membrane (BioMesh-s, Samyang Biopharma) was trimmed in order to conceal the lesion, extending approximately 2 mm beyond the edges of the furcation defect. The membrane was positioned over the tooth and sutured over the defect with the help of sling sutures. The rhBMP-2 solution (BMP-2, Life technologies) was prepared following the manufacturer's directions (the vial was briefly centrifuged before opening so as to bring the entire contents to the bottom). The lyophilized rhBMP-2 was reconstituted with sterile 20 mmol/L acetic acid (Aceto, Alfachemicals) to a concentration of 0.1 mg/mL. Using an insulin syringe (Accu point, AdvaCare), 0.01 mL was drawn up from the control rhBMP2 solution with a concentration of 0.1 mg/mL, and was injected into the inner side of the membrane facing the defect (Fig 2).

In the control group (PLA/PGA alone), the membrane was trimmed and placed over the defect in a manner similar to the test group, except for the application of rhBMP-2. The flap was relocated and sutured in a coronal direction, with its margin

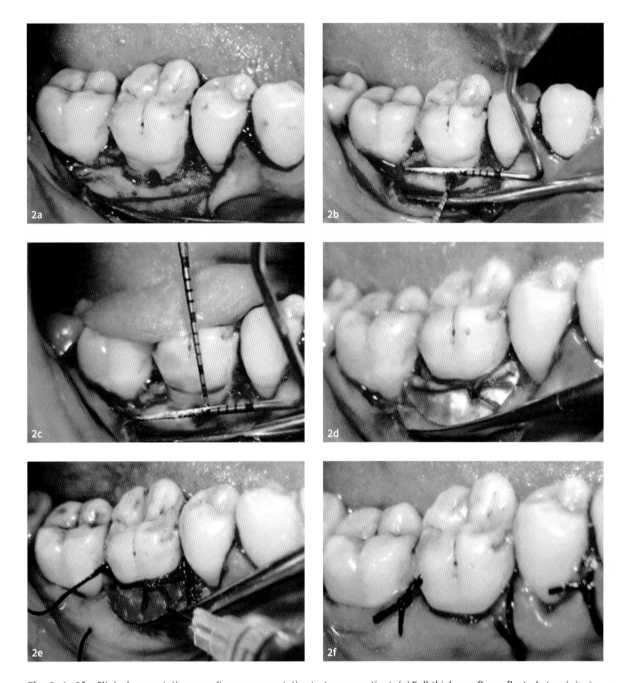

Figs 2a to 2f Clinical presentation revealing a representative test group patient. *(a)* Full-thickness flap reflected at recipient site. *(b)* Intrasurgical horizontal defect depth measurement. *(c)* Intrasurgical vertical defect depth measurement. (d) PLA/PGA sutured over the furcation defect. *(e)* Insertion of rhBMP-2 on inner surface of the membrane. *(f)* Flap sutured 1 mm coronal to the cementoenamel junction, covering the PLA/PGA membrane.

1 to 2 mm coronal to the cementoenamel junction, thus entirely covering the PLA/PGA membrane. To keep the flap in place, an interproximal suture (Vicryl Plus, Ethicon) was employed. For about 2 minutes, gentle compression was applied to the concerned area using a saline-soaked gauze to adapt the soft tissues to the tooth/root surface and minimize any space where a clot could develop and impair regeneration. A periodontal surgical dressing (Coe-Pak, GC) was applied to the surgical site. Again, all 24 patients were blinded to the respective treatment groups. The treatment was provided by an experienced periodontist (AAA), and all the clinical measurements were recorded by the co-investigators (BVK and KRB).

Postoperative care

During the postsurgical phase, an analgesic combination of ibuprofen 400 mg (Avibru, Bhavishya Pharmaceuticals) and acetaminophen 325 mg (A-Mol, Aan Pharma; three times a day), as well as an antibiotic (containing amoxicillin 500 mg; Blumox-500DT, Blue Cross Laboratories; three times a day) were administered for 5 days. Patients were instructed to avoid brushing their teeth at the treated site. For 4 weeks, patients were directed to rinse twice daily with 0.12% chlorhexidine gluconate (Orahex, Nicholas Piramal) for 1 minute. Patients were advised not to disturb the periodontal dressing and to prevent causing any unnecessary damage to the treated area. The periodontal dressing and stitches were removed 10 days postsurgery. After saline irrigation, careful polishing was performed with polishing paste (Detartrine, Septodont). Subjects were advised to clean the treated area with a cotton pellet that was saturated with 0.2% chlorhexidine gluconate (Orahex, Nicholas Piramal) for 2 to 3 weeks following an apicocoronal direction, and, subsequently, brushing was reinstalled. The recall appointments were after 1, 3, and 6 months following surgery. Both supra- and subgingival air polishing (as well as scaling, if necessary) were performed at each recall appointment. Clinical parameters were evaluated after 6 months using the previously made acrylic stents (but without surgical re-entry). Primary outcome was rCAL, and secondary outcomes were VPD as well as HPD, and relative gingival marginal levels (rGML).

With the follow-ups, patients were asked to report potential side effects, to enlighten any possible adverse reactions, and whether they would be satisfied with the outcomes. Special focus was given to postsurgical pain or other complications, and subjective perception was evaluated.

Statistical analysis

After having checked for normal distribution and homoscedasticity, comparison of PI as well as PBI at baseline and after 6 months was done applying the Student paired t test. The means and standard deviations (SDs) were determined for all clinical measurements comprising rCAL, VPD, HPD, and rGML. The obtained data were then assessed for statistical implication by standard methods using statistical software (SPSS version 25, IBM). The statistician performing the analysis (PB) was blinded to the treatment groups. The primary endpoint was the clinical attachment level 6 months postsurgery. The Student paired t test was used for all comparisons of the baseline data to that obtained at 6 months for both treatment groups. Com-

parison between test and control groups at baseline and after 6 months was carried out using the Student unpaired t test. With all statistical comparisons, significance levels of 5% ($\alpha = .05$) indicated statistically significant differences that were unlikely to have arisen by chance. Statistical evaluation was performed to see outcome trends considered to be helpful regarding the final decision to proceed with a larger full-scale clinical trial. With the outcome of the current investigation, the study was registered (International Standard Randomized Controlled Trial Number ISRCTN10907678), to schedule the clinical controlled trial.

Results

A total of 24 participants (aged 25 to 55 years, with 14 female patients; mean ± SD age was 38.1 ± 7.6 years were enrolled in this trial, and all patients were available for the subsequent follow-ups. Along with a high acceptance of the intervention, all treated cases showed uneventful healing during the study period, and no tooth was lost. None of the treated sites was eliminated (due to data loss), and no patients were lost until the termination of the study, thus indicating the feasibility of both the chosen set-up and the larger definitive trial. The mean ± SD PI scores were comparable, and remained low (< 0.8) in both groups throughout the study period (Table 1). Moreover, a decreased PBI score indicating a satisfactory enhancement of the gingival conditions was noted throughout the study period. The differences in PI scores and PBI scores between baseline and 6 months after surgical treatment were compared using a paired t test, and a statistically noteworthy decrease ($P = .001$) was observed (Table 1). According to the outcomes apparent from Table 2 and Table 3, the mean baseline defect characteristics and intrasurgical measurements did not show any statistically significant differences ($P > .05$), thus indicating an effective randomization process.

Regarding the primary (rCAL) and secondary outcomes (VPD, HPD, and rGML), the treatment effects revealed highly significant improvements from baseline to 6-month follow-ups for both groups ($P < .001$; Table 4). It is remarkable that all investigated categories seemed to benefit from the test group treatment (PLA/PGA membrane plus rhBMP-2).

Consequently, the mean differences between baseline and 6-month data were calculated, and the respective results are shown in Table 5. With reference to rCAL and HPD, comparable values between the test and the control groups could be observed. The mean ± SD CAL gains in the PLA/PGA + rhBMP-2 group and the PLA/PGA group amounted to 3.08 ± 0.99 mm and 2.91 ± 1.67 mm, respectively; with a difference of 0.16 ± 0.03 mm (slightly favoring the test group), these results were nonsignificant ($P=.76$). A similar trend could be revealed with the HPD reduction; here, the mean ± SD difference in HPD between both groups at the 6-month follow-up was 0.50 ± 0.90 mm, thus again suggesting an increased HPD reduction with the test group, but this just missed a significant difference ($P=.05$; Table 5).

In contrast, the mean ± SD VPD reduction at 6 months showed clearly improved values for the test group (2.00 ± 0.60 mm) when compared with the VPD reduction for PLA/PGA alone (0.83 ± 0.38 mm); the difference amounted to 1.16 ± 0.60 mm, and was significant ($P=.01$). A similar trend could be observed with the R-GML parameters; here, improved values for the control group (1.58 ± 1.44 mm) were found, while only a small recession (0.50 ± 0.9 mm) was revealed with the PLA/PGA + rhBMP-2 group; the difference (1.08 ± 1.16 mm) indicated less reduction of gingival recession in the control group, and this, again, was significant ($P=.03$; Table 5).

Frequency analysis performed for furcation changes revealed complete closure with five studied sites (41.66%) in the test group, if compared to two sites (16.66%) in the control group. Changes from Class II to Class I furcation defects were observed with seven sites (58.33%) in the PLA/PGA + rhBMP-2 group, and with 10 sites (83.33%) in the PLA/PGA group.

Except for postsurgical pain experienced on the day of intervention, as well as for temporary impairment due to the wound dressing, no adverse reactions were reported. In particular, none of the participants complained about signs of inflammation like swelling or suppuration. All patients could resume their personal oral hygiene as scheduled, and were satisfied with the healing progress.

Discussion

The present research aimed to determine the efficacy of rhBMP-2 in combination with a PLA/PGA membrane as a carrier for periodontal regenerative treatment in Class II furcation defects. Current systematic reviews[2,30-34] evaluating the treatment outcomes of furcation type defects are consistent in their conclusion that nonregenerative surgical approaches are less effective than regenerative therapies. Furthermore, studies comparing nonsurgical or open debridement alone approaches to GTR reported significantly superior results with the use of GTR,[35,36] with resorbable membranes revealing slightly superior outcomes if compared to nonresorbable membranes.[37] Clinically, bone fill obtained in horizontal and vertical components of the furcation defects and improvement in the overall clinical parameters have been used to reveal successful regeneration. Following GTR therapy in multirooted teeth presenting furcation defects, the survival rate has been reported to be as high as 83% to 100% after an observation period of 5 to 12 years (and even longer).[23,25,30,38-40]

In a meta-analysis evaluating clinical regeneration with GTR membranes in furcation defects, the best clinical results were reported for PLA/PGA membranes.[41] Hence, a PLA/PGA membrane was used for treating Class II furcation defects in the present study. In a histologic study[42] evaluating the osteoinductive potential of PLA/PGA combined with BMP in rats, complete replacement of PLA/PGA disks with new bone after a period of 2 weeks was reported. Additionally, radiographically dense radiopacities were seen for disks impregnated with BMP.[42] Substantial increase in alveolar ridge bone heights[43] and widths[43] in extraction sockets with the use of rhBMP-2 have been reported. Thus, the mentioned literature provides evidence for enhanced bone formation using rhBMP-2 in both animals and humans.[44,45] However, even if considered promising, there is scant evidence in the literature regarding the use of rhBMP-2 for furcation treatment in humans. With this scientific background in mind, a clear rationale and justification for the present pilot trial was given, and potential exposures to unnecessary risks of research were considered negligible.

The current pilot investigation was undertaken to preevaluate any possible efficacy of rhBMP-2 in combination with a PLA/PGA membrane in Class II furcation lesions; PLA/PGA membrane treatment alone was used as control, since open flap debridement (without any regenerative procedures) was considered unethical, due to the lack of improvement of the furcation status.[35] Based on the findings of the present study, both null hypotheses were at least partially rejected; clinically relevant horizontal and vertical defect depth reductions, along with gains in clinical attachment levels (primary endpoint) and reduction of gingival recessions, were evident for Class II furcation type defects. There was a strong tendency that the use of rhBMP-2 in combination with a PLA/PGA membrane was more efficacious when compared to the sole use of PLA/PGA membranes for treating Class II furcation type defects.

However, the outcome presented above must be viewed with care and a degree of restraint. Since no data on the efficacy of PLA/PGA + rhBMP-2 were available, no sample case calculation was possible, and a pilot study was deemed mandatory. The aim of a pilot trial should not be to focus on efficacy of a treatment only, but rather to decide whether a larger definitive trial is worthwhile and feasible; while statistical significance in a pilot study does not mean that the main trial is not required,[26] this will help with the final decision, and the exploratory outcome of the present study seems promising enough to justify a large-scale randomized clinical trial.

Table 1 Comparison of the mean ± SD PI and PBI scores between baseline and 6-month follow-up in both the PLA/PGA and the PLA/PGA + rhBMP-2 groups

Parameters	Group	Baseline	6 months	Difference	P value
PI	PLA/PGA (control)	0.75±0.06[a]	0.51±0.05[a]	0.23±0.04	<.001
	PLA/PGA + rhBMP-2 (test)	0.77±0.07[a]	0.54±0.05[a]	0.23±0.08	<.001
PBI	PLA/PGA (control)	0.67±0.06[a]	0.43±0.04[a]	0.24±0.07	<.001
	PLA/PGA + rhBMP-2 (test)	0.70±0.08[a]	0.47±0.06[a]	0.22±0.10	<.001

[a]Same superscript letter indicates nonsignificant differences (P>.05) between groups, both at baseline and 6 months postsurgery.

Table 2 Baseline characteristics of the sites for PLA/PGA and PLA/PGA + rhBMP-2 groups (mean ± SD; in mm)

Parameters	Control group (PLA/PGA)	Test group (PLA/PGA + rhBMP-2)	Difference	P value
Relative clinical attachment level (rCAL)	9.75±1.81	9.33±1.37	0.41±1.92	.520
Vertical probing depth (VPD)	4.58±0.66	3.75±0.49	0.83±0.79	.730
Horizontal probing depth (HPD)	3.25±0.45	3.16±0.38	0.08±0.66	.630
Relative gingival marginal level (rGML)	5.16±1.52	4.66±1.49	0.50±1.73	.420

Table 3 Intrasurgical hard tissue (baseline) measurements of the sites for PLA/PGA and PLA/PGA + rhBMP-2 groups (mean ± SD; in mm)

Parameters	Control group (PLA/PGA)	Test group (PLA/PGA + rhBMP-2)	Difference	P value
Horizontal defect depth (HDD)	3.00±0.60	3.08±0.51	0.08±0.99	.710
Vertical defect depth (fornix to base of defect) (VDD)	3.25±0.45	2.91±0.66	0.33±0.49	.160

Notwithstanding, a recent systematic review on furcation treatment revealed that most of the studies that were finally included had an unclear risk of bias;[33] this drawback seems a widespread phenomenon, since there is a vast number of poorly designed and/or reported studies,[27] and this does not only refer to dentistry. Consequently, an equally relevant aim of the current investigation (if compared to any statistically relevant issues) was to clarify various feasibility aspects (like recruitment rates, allocation concealment, randomization and retention of patients, pretreatment and intervention management, adherence as well as engagement, and acceptance rates).[27] In particular with regard to data acquisition (baseline and postsurgical measurements), the current set-up confirmed the practicability of the applied methods (see Fig 2). However, statements referring to safety of the studied treatment options do not seem adequate with the small sample size of the current investigation. Moreover, it must be reemphasized that the latter aspect does not allow for any definite or conclusive statements

on efficacy, due to the poor power of the current pilot trial. Finally, it should be kept in mind that every efficacy trial only will evaluate interventional achievements under optimum conditions (in the present trial, this would refer to nonsmokers with good general health, with antibiotic protection, and with good compliance/good and regularly controlled oral hygiene), while, notably, effectiveness trials will confirm treatment benefits of the intervention when delivered via a real-world program.

The present research was conducted over a period of 6 months, and this might be considered critical for the evaluation of the outcomes of periodontal regeneration.[32,35] Nonetheless, it should be kept in mind that PLA/PGA + rhBMP-2 efficacy was not the only aspect of the current investigation. At baseline, the investigated parameters at the sites treated with PLA/PGA or PLA/PGA + rhBMP-2 displayed no statistical differences, thus revealing comparable starting points for both groups. There were no signs of allergy, infection, or any other adverse complications in patients treated using PLA/PGA with or

Table 4 Comparison of the clinical parameters between baseline and 6-month follow-up in the PLA/PGA group and the PLA/PGA+ rhBMP-2 groups (mean ± SD; in mm)

Parameters	Group	Baseline	6 months	P value
rCAL	PLA/PGA (control)	9.75±1.81	6.81±1.19	<.001
	PLA/PGA + rhBMP-2 (test)	9.33±1.37	6.25±1.35	<.001
VPD	PLA/PGA (control)	4.58±0.66	3.75±0.45	<.001
	PLA/PGA + rhBMP-2 (test)	4.66±0.49	2.66±0.49	<.001
HPD	PLA/PGA (control)	3.25±0.45	1.16±0.71	<.001
	PLA/PGA + rhBMP-2 (test)	3.16±0.38	0.58±0.51	<.001
rGML	PLA/PGA (control)	5.16±1.52	3.58±0.99	<.001
	PLA/PGA + rhBMP-2 (test)	4.66±1.49	4.16±1.19	<.001

HPD, horizontal probing depth; rCAL, relative clinical attachment level; rGML, relative gingival marginal level; VPD, vertical probing depth.

without rhBMP-2. During the 6-month period of observation, no tooth was lost, and uneventful wound healings could not be observed; in particular, no incidence of exposure of the bioresorbable membrane was observed, and this at least partially was due to the sufficient volume[46,47] of keratinized marginal gingiva. As indicated by PI and PBI scores, all the enrolled patients exhibited good oral hygiene and clinically healthy gingival conditions throughout the study interval. This may be the result of repeated oral hygiene reinforcement and a regular supportive periodontal health care program reinforced by air-polishing followed throughout the study period, thus resulting in a repeated reduction of the periodontal pathogens,[48] and elucidating the evidence from the literature.[49,50] On the other side, due to the inclusion criteria and the provided preventive support, the investigated small cohort must not be viewed as representative, and the current outcome should be weighed up carefully (but is not considered generalizable). Similar caution would seem mandatory with the intrinsic limitations of manually assessing probing depths; though the investigators involved in the current trial both had several years of experience, and even if acrylic stents were used to standardize the measurement, systemic or random errors could not be totally ruled out. Such limitations will also be reduced with a larger sample size.

A few study reports grounded on both short-term[51] and long-term[52] data have indicated that good oral hygiene (as assessed per low plaque scores) was related to long-term stability of the clinical attachment gain; notwithstanding, an accelerated clinical attachment loss can occur following surgery in biofilm-infected dentitions.[52] Traditionally, periodontal therapy has focused on VPD reduction, since increased pockets depths at the treated areas act as indicators of risk for progression of periodontal disease.[53] In the current study, a satisfactory reduction of the mean VPD was found in both groups; however, a difference between the test group and the membrane-only group (1.16±0.57 mm) was observed, and this statistically significant improvement (P<.001) was considered clinically relevant.

When keeping in mind that, with reference to furcation treatment, there are no studies reporting on the efficacy of a combination of PLA/PGA and rhBMP-2 available in the accessible literature, no comparisons can be made on the effects of rhBMP-2 in Class II furcation defects. The mean VPD reduction attained in the control group (0.83±0.79 mm), however, is in accordance with the available studies using bioresorbable membranes in treating Class II furcation type defects.[8,23,54] The mean VPD reduction in the control group noted in the present study could be explained by the somewhat higher mean initial VPD (4.58± 0.66 mm). It has been demonstrated that VPD reduction following periodontal regenerative surgery is strongly dependent on the initial VPDs.[55]

The principal parameter for validation of effective clinical defect fill after periodontal therapy is CAL gain.[54,56,57] As outcome measures to assess periodontal defect fill of furcation-treated sites, it has become progressively common to determine the gain in attachment both in vertical and in horizontal directions, since the primary goal of furcation treatment is the reduction of the defect magnitude to a size which can be maintained by routine oral hygiene methods and mechanical/hand instrumentation.[54,56] In the current study, significant CAL gain was noted in both groups. When comparing the two groups, a slightly greater gain in CAL was observed in the PLA/PGA + rhBMP-2 group, which was, however, nonsignificant (P=.76). Similar findings were observed in a study in rats conducted to

Table 5 Comparison of the clinical parameters between PLA/PGA and PLA/PGA + rhBMP-2 groups at the 6-month follow-up (mean ± SD; in mm)

Parameters	Control group (PLA/PGA)	Test group (PLA/PGA + rhBMP-2)	Difference	P value
CAL gain	2.91 ± 1.67	3.08 ± 0.99	0.16 ± 0.03	.760
VPD reduction	0.83 ± 0.38	2.00 ± 0.60	1.16 ± 0.57	.010
HPD reduction	2.08 ± 0.66	2.58 ± 0.51	0.50 ± 0.90	.050
GR	1.58 ± 1.44	0.50 ± 0.90	1.08 ± 0.16	.030

CAL, clinical attachment level; GR, gingival recession; HPD, horizontal probing depth; VPD, vertical probing depth.

evaluate the osteoinductive potential of PLA/PGA disks incorporated with BMP. New bone formation after a period of 4 weeks with complete replacement of PLA/PGA disks was seen in sites with BMP, whereas sites receiving PLA/PGA disks without BMP were occupied with fibrous connective tissue histologically.[42]

The observations made in the current study with regards to CAL gain in the PLA/PGA group are comparable with the results stated in previous studies.[23,35,58] The main clinical end point for the treatment of furcation lesions would be the complete closure of furcation areas; if this outcome cannot be obtained, at least a conversion of deep lesions into shallow lesions would seem desirable.[59] In the present study, the PLA/PGA + rhBMP-2 group showed significant HPD reductions of 2.58 ± 0.51 mm, compared to PLA/PGA alone (2.08 ± 0.71 mm), after 6 months, and the number of Class II furcation defects that were closed/converted to Class I lesions was higher in the PLA/PGA + rhBMP-2 group. An overall partial closure of furcation lesions was predominantly observed, whereas complete closures of furcation areas were found to be less common. Comparable results have been reported in previous studies[57,60] using PLA/PGA membranes only. In the present investigation, this could be due to greater reduction in VPD in the PLA/PGA + rhBMP-2 group (if compared to the PLA/PGA alone group); moreover, enhanced bone formation due to BMP addition has been observed previously,[42] and this might have positively influenced the present outcome.

It has been stated that the management of Class II furcation involvement presents a unique clinical problem, due to the complex anatomy at the furcation area,[28] considered hard to standardize with respect to clinical trials (and, thus, lowering the predictability of each treatment approach[61]); nevertheless, the primary aim of each furcation treatment approach should be to clean the furcation and to facilitate (or even enable) patients' oral hygiene.[47] In the current trial, all Class II furcation type defects were either closed or converted to Class I lesions in both groups. However, the certainty of these treatment goals should be interpreted carefully since the influence of several factors like presurgical probing depths, patient compliance, complexity of defects, root morphology, surgical techniques used, and level of maintenance and home care cannot be denied.[52,60,62] Therefore, there is a need to better understand the factors and conditions that may have an impact upon treatment outcomes. Although there is a paucity of data on gingival recession following regenerative therapy with the use of PLA/PGA + rhBMP-2 with regard to the treatment of furcation defects, the present study showed a minimal gingival recession of 0.50 mm in the PLA/PGA + rhBMP-2 group (compared to 1.58 mm in the PLA/PGA alone group) at 6 months. When gingival recession was compared between the groups, a significantly decreased (P = .03) gingival recession in the test group could be revealed. This could be attributed to variations with the coronal positioning of the flaps, even if this was performed similarly in all cases. Notwithstanding, with a full-scale clinical trial, this possible source of imprecision should attract vigilance regarding the complete adherence to the study protocol.

The most consistent parameter for evaluating periodontal tissue regeneration is a histologic evaluation. However, owing to certain ethical deliberations and patient-associated limitations, neither a surgical reentry nor a histologic verification of any periodontal regeneration was possible with the current study (as with other investigations including patients); thus, neither the nature nor the quality of the regenerated tissues can be commented upon. Notwithstanding, from the current outcome, the application of PLA/PGA + rhBMP-2 seems to be a promising treatment mode of Class II furcation type defects. Moreover, a period of 6 months could be considered short to evaluate the effectiveness of periodontal therapy, particularly when dealing with biomaterials and barrier techniques. However, the present investigation focused on the primary biologic reactions, and aimed to exclude other potentially negative patient-centered factors (including limited retention, adherence, and engagement) usually observed in the long term. It should be kept in mind that in a long-term study running for 3 years,[6] it was stated that the majority of clinical changes obtained were achieved with the 6-month reentry, and no significant changes thereafter for up to 3 years were reported.

Nevertheless, the 6-month evaluation period in the present study would be considered as one of the major limitations,[35] even if the clinical results revealed some preliminary evidence on the clinical efficacy of using PLA/PGA + rhBMP-2 in improving the clinical variables; indeed, this supports the concept that the use of rhBMP-2 in combination with a PLA/PGA membrane provided additional benefits of statistical significance and, more important, of clinical relevance when treating Class II furcation type defects. In fact, the vertical as well as the horizontal probing depth reductions were consistently greater in the PLA/PGA + rhBMP-2 group, compared to the sites treated with PLA/PGA alone, thus highlighting a clinically meaningful difference, the more so as this has been considered a highly important aspect regarding the survival rate of molars.[47]

With the present investigation, several aspects of practical operability (like recruitment, randomization, acceptance and retention of patients, as well as adherence to the study protocol) have been shown to be satisfactory; thus, the current pilot study investigating the feasibility of a future definitive RCT clearly has provided answers to the question whether such a full-scale trial can be done, should be done, and, if so, how.[27] Consequently, with regard to the improvements of clinical parameters assessed in the present pilot RCT, further longitudinal investigations seem mandatory, in particular when reflecting on the documented radiographic evidence of rhBMP-2 use and its clinical long-term efficacy.[41-45] With the proven practicability of the present set-up in mind, and when facing the current

clinically meaningful outcome, such a large-scale RCT clearly seems justified. Finally, the present pilot RCT allows for tentative empirical estimates of treatment effect sizes[63] and confidence intervals;[64] if done carefully, by prespecifying clinically meaningful differences,[65] and by avoiding any potential trial underpowering,[65] this would provide a sound basis for sample size calculations of future clinical trials with long-term follow-ups. ⊞

Conclusion

With regards to the aims of the current pilot trial studying the treatment of Class II furcation defects, the use of rhBMP-2 in combination with a PLA/PGA membrane has provided some preliminary evidence (deemed to be carefully assessed) on the clinical efficacy of the intervention when compared to the use of PLA/PGA membranes alone; the clinically relevant improvements strongly call for a definitive full-scale main trial to confirm the present provisional outcome. The set-up presented has provided support for the trial design, the more so as, overall, the applied methodology has been considered acceptable and eligible among the cohort under investigation.

Acknowledgments

The authors thank Dr Pavan Bajaj (Sharad Pawar Dental College & Hospital, Wardha, Maharashtra, India), for his support with the statistical analysis, and with the interpretation of the studied data. This investigator-driven study was supported by the authors and their respective institutions only, without any external funding. The authors declare no potential conflict of interest with respect to authorship and/or publication of this study.

References

1. Matia J. Efficiency of scaling of molar furcation area with and without surgical access. Int J Periodontics Restorative Dent 1986;6:25–35.

2. Jepsen S, Eberhard J, Herrera D, Needleman I. A systematic review of guided tissue regeneration for periodontal furcation defects. What is the effect of guided tissue regeneration compared with surgical debridement in the treatment of furcation defects? J Clin Periodontol 2002;29:103–116.

3. Calongne KB, Aichelmann-Reidy ME, Yukna RA, Mayer ET. Clinical comparison of microporous biocompatible composite of PMMA, PHEMA and calcium hydroxide grafts and expanded poly-tetrafluoroethylene barrier membranes in human mandibular molar Class II furcations. A case series. J Periodontol 2001;72:1451–1459.

4. Yukna RA, Evans GH, Aichelmann-Reidy MB, Mayer ET. Clinical comparison of bioactive glass bone replacement graft material and expanded polytetrafluoroethylene barrier membrane in treating human mandibular molar class II furcations. J Periodontol 2001;72:125–133.

5. Müller HP, Eger T, Lange D. Management of furcation-involved teeth: a retrospective analysis. J Clin Periodontol 1995;22:911–917.

6. Yukna RA, Evans GH, Aichelmann-Reidy MB, Mayer ET. Clinical comparison of bioactive glass bone replacement graft material and expanded polytetrafluoroethylene barrier membrane in treating human mandibular molar class II furcations. J Periodontol 2001;72:125–133.

7. de Obarrio JJ, Arauz-Dutari JI, Chamberlain TM, Croston A. The use of autologous growth factors in periodontal surgical therapy: platelet gel biotechnology – case reports. Int J Periodontics Restorative Dent 2000;20:487–497.

8.	Reddy MS, Aichelmann-Reidy ME, Avila-Ortiz G, et al. Periodontal regeneration – furcation defects: a consensus report from the AAP regeneration workshop. J Periodontol 2015;86: S131–S133.

9.	Urist MR. Bone: formation by autoinduction. Science 1965;150:893–899.

10.	Sigurdsson TJ, Lee MB, Kubota K, Turek TJ, Wozney JM, Wikesjö UM. Periodontal repair in dogs: recombinant human bone morphogenetic protein-2 significantly enhances periodontal regeneration. J Periodontol 1995;66: 131–138.

11.	Boyne P, Nakamura A, Shabahang S. Evaluation of the long-term effect of function on rhBMP-2 regenerated hemimandibulectomy defects. Br J Oral Maxillofac Surg 1999;37:344–352.

12.	Sykaras N, Triplett RG, Nunn ME, Iacopino AM, Opperman LA. Effect of recombinant human bone morphogenetic protein-2 on bone regeneration and osseointegration of dental implants. Clin Oral Implants Res 2001;12:339–349.

13.	Boyne PJ, Marx RE, Nevins M, et al. A feasibility study evaluating rhBMP-2/absorbable collagen sponge for maxillary sinus floor augmentation. Int J Periodontics Restorative Dent 1997;17:11–25.

14.	Howell TH, Fiorellini J, Jones A, et al. A feasibility study evaluating rhBMP-2/absorbable collagen sponge device for local alveolar ridge preservation or augmentation. Int J Periodontics Restorative Dent 1997;17:124–139.

15.	Geiger M, Li R, Friess W. Collagen sponges for bone regeneration with rhBMP-2. Adv Drug Deliv Rev 2003;55:1613–1629.

16.	McKay WF, Peckham SM, Badura JM. A comprehensive clinical review of recombinant human bone morphogenetic protein-2 (INFUSE Bone Graft). Int Orthop 2007;31:729–734.

17.	Sigurdsson TJ, Nygaard L, Tatakis DN, et al. Periodontal repair in dogs: evaluation of rhBMP-2 carriers. Int J Periodontics Restorative Dent 1996;16:524–537.

18.	Barboza EP, Caúla AL, de Oliveira Caúla F, et al. Effect of recombinant human bone morphogenetic protein-2 in an absorbable collagen sponge with space-providing biomaterials on the augmentation of chronic alveolar ridge defects. J Periodontol 2004;75:702–708.

19.	Boyan B, Lohmann C, Somers A, et al. Potential of porous poly-D, L-lactide-co-glycolide particles as a carrier for recombinant human bone morphogenetic protein-2 during osteoinduction in vivo. J Biomed Mater Res 1999;46:51–59.

20.	Zegzula HD, Buck DC, Brekke J, Wozney JM, Hollinger JO. Bone formation with use of rhBMP-2 (recombinant human bone morphogenetic protein-2). J Bone Joint Surg Am 1997;79:1778–1790.

21.	Isobe M, Yamazaki Y, Mori M, Ishihara K, Nakabayashi N, Amagasa T. The role of recombinant human bone morphogenetic protein-2 in PLGA capsules at an extraskeletal site of the rat. J Biomed Mater Res 1999;45:36–41.

22.	Gao Y, Wang S, Shi B, et al. Advances in modification methods based on biodegradable membranes in guided bone/tissue regeneration: a review. Polymers 2022;14:871.

23.	Eickholz P, Pretzl B, Holle R, Kim TS. Long-term results of guided tissue regeneration therapy with non-resorbable and bioabsorbable barriers. III. Class II furcations after 10 years. J Periodontol 2006;77:88–94.

24.	Whitehead AL, Julious SA, Cooper CL, Campbell MJ. Estimating the sample size for a pilot randomised trial to minimise the overall trial sample size for the external pilot and main trial for a continuous outcome variable. Stat Methods Med Res 2016;25:1057–1073.

25.	Chowdhary Z, Mohan R. Furcation involvement: still a dilemma. Indian J Multidiscip Dent 2017;7:34–40.

26.	Eldridge SM, Chan CL, Campbell MJ, et al. CONSORT 2010 statement: extension to randomised pilot and feasibility trials. BMJ 2016; 355:i5239.

27.	Thabane L, Ma J, Chu R, et al. A tutorial on pilot studies: the what, why and how. BMC Med Res Methodol 2010;10:1–10.

28.	Bhatnagar MA, Deepa D. Management of grade II furcation defect in mandibular molar with alloplastic bone graftand bioresorbable guided tissue regeneration membrane: a case report. Int J Periodontol Implantol 2016;1:96–99.

29.	Oringer RJ, Fiorellini JP, Koch GG, et al. Comparison of manual and automated probing in an untreated periodontitis population. J Periodontol 1997;68:1156–1162.

30.	Huynh-Ba G, Kuonen P, Hofer D, Schmid J, Lang NP, Salvi GE. The effect of periodontal therapy on the survival rate and incidence of complications of multirooted teeth with furcation involvement after an observation period of at least 5 years: a systematic review. J Clin Periodontol 2009;36:164–176.

31.	Murphy KG, Gunsolley JC. Guided tissue regeneration for the treatment of periodontal intrabony and furcation defects. A systematic review. Ann Periodontol 2003;8:266–302.

32.	Reynolds MA, Aichelmann-Reidy ME, Branch-Mays GL, Gunsolley JC. The efficacy of bone replacement grafts in the treatment of periodontal osseous defects. A systematic review. Ann Periodontol 2003;8:227–265.

33.	Kinaia BM, Steiger J, Neely AL, Shah M, Bhola M. Treatment of Class II molar furcation involvement: meta-analyses of reentry results. J Periodontol 2011;82:413–428.

34.	Avila-Ortiz G, De Buitrago JG, Reddy MS. Periodontal regeneration–furcation defects: a systematic review from the AAP regeneration workshop. J Periodontol 2015;86:S108–S130.

35.	Jepsen S, Gennai S, Hirschfeld J, Kalemaj Z, Buti J, Graziani F. Regenerative surgical treatment of furcation defects: a systematic review and Bayesian network meta-analysis of randomized clinical trials. J Clin Periodontol 2020;47:352–374.

36.	Khanna D, Malhotra S, Naidu DV. Treatment of grade II furcation involvement using resorbable guided tissue regeneration membrane: a six-month study. J Indian Soc Periodontol 2012;16:404–410.

37.	da Silva Pereira SL, Sallum AW, Casati MZ, et al. Comparison of bioabsorbable and non-resorbable membranes in the treatment of dehiscence-type defects. A histomorphometric study in dogs. J Periodontol 2000;71:1306–1314.

38.	Eickholz P, Hausmann E. Evidence for healing of periodontal defects 5 years after conventional and regenerative therapy: digital subtraction and bone level measurements. J Clin Periodontol 2002;29:922–928.

39.	Yukna RA, Yukna CN. Six-year clinical evaluation of HTR synthetic bone grafts in human grade II molar furcations. J Periodontal Res 1997;32:627–633.

40.	Dannewitz B, Krieger JK, Hüsing J, Eickholz P. Loss of molars in periodontally treated patients: a retrospective analysis five years or more after active periodontal treatment. J Clin Periodontol 2006;33:53–61.

41.	Evans G, Yukna R, Cambre K, Gardiner D. Clinical regeneration with guided tissue barriers. Curr Opin Periodontol 1997;4:75–81.

42.	Miki T, Imai Y. Osteoinductive potential of freeze-dried, biodegradable, poly (glycolic acid-co-lactic acid) disks incorporated with bone morphogenetic protein in skull defects of rats. Int J Oral Maxillofac Surg 1996;25:402–406.

43.	Kelly MP, Vaughn OLA, Anderson PA. Systematic review and meta-analysis of recombinant human bone morphogenetic protein-2 in localized alveolar ridge and maxillary sinus augmentation. J Oral Maxillofac Surg 2016; 74:928–939.

44.	de Freitas RM, Spin-Neto R, Junior EM, Pereira LAVD, Wikesjö UM, Susin C. Alveolar ridge and maxillary sinus augmentation using rh BMP-2: a systematic review. Clin Implant Dent Relat Res 2015;17:e192–e201.

45.	Hsu YT, Al-Hezaimi K, Galindo-Moreno P, O'valle F, Al-Rasheed A, Wang HL. Effects of recombinant human bone morphogenetic protein-2 on vertical bone augmentation in a canine model. J Periodontol 2017;88:896–905.

46.	Saida H, Fukuba S, Shiba T, Komatsu K, Iwata T, Nitta H. Two-stage approach for class II mandibular furcation defect with insufficient keratinized mucosa: a case report with 3 years' follow-up. J Int Med Res 2021;49:1–9.

47.	Rasperini G, Majzoub J, Limiroli E, et al. Management of furcation-involved molars: recommendation for treatment and regeneration. Int J Periodontics Restorative Dent 2020;40:e137–e146.

48.	Derdilopoulou FV, Nonhoff J, Neumann K, Kielbassa AM. Microbiological findings after periodontal therapy using curettes, Er:YAG laser, sonic, and ultrasonic scalers. J Clin Periodontol 2007;34:588–598.

49.	Löe H, Anerud A, Boysen H, Smith M. The natural history of periodontal disease in man: the rate of periodontal destruction before 40 years of age. J Periodontol 1978;49:607–620.

50.	Wolgin M, Frankenhauser A, Shakavets N, Bastendorf K-D, Lussi A, Kielbassa AM. A randomized controlled trial on the plaque-removing efficacy of a low-abrasive air-polishing system to improve oral health care. Quintessence Int 2021;52:752–762.

51. Selvig KA, Kersten BG, Chamberlain AD, Wikesjo UM, Nilveus RE. Regenerative surgery of intrabony periodontal defects using ePTFE barrier membranes: scanning electron microscopic evaluation of retrieved membranes versus clinical healing. J Periodontol 1992;63:974–978.

52. Cortellini P, Pini-Prato G, Tonetti M. Periodontal regeneration of infrabony defects (V). Effect of oral hygiene on long-term stability. J Clin Periodontol 1994;21:606–610.

53. Armitage GC. Periodontal diseases: diagnosis. Ann Periodontol 1996;1:37–215.

54. Polson AM, Southard GL, Dunn RL, Polson AP, Billen JR, Laster LL. Initial study of guided tissue regeneration in Class II furcation defects after use of a biodegradable barrier. Int J Periodontics Restorative Dent 1995;15:42–55.

55. Cortellini P, Prato GP, Tonetti MS. Periodontal regeneration of human infrabony defects. I. Clinical measures. J Periodontol 1993;64:254–260.

56. Gottlow J, Nyman S, Lindhe J, Karring T, Wennström J. New attachment formation in the human periodontium by guided tissue regeneration: case reports. J Clin Periodontol 1986;13:604–616.

57. Becker W, Becker BE, Mellonig J, et al. A prospective multi-center study evaluating periodontal regeneration for Class II furcation invasions and intrabony defects after treatment with a bioabsorbable barrier membrane: 1-year results. J Periodontol 1996;67:641–649.

58. Bouchard P, Giovannoli JL, Mattout C, Davarpanah M, Etienne D. Clinical evaluation of a bioabsorbable regenerative material in mandibular class II furcation therapy. J Clin Periodontol 1997;24:511–518.

59. Sanz M, Giovannoli JL. Focus on furcation defects: guided tissue regeneration. Periodontol 2000 2000;22:169–189.

60. Friedmann A, Stavropoulos A, Bilhan H. GTR treatment in furcation grade II periodontal defects with the recently reintroduced guidor PLA matrix barrier: a case series with chronological step-by-step illustrations. Case Rep Dent 2020;2020:8856049.

61. Verma PK, Srivastava R, Gautam A, Chaturvedi TP. Multiple regenerative techniques for class II furcation defect. Eur J Gen Dent 2012;1:90–93.

62. Chiu M-Y, Lin C-Y, Kuo P-Y. The predictive performance of surgical treatment in upper molars with combined bony defect and furcation involvement: a retrospective cohort study. BMC Oral Health 2022;22:1–12.

63. In J. Introduction of a pilot study. Korean J Anesthesiol 2017;70:601–605.

64. Teresi JA, Yu X, Stewart AL, Hays RD. Guidelines for designing and evaluating feasibility pilot studies. Med Care 2022;60:95–103.

65. National Center for Complementary and Integrative Health. Pilot studies: common uses and misuses. https://www.nccih.nih.gov/grants/pilot-studies-common-uses-and-misuses. Accessed 14 November 2022.

Ankita A. Agrawal

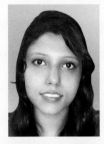

Ankita A. Agrawal   Postgraduate student, Department of Periodontology and Oral Implantology, Sharad Pawar Dental College, Datta Meghe Institute of Medical Sciences, Wardha, Maharashtra, India

Prasad V. Dhadse   Professor and Head, Department of Periodontology and Oral Implantology, Sharad Pawar Dental College, Datta Meghe Institute of Medical Sciences, Wardha, Maharashtra, India

Bhairavi V. Kale   Postgraduate student, Department of Periodontology and Oral Implantology, Sharad Pawar Dental College, Datta Meghe Institute of Medical Sciences, Wardha, Maharashtra, India

Komal R. Bhombe   Postgraduate student, Department of Periodontology and Oral Implantology, Sharad Pawar Dental College, Datta Meghe Institute of Medical Sciences, Wardha, Maharashtra, India

Kiran K. Ganji   Assistant Professor, Department of Preventive Dentistry, College of Dentistry, Jouf University, Saudi Arabia; and Department of Periodontology and Oral Implantology, Sharad Pawar Dental College, Datta Meghe Institute of Medical Sciences, Wardha, Maharashtra, India

Andrej M. Kielbassa   Professor and Head, Center for Operative Dentistry, Periodontology, and Endodontology, Department of Dentistry, Faculty of Medicine and Dentistry, Danube Private University (DPU), Krems, Austria

Correspondence: Prof Dr Dr h c Andrej M. Kielbassa, Center for Operative Dentistry, Periodontology, and Endodontology, Department of Dentistry, Faculty of Medicine and Dentistry, Danube Private University (DPU), Steiner Landstraße 124, A – 3500 Krems, Austria. Email: andrej.kielbassa@dp-uni.ac.at

First submission: 14 Nov 2022
Acceptance: 19 Nov 2022
Online publication: 29 Nov 2022

Ferric sulfate pulpotomy in primary teeth with different base materials: a 2-year randomized controlled trial

Burak Aksoy, DDS, PhD/Hamdi Cem Güngör, DDS, PhD/Serdar Uysal, DDS, PhD/Cesar D. Gonzales, DDS, MS/ Seval Ölmez, DDS, PhD

Objective: To evaluate the effects of zinc oxide–eugenol, calcium hydroxide, and mineral trioxide aggregate as base materials on the clinical and radiographic success of ferric sulfate pulpotomies in primary molars. **Method and materials:** Following hemostasis with 15.5% ferric sulfate, 105 teeth were randomly allocated to three groups: Group 1, zinc oxide–eugenol; Group 2, calcium hydroxide; and Group 3, mineral trioxide aggregate. All teeth were restored with stainless-steel crowns. Clinical and radiographic examinations were conducted at 6, 12, 18, and 24 months. **Results:** After 24 months, clinical success rates for Groups 1 to 3 were 97.1% (34/35 teeth), 94.2% (33/35 teeth), and 97.1% (34/35 teeth), respectively ($P > .05$). Radiographic success rates were 65.7% (23/35 teeth), 65.7% (23/35 teeth), and 77.1% (27/35 teeth), respectively ($P > .05$). Internal resorption was the most observed radiographic finding (15/105 teeth). **Conclusions:** The choice of zinc oxide–eugenol, calcium hydroxide, and mineral trioxide aggregate, as base materials, did not affect the clinical and radiographic success of ferric sulfate pulpotomies in primary teeth. (Quintessence Int 2022;53:782–789; doi: 10.3290/j.qi.b3149429)

Key words: calcium hydroxide, ferric sulfate, mineral trioxide aggregate, primary teeth, pulpotomy, stainless steel crown, zinc oxide–eugenol

Vital pulpotomy becomes the choice of treatment when complete removal of carious dentin results in exposure of the inflamed pulp in a primary tooth.[1] The goal is to preserve the arch integrity and normal oral function, by retaining the tooth until its natural exfoliation time and replacement by its permanent successor. However, with the number of available studies in the field, the American Academy of Pediatric Dentistry (AAPD) guidelines base its recommendation on moderate-quality evidence at 24 months.[1,2]

Formocresol (FC) is a devitalizing medicament that has been used in dentistry for over 80 years.[3] It is one of the medicaments recommended for pulpotomy of primary teeth expected to be retained for at least 24 months.[1,4] The pulpotomy technique utilizing FC has a history of overall clinical success ranging from 55% to 98%.[5] However, potential carcinogenecity of one of its components (formaldehyde)[3] has posed a major setback for its clinical use and has led to searches for more biocompatible materials with the same or better success as FC. In this context, ferric sulfate (FS) has drawn attention as an alternative, which enables hemostasis by forming a ferric ion-protein clot on the pulp surface following a chemical reaction with blood.[6] It has been proposed that this formation might act as a barrier to the irritative substances that cause inflammation and internal resorption in the underlying pulp.[7]

Zinc oxide and eugenol (ZOE) paste is a commonly used dressing in primary tooth pulpotomies. Free eugenol in contact with vital pulp tissue causes a moderate to severe inflammatory response, which results in chronic inflammation and necrosis.[8,9] Internal resorption is a frequently reported finding in pulpotomies of primary teeth.[5,10] Some researchers have stated that eugenol could leach through the underlying blood clot and might cause the inflammatory reaction of the pulp.[8,11] Smith et al[5] suggest that ZOE paste might not be an ideal base material for FS pulpotomies. Another pulpotomy dressing for primary teeth is calcium hydroxide (CH) paste. It has been claimed that CH also leads to internal resorption when it is placed over the pulp in the presence of inflammation or without sufficient hemorrhage control.[12,13] Uncontrolled hemorrhage may have an impact on the success rate as it can prevent the contact between the medicament and the pulp tissue.[13-16]

Due to its properties such as biocompatibility, high alkalinity, radiopacity, and induction of dentin bridge formation, mineral trioxide aggregate (MTA) has been suggested as a suitable medicament for pulpotomies of primary teeth.[4,17] Its antimicrobial properties are similar to ZOE, while the sealing ability is better than ZOE.[18]

The effect of base materials on the outcome of FS pulpotomy in primary teeth has not been largely studied.[19-22] The present study aimed to evaluate the effects of ZOE, CH, and MTA on the success of primary molar pulpotomies with FS. The tested null hypothesis was that there are no statistically significant differences between ZOE, CH, and MTA in terms of clinical and radiographic outcomes.

Method and materials

The protocol of the present randomized clinical trial was reviewed and approved by the Clinical Researches Ethics Board of the Hacettepe University (Protocol Number: HEK 09/94-43). Each patient's parent/guardian received detailed information regarding the study protocol explaining the procedures, possible discomforts, and risks versus benefits. A signed informed consent form was obtained for each of the participants. The study design followed the CONSORT 2010 Statement: Updated guidelines for reporting parallel group randomized trials.[23]

Participants

The power analysis considering α = .05, power equal to 80% and the 10% outcome difference (one group is 10%, and another 0%) led to a required sample size of 30 for each group. It was further increased to 35 (teeth/group) to improve the validity of the study and compensate for the probable loss during follow-up visits.

The study population comprised patients who were seen for routine exams in the pediatric dentistry clinics of Hacettepe University Faculty of Dentistry in Ankara, Turkey. Healthy and cooperative children with primary molars that met the following criteria were invited to participate in the study:

- asymptomatic with deep caries lesions
- no mobility and tenderness to palpation/percussion tests
- no pathologic signs of pulpal infection, (ie, tooth mobility, parulis/fistula, and soft tissue swelling)
- carious exposure of the pulp during caries excavation

- no pulpal necrosis (excessive or no bleeding at all) or infectious exudate (pus) after entry into the pulp chamber
- attainment of radicular pulp hemostasis after compression with a sterile cotton pellet
- restorable with a stainless-steel crown
- no radiographic evidence of pulp degeneration (ie, internal root resorption, interradicular and/or furcal bone destruction, widened periodontal ligament space, pathologic root resorption)
- physiologic root resorption of less than one-third.

All radiographs were taken with size 0 ultra-speed dental film (Eastman Kodak) using a Phot-X II x-ray unit (Belmont Dental) set at 70 kV, 8 mA, with an exposure time of 0.32 seconds. Patients were fitted with a lead apron and thyroid collar before radiation exposure. The dental film was positioned intraorally with a positioning device (Dentsply Rinn).

Clinical procedure

One pediatric dental practitioner (BA) treated all primary molars according to the following protocol: After topical analgesia obtained with 20% benzocaine gel (Vision Paste), local anesthesia containing 2% articaine with 1:100,000 epinephrine (Ultracain D-S Fort, Sanofi Aventis) was administered. Under rubber dam isolation, the cavity outline was established with diamond round and fissure burs working on a high-speed handpiece. Carious dentin was removed with a slow-speed handpiece using a large round stainless-steel bur. Following pulp exposure, the pulp chamber was accessed with a high-speed diamond fissure bur. The coronal pulpal tissue was then removed using a sterile slow-speed round bur which was followed by irrigation with saline solution to clear the debris. Hemostasis was achieved with sterile dry cotton pellets under slight pressure.

A 15.5% ferric sulfate solution (Astringedent, Ultradent Products) was applied on the pulp stumps for 15 seconds with the dental infuser supplied by the manufacturer. The pulp chamber was then rinsed thoroughly with saline and dried with cotton pellets. If the bleeding had not stopped after this initial application of ferric sulfate, the tooth was excluded from the study. If hemostasis was achieved, the teeth were divided into three groups and the pulp stumps were covered with one of the following base materials. In Group 1, the pulp chamber floor was covered with ZOE paste. In Group 2, CH powder (Merck) was mixed with sterile saline at 1:1 ratio and was placed in the pulp chamber. In Group 3, the pulp stumps were covered with MTA

(MTA Angelus, Angelus) paste prepared by mixing powder and sterile saline at 3:1 ratio. The choice of base material was made by drawing sequentially numbered, opaque sealed envelopes (allocation concealment).[24]

In all groups, a glass-ionomer cement (Kavitan Pro, Spofa Dental) was placed over the base materials to completely cover the pulp chamber. The procedures were terminated by restoration of all teeth with stainless-steel crowns (SSC). Immediate postoperative periapical radiographs were taken to assure that the dressing agents were correctly placed over the remaining radicular pulp and to serve as baseline evaluation data for further postoperative evaluations.

Follow-up

The patients were scheduled for clinical examinations at 6, 12, 18, and 24 months. A follow-up radiograph was taken every 6 months during recall appointments (a total of four radiographs). Clinical examinations were performed by two pediatric dental practitioners who were blinded to study groups and were previously calibrated (intra-examiner reproducibility, κ=.94; inter-examiner reproducibility, κ=.88). A standardized evaluation form was used to record the following signs and symptoms:

- history of spontaneous pain
- tenderness to percussion/palpation
- mobility
- swelling
- pus/fistula formation.

The restorations (SSCs) were also evaluated with respect to marginal adaptation and loss of the crown.

The radiographs taken during recall visits were evaluated by two investigators using the same standard view box. They were also blinded to the study protocol and had been previously calibrated. Cohen unweighted kappa statistics for intra- and inter-examiner reproducibility were κ=.91 and κ=.84, respectively. If a discrepancy occurred between examiners, a consensus was reached by having both examiners view the radiographs again and come to an agreement. Radiographic evaluation comprised observation of:

- peri- or interradicular radiolucency
- loss of lamina dura
- pathologic/abnormal root resorption
- internal/external root resorption.

Internal root resorption was not regarded as a failure unless the inflammatory process resulted in significant destructive changes in the tissues surrounding the root.[5,25]

Statistical analysis

Data analyses were performed by using SPSS 11.5 software for Windows (IBM). The difference between the groups regarding radiographic and clinical success was compared using log-rank test with Kaplan-Meier survival analysis, and cumulative survival rates were calculated. The level of significance was set at $P < .05$. The Bonferroni correction was used to reduce type one errors.

Results

The final study sample consisted of 105 primary molars of 19 females and 21 males. The patients' mean age at the time of treatment was 69.6±10.4 months. Fifty-five primary first and fifty primary second molars were treated. Of those, 55 were in the maxilla and 50 were in the mandible.

The flow of participants and pulpotomies that were followed from allocation to final data analysis is presented in Fig 1. All patients attended the follow-up visits, resulting in no dropouts. It was also observed that all SSCs remained in function with optimum marginal adaptation (no restorative failure).

Two teeth in Group 1 (ZOE) and one tooth in Group 2 (CH) exfoliated at 12 and 18 months, respectively. During the 24-month study period, a total of four teeth were extracted due to the symptoms observed. The extractions were done at the 12-month (one tooth from Group 2) and 18-month (three teeth; one tooth from each group) recall visits.

Clinical and radiographic findings

The clinical and radiographic findings observed within the study groups are presented in Table 1. During the 2-year study period, no teeth presented with a history of spontaneous pain ($P > .05$). Tenderness to percussion/palpation was observed in seven teeth (6.67%). Teeth with this finding continued to follow-up visits, unless there were other clinical or radiographic signs that were indicative of irreversible pulpitis and necessitated an extraction. Eventually, two of those teeth with tenderness to percussion (one from Group 2 and one from Group 3) were extracted at 18 months due to abnormal mobility. The space maintainers were fabricated and delivered to the patients. The percentages of cases in the groups with tenderness to percussion/palpation after 24 months were 8.57% (3/35), 5.71% (2/35), and 5.71% (2/35), respectively ($P > .05$).

Eight teeth (7.62%) were registered for presenting mobility. The percentages of observed cases in the groups were 5.71% (2/35), 11.42% (4/35), and 5.71% (2/35), respectively ($P > .05$). Of

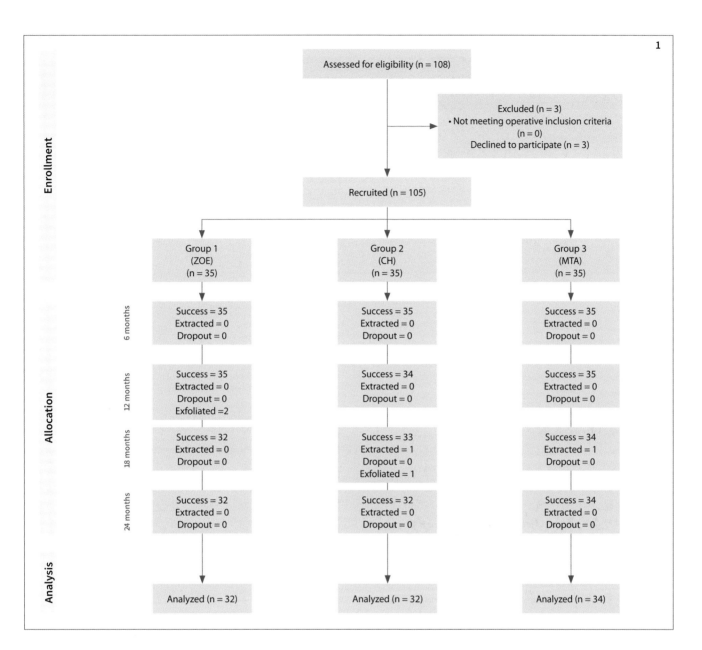

Fig 1 Flowchart of participants in the study.

those, two teeth (one in Group 2 and one in Group 3) were extracted at 18 months due to also presenting tenderness to percussion. The remaining six teeth continued to recall appointments with no adverse events occurring.

Mucosal swelling was observed in four teeth (3.81%). One tooth was in Group 1 (2.85%) and was extracted at 18 months. Two teeth were in Group 2 (5.71%); one was extracted at 12 months, and the other extracted at 18 months due to associated symptoms (tenderness to percussion and mobility). In Group 3, one tooth (2.85%) was extracted at 18 months due

also to the presence of tenderness to percussion and mobility. All extractions were followed by space maintainer placement. No statistically significant difference was observed between the groups regarding this finding ($P > .05$).

Pus/fistula formation was noted in two teeth (1.9%). One tooth in Group 1 (2.86%) also presented mucosal swelling, and was extracted at 18 months. The other tooth (2.86%) was in Group 2 and was extracted at 12 months, also with mucosal swelling. The study groups did not differ significantly with respect to pus/fistula formation ($P > .05$).

Table 1 The clinical and radiographic findings observed within the study groups at follow-up

Parameter		Group 1: ZOE (N = 35)				Group 2: CH (N = 35)				Group 3: MTA (N = 35)				Total	P
Finding observed (months)		6	12	18	24	6	12	18	24	6	12	18	24		
Clinical	Spontaneous pain	0	0	0	0	0	0	0	0	0	0	0	0	0	.688
	Percussion/palpation	0	1	1	1	0	1	1[a]	0	0	1	1[b]	0	7	.362
	Mobility	0	0	1	1	0	2	1[a]	1	0	1	1[b]	0	8	.228
	Swelling	0	0	1[c]	0	0	1[d]	1[a]	0	0	0	1[b]	0	4	.126
	Pus/fistula formation	0	0	1[c]	0	0	1[d]	0	0	0	0	0	0	2	.355
Radio-graphic	Peri-/interradicular RL	0	0	2[*]	1	0	1[†]	1	0	0	0	2	0	7	.085
	Loss of lamina dura	0	0	2	1	0	1[†]	2[‡]	1	0	0	1[§]	1	9	.256
	Pathologic/abnormal RR	0	1	2[*]	0	0	1[†]	2[‡]	1	0	0	2[§]	0	9	.155
	Internal/external RR	0	0	2[*]	3	0	2	2[‡]	2	0	0	2[§]	2	15	.573

The same superscript letters ([a,b,c,d]) indicate the teeth with multiple clinical findings which were extracted. The superscripts ([*,†,‡,§]) indicate the same tooth with multiple radiographic findings. RL, radiolucency; RR, root resorption.

During the entire study period no teeth presented periradicular radiolucency. However, interradicular radiolucency was noted in 6.67% of teeth (7/105). This finding was observed in the Groups 1 to 3 with the following percentages: 8.57% (3/35), 5.71% (2/35), and 5.71% (2/35), respectively (P>.05). Loss of lamina dura was observed in 8.57% of teeth (9/105). The rates in the groups were 8.57% (3/35), 11.42% (4/35), and 5.71% (2/35), respectively (P>.05). Pathologic/abnormal root resorption was observed in 8.57% of teeth (9/105). The rates were 8.57% (3/35), 11.42% (4/35), and 5.71% (2/35) for the groups, respectively (P>.05). The progression of pathologic and internal/external root resorption in Group 2 is presented in Fig 2. Internal/external root resorption was observed in 14.28% of teeth (15/105). The finding was observed in 14.28% (5/35), 14.14% (6/35), and 11.42% (4/35) of teeth in respective groups (P>.05). Of those, four teeth were extracted due to the accompanying clinical symptoms mentioned above (under the sections related to tenderness to percussion, mobility, mucosal swelling, and pus/fistula formation).

After 24 months, overall clinical success rate of FS pulpotomies was 96.18% (101/105). Clinical success rates in Group 1 to 3 were 97.14% (34/35), 94.28% (33/35), and 97.14% (34/35), respectively. Regarding the radiographic success at 24 months, 12 teeth in Group 1 (one tooth with multiple findings), 12 teeth in Group 2 (two teeth with multiple findings), and 8 teeth in Group 3 (one tooth with multiple findings) showed signs of radiographic failure. Therefore, radiographic success rates in the groups were 65.71% (23/35), 65.71% (23/35), and 77.14% (27/35), respectively. The study groups did not differ significantly with respect to clinical and radiographic success rates (P=.234 and P=.216, respectively). Cumulative success probabilities in the study groups with respect to at least one clinical and radiographic failure parameter are presented in Table 2.

Discussion

The AAPD recommends MTA and FC as the medicaments of choice for pulpotomies in primary teeth expected to be retained for at least 24 months.[1] Both materials have gained strong recommendations with moderate-quality evidence, while FS received a conditional recommendation due to the low-quality evidence.[4] However, a recent systematic review and meta-analysis reported that both FC and FS were comparable pulpotomy materials for primary molars in terms of clinical and radiographic success at 24 months.[26]

The control of pulpal hemorrhage is a critical and indispensable step in pulpotomy procedures. FS is an effective hemostatic agent which seals the severed blood vessels mechanically by forming a ferric ion-protein complex on the pulp surface.[3] The studies have reported comparable and/or beneficial effects in primary teeth where FS yielded success rates ranging between 75.86% and 99%.[5,10,27-29] The overall clinical success rate of the present study (96.18%) was in line with those previously reported.[5,27,28]

Watts and Paterson[8] claimed that, when used as a base material in pulpotomies, zinc eugenolate in ZOE could undergo hydrolysis. It forms free eugenol that may leach into the pulp over time and causes a moderate to severe inflammatory response.[8] One common response of the pulp to chronic inflammation is internal resorption.[5] Ranly[30] hypothesized that ferric ion–protein complex at the pulp surface formed by FS might act as a barrier between the pulp tissue and ZOE. This could pre-

Figs 2a to 2d Periapical radiographs showing progression of pathologic root resorption in teeth of Group 2. *(a)* Preoperative view. *(b)* 6 months. *(c)* 12 months. *(d)* 18 months.

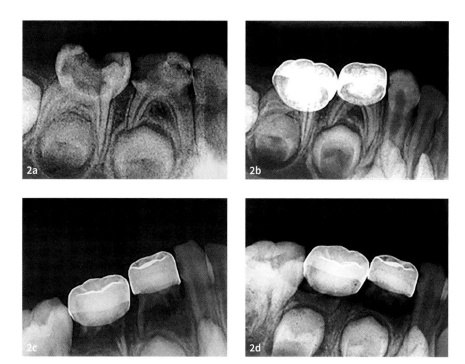

vent the chronic inflammation and/or necrosis of the pulp.[30] However, previous studies with FS[5] and FC[15] have associated internal resorption with the use of ZOE. Following the lower radiographic success rate observed, Smith et al[5] concluded that ZOE might not be an ideal base material for FS pulpotomies. They argued that, compared to the fixed tissue barrier obtained with FC, ferric ion–protein complex obtained with FS was not sufficient to separate eugenol completely from the pulp. On the other hand, Doyle et al[21] evaluated the use of eugenol-free and eugenol-based materials after hemostasis with FS. Interestingly, eugenol-free base resulted in significantly lower survival rates and the authors did not recommend it for pulpotomies.

When compared to other materials such as FC and MTA, relatively lower success rates have been reported for CH in primary teeth pulpotomies.[12,13,16] These results have been ascribed to the lack of sufficient hemorrhage control, without which any excessive oozing of serum or plasma would occupy, fill, or create a space between the capping agent and the pulp.[31] According to Stanley,[31] the formation of a blood clot or a thick fibropurulent membrane over the pulp wound could be subject to secondary infection and lead to complete loss of pulp vitality. Markovic et al[19] used CH as a base material in pulpotomies where hemostasis was obtained with FS or FC. Their overall clinical and radiographic success rates were 90.9% and 84.8% for FC; 89.2% and 81.1% for FS, respectively. With clinical and radiographic suc-

cess rates of 94.2% and 65.7%, respectively, CH was not statistically different from the other groups of the present study.

In terms of biocompatibility and efficacy, Smail-Faugeron et al[17] suggested that MTA was the best material to be in contact with the remaining root dental nerve after a pulpotomy. Their meta-analysis indicated that MTA was less likely to fail than either CH or FC. The studies with MTA have yielded superior clinical success rates, but also satisfactory radiographic outcomes.[10,18,25,32] In the study by Doyle et al[21] applying MTA to FS-treated pulp resulted in better outcomes than FS pulpotomy with a ZOE base. However, the difference in radiographic outcomes between the two groups was not statistically significant. The present study was also not able to report significantly different clinical and radiographic outcomes for MTA. However, with a longer follow-up period, a change in the outcomes cannot be ruled out.

Internal resorption has been the most commonly reported radiographic finding in primary tooth pulpotomy studies.[5,32,33] During the present study period, a total of 15 teeth (14.28%) showed signs of internal resorption. Fei et al[34] observed 56 primary molars treated with FS and reported a 96% radiographic success at 12 months, while Fuks et al[10] reported a 93% success rate of 41 pulpotomized teeth after 24 to 34 months. The observation period of the present study was greater than that of Fei et al,[34] while the number of teeth included were also greater than both studies. This may explain the differences between the findings.

Table 2 Cumulative success probabilities in the study groups with respect to at least one clinical and radiographic failure parameter

Follow-up interval (months)	Group 1: ZOE		Group 2: CH		Group 3: MTA	
	Clinical	Radiographic	Clinical	Radiographic	Clinical	Radiographic
6	100.0% (35/35)	100.0% (35/35)	100.0% (35/35)	100.0% (35/35)	100.0% (35/35)	100.0% (35/35)
12	100.0% (35/35)	97.1% (34/35)	97.1% (34/35)	91.4% (32/35)	100.0% (35/35)	100.0% (35/35)
18	97.1% (34/35)	80.0% (28/35)	94.2% (33/35)	77.1% (27/35)	97.1% (34/35)	82.9% (30/35)
24	97.1% (34/35)	65.7% (23/35)	94.2% (33/35)	65.7% (23/35)	97.1% (34/35)	77.1% (27/35)

The failures of pulpotomy in primary teeth have been attributed to misdiagnosis of radicular pulp inflammation prior to treatment[16] and due to microleakage of multisurface restorations with amalgam[15] or composite.[35] The lack of short-term failure (ie, during the first 6 months) in the present study can be attributed to the meticulous effort in the proper diagnosis of the teeth selected to be included in the study. Additionally, the teeth were restored with SSC to rule out the possibility of poor restoration seal, which might have contributed to the clinical outcome.[35]

The present study was not able show significant differences between ZOE, CH, and MTA with regard to clinical and radiographic success of FS pulpotomy in primary molars. Hence, the study failed to reject the null hypothesis. The lack of another hemostatic agent group to compare with FS could be one of the limitations of the present study. Since the aim was to evaluate the effect of base materials on the outcome of FS pulpotomy, the methodology did not comprise such a study plan. There is no doubt that an increase in sample size and follow-up period could lead to more precise results. However, the number of teeth included in this study and the duration of observation were consistent with most studies published in the literature.[19,36,37] ▦

Conclusion

Within the limitations of the present study, the following conclusion could be drawn: The choice of base materials as ZOE, CH, or MTA did not affect the clinical and radiographic success of FS pulpotomies in primary teeth.

Acknowledgments

The present study was conducted as Dr Aksoy's thesis, under the supervision of Prof Dr Ölmez, to fulfill the requirements of the pediatric dentistry specialty program in Turkey. The authors thank Hacettepe University Scientific Research Unit, Ankara, Turkey, for its support to this study via a grant, THD-2017-14387. Assistant Professor Dr Shentong Han from Marquette University School of Dentistry is gratefully acknowledged for his help with the statistical analysis. The authors report no conflicts of interest.

References

1. American Academy of Pediatric Dentistry. Pulp therapy for primary and immature permanent teeth. The Reference Manual of Pediatric Dentistry. 2018/10/15 ed. Chicago: American Academy of Pediatric Dentistry, 2020:384–392.

2. Coll JA, Seale NS, Vargas K, Marghalani AA, Al Shamali S, Graham L. Primary tooth vital pulp therapy: a systematic review and meta-analysis. Pediatr Dent 2017;39:16–123.

3. Fuks AB, Guelmann M, Kupietzky A. Current developments in pulp therapy for primary teeth. Endod Topics 2012;23:50–72.

4. Dhar V, Marghalani AA, Crystal YO, et al. Use of vital pulp therapies in primary teeth with deep caries lesions. Pediatr Dent 2017; 39:E146–E159.

5. Smith NL, Seale NS, Nunn ME. Ferric sulfate pulpotomy in primary molars: a retrospective study. Pediatr Dent 2000;22:192–199.

6. Vargas KG, Packham B, Lowman D. Preliminary evaluation of sodium hypochlorite for pulpotomies in primary molars. Pediatr Dent 2006;28:511–517.

7. Fuks AB. Vital pulp therapy with new materials for primary teeth: new directions and treatment perspectives. J Endod 2008;34:S18–S24.

8. Watts A, Paterson RC. Pulpal response to a zinc oxide-eugenol cement. Int Endod J 1987; 20:82–86.

9. Hansen HP, Ravn JJ, Ulrich D. Vital pulpotomy in primary molars. A clinical and histologic investigation of the effect of zinc oxide-eugenol cement and Ledermix. Scand J Dent Res 1971;79:13–25.

10. Fuks AB, Holan G, Davis JM, Eidelman E. Ferric sulfate versus dilute formocresol in pulpotomized primary molars: long-term follow up. Pediatr Dent 1997;19:327–330.

11. Gonzalez-Lara A, Ruiz-Rodriguez MS, Pierdant-Perez M, Garrocho-Rangel JA, Pozos-Guillen AJ. Zinc oxide-eugenol pulpotomy in primary teeth: a 24-month follow-up. J Clin Pediatr Dent 2016;40:107–112.

12. Percinoto C, de Castro AM, Pinto LM. Clinical and radiographic evaluation of pulpotomies employing calcium hydroxide and trioxide mineral aggregate. Gen Dent 2006;54: 258–261.

13. Schroder U. A 2-year follow-up of primary molars, pulpotomized with a gentle technique and capped with calcium hydroxide. Scand J Dent Res 1978;86:273–278.

14. Hafez AA, Cox CF, Tarim B, Otsuki M, Akimoto N. An in vivo evaluation of hemorrhage control using sodium hypochlorite and direct capping with a one- or two-component adhesive system in exposed nonhuman primate pulps. Quintessence Int 2002;33:261–272.

15. Holan G, Fuks AB, Ketlz N. Success rate of formocresol pulpotomy in primary molars restored with stainless steel crown vs amalgam. Pediatr Dent 2002;24:212–216.

16. Waterhouse PJ, Whitworth JM. Pediatric endodontics: Endodontic treatment for the primary and young permanent dentition. In: Berman LH, Hargreaves KJ (eds). Cohen's Pathways of the Pulp. 11th ed. St Louis: Elsevier, 2016:e1–e44.

17. Smail-Faugeron V, Glenny AM, Courson F, Durieux P, Muller-Bolla M, Fron Chabouis H. Pulp treatment for extensive decay in primary teeth. Cochrane Database Syst Rev 2018;5: CD003220.

18. Mettlach SE, Zealand CM, Botero TM, Boynton JR, Majewski RF, Hu JC. Comparison of mineral trioxide aggregate and diluted formocresol in pulpotomized human primary molars: 42-month follow-up and survival analysis. Pediatr Dent 2013;35:E87–E94.

19. Markovic D, Zivojinovic V, Vucetic M. Evaluation of three pulpotomy medicaments in primary teeth. Eur J Paediatr Dent 2005;6: 133–138.

20. Mohamed N. A comparison of two liner materials for use in the ferric sulfate pulpotomy. SADJ 2008;63:338–342.

21. Doyle TL, Casas MJ, Kenny DJ, Judd PL. Mineral trioxide aggregate produces superior outcomes in vital primary molar pulpotomy. Pediatr Dent 2010;32:41–47.

22. Atasever G, Keceli TI, Uysal S, Gungor HC, Olmez S. Primary molar pulpotomies with different hemorrhage control agents and base materials: A randomized clinical trial. Niger J Clin Pract 2019;22:305–312.

23. Schulz KF, Altman DG, Moher D, Group C. CONSORT 2010 statement: updated guidelines for reporting parallel group randomized trials. Ann Intern Med 2010;152:726–732.

24. Doig GS, Simpson F. Randomization and allocation concealment: a practical guide for researchers. J Crit Care 2005;20:187–191.

25. Oliveira TM, Moretti AB, Sakai VT, et al. Clinical, radiographic and histologic analysis of the effects of pulp capping materials used in pulpotomies of human primary teeth. Eur Arch Paediatr Dent 2013;14:65–71.

26. Jayaraman J, Nagendrababu V, Pulikkotil SJ, Veettil SK, Dhar V. Effectiveness of formocresol and ferric sulfate as pulpotomy material in primary molars: a systematic review and meta-analysis with trial sequential analysis of randomized clinical trials. Quintessence Int 2020;51:38–48.

27. Ibricevic H, Al-Jame Q. Ferric sulphate and formocresol in pulpotomy of primary molars: long term follow-up study. Eur J Paediatr Dent 2003;4:28–32.

28. Brar KA, Kratunova E, Avenetti D, da Fonseca MA, Marion I, Alapati S. Success of Biodentine and ferric sulfate as pulpotomy materials in primary molars: a retrospective study. J Clin Pediatr Dent 2021;45:22–28.

29. Guven Y, Aksakal SD, Avcu N, Unsal G, Tuna EB, Aktoren O. Success rates of pulpotomies in primary molars using calcium silicate-based materials: a randomized control trial. Biomed Res Int 2017;2017:4059703.

30. Ranly DM. Pulpotomy therapy in primary teeth: new modalities for old rationales. Pediatr Dent 1994;16:403–409.

31. Stanley HR. Pulp capping: conserving the dental pulp: can it be done? Is it worth it? Oral Surg Oral Med Oral Pathol 1989;68: 628–639.

32. Moretti AB, Sakai VT, Oliveira TM, et al. The effectiveness of mineral trioxide aggregate, calcium hydroxide and formocresol for pulpotomies in primary teeth. Int Endod J 2008;41:547–555.

33. Fuks AB, Kupietzky A, Guelmann M. Pulp therapy for the primary dentition. In: Casamassimo PS, Fields HW, McTigue DJ, Nowak AJ (eds). Pediatric dentistry: infancy through adolescence. 5th ed. St Louis: Elsevier, 2013.

34. Fei AL, Udin RD, Johnson R. A clinical study of ferric sulfate as a pulpotomy agent in primary teeth. Pediatr Dent 1991;13:327–332.

35. Hutcheson C, Seale NS, McWhorter A, Kerins C, Wright J. Multi-surface composite vs stainless steel crown restorations after mineral trioxide aggregate pulpotomy: a randomized controlled trial. Pediatr Dent 2012;34:460–467.

36. Erdem AP, Guven Y, Balli B, et al. Success rates of mineral trioxide aggregate, ferric sulfate, and formocresol pulpotomies: a 24-month study. Pediatr Dent 2011;33: 165–170.

37. Akcay M, Sari S. The effect of sodium hypochlorite application on the success of calcium hydroxide and mineral trioxide aggregate pulpotomies in primary teeth. Pediatr Dent 2014;36:316–321.

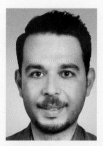

Burak Aksoy

Burak Aksoy Private Practice in Pediatric Dentistry, Antalya, Turkey

Hamdi Cem Güngör Associate Professor, Division of Pediatric Dentistry, Department of Developmental Sciences, Marquette University School of Dentistry, Milwaukee, WI, USA

Serdar Uysal Associate Professor, Department of Dentomaxillofacial Radiology at Hacettepe University Faculty of Dentistry, Ankara, Turkey

Cesar D. Gonzales Associate Professor, Director Division of Pediatric Dentistry, Department of Developmental Sciences, Marquette University School of Dentistry, Milwaukee, WI, USA

Seval Ölmez Professor, Department of Pediatric Dentistry at Hacettepe University Faculty of Dentistry, Ankara, Turkey

Correspondence: H. Cem Güngör, Division of Pediatric Dentistry, Department of Developmental Sciences, Marquette University School of Dentistry, 1801 W Wisconsin Ave., Milwaukee, WI 53233, USA. Email: hcem.gungor@marquette.edu

Influence of treatment setting on success of pulpectomy in primary molars: a retrospective analysis up to 4 years

Haneen Al-Attiya, MSc/Mhd Said Mourad, Dr med dent, MSc/Christian H. Splieth, Prof Dr med dent/ Julian Schmoeckel, Dr med dent, MSc

Objectives: The objective of this study was to analyze the success of primary molar pulpectomy with a minimum of 1 year and up to 4 years follow-up with focus on the treatment setting (general anesthesia, sedation, local anesthesia alone). **Method and materials:** Data were retrieved from 92 patients' records between 2012 and 2020. The pulpectomy treatment using calcium-hydroxide/iodoform paste was performed under general anesthesia (n = 45), nitrous oxide sedation (n = 21), or local anesthesia alone (n = 39). Bivariate and multivariate analyses were performed. **Results:** The overall success of pulpectomy was 59.5% 4 years post-treatment. The 4-years clinical success rate was clinically relevantly higher under general anesthesia (78.6% vs 57.1% under nitrous oxide sedation, 43.8% with local anesthesia only) and in the mandibular arch (70.8% vs 38.5% in the maxillary arch). This could be related to the strict case selection under sedation and especially general anesthesia. Despite statistically significant differences in the bivariate analysis for most outcomes and follow-up periods, this was not the case in multivariate regression. **Conclusion:** Pulpectomy performed in primary molars offers a successful long-term treatment option especially with a strict case selection as under general anesthesia. *(Quintessence Int 2023;54:6–15; doi: 10.3290/j.qi.b3512239)*

Key words: general anesthesia, nitrous oxide sedation, primary molars, pulpectomy, success rate

ECC (early childhood caries) remains a major health problem globally with relevant consequences on both children's and their caregivers' quality of life,[1] such as premature loss of primary teeth, especially primary molars, and negatively influences normal development and occlusion.[2] The prevalence of more than 50% in most countries worldwide (prevalence range of 23% to 90%) is reported.[3] In addition, the oral health-related quality of life (OHRQoL) is also negatively affected by the early loss of primary teeth.[4] Thus, retaining primary teeth until their physiologic exfoliation is crucial when treating those teeth as they influence the occlusion, articulation, mastication, and esthetics. They also guide the eruption of the permanent successors.[5] Correspondingly, many studies have found a relationship between caries and the risk for early loss of primary teeth and the need for early orthodontic intervention, and also the need for complex orthodontic treatments later on.[6] Despite all the well-known negative consequences of premature loss of primary teeth, extraction of the severely decayed or necrotic primary teeth, as well as those

with irreversible pulpitis, is preferred by many practitioners as opposed to retaining them.[7] Refrainment from trying to retain such teeth through pulpectomy is perhaps due to the disadvantages of this procedure in primary molars. The lengthy and challenging procedure due to the unpredictable and complex anatomy of the primary molar canal system, the possible negative effect of root canal filling materials, and instrumentation on the tooth bud of succedaneous teeth[8] are among the disadvantages of such a procedure. In addition, there is no ideal root canal filling material,[9] and behavior management skills are required to deal with the low compliance and relatively short attention span of children.[7] One of the key factors in delivering high-quality successful dental treatments in pediatric patients is increasing the compliance through various pharmacologic and nonpharmacologic behavior management techniques.[10]

Although success of pulpectomy has been reported in the literature, long-term success over several years has rarely been reported; follow-up in most of the studies ranged from 12 to 18 or 30 months.[9,11-13] Also, there is a large variation (53.6% to 97%) in the reported success rates of pulpectomy in primary teeth.[11,12] Therefore, the main aim of the present study was to retrospectively assess clinically the success of pulpectomies in primary molars performed with a calcium-hydroxide/iodoform paste along with the potential effect of different behavior management techniques on the success (general anesthesia [GA], nitrous oxide [N$_2$O] sedation, and local anesthesia [LA]) of a specialized pediatric dental service up to 4 years.

Method and materials

The ethical approval for this study was obtained through the Greifswald University Ethics Committee in order to approve the retrospective evaluation of clinical interventions carried out in the Department of Preventive and Pediatric Dentistry at the University of Greifswald (Internal RegNo BB 028/16). For data collection purposes, patients' digital records were searched using the key words "vitapex" and "pulpectomy" between 1 January 2012 and 14 September 2020. Furthermore, to ensure complete data extraction, a second search of the database was carried out utilizing the billing abbreviations used by the German health insurance system for pulpectomy ("WK" and "WF" in primary teeth) carried out by all dental practitioners working in the Department of Preventive and Pediatric Dentistry (pediatric dentists or general dental practitioners before completing the master program), as well as the students of the master program in pediatric dentistry offered by the department during the same time period. In total, 92 dental records could be identified of patients (Fig 1) who underwent pulpectomy treatment, in 117 primary teeth. Those 117 primary teeth were screened for eligibility by applying the following inclusion criteria:

- primary molars that underwent pulpectomy treatment between 1 January 2012 and 14 September 2020
- with the use of calcium-hydroxide/iodoform paste as root canal filling material
- having a minimum follow-up period of 1 year.

Primary molars treated during this period that had not completed a follow-up time of 1 year posttreatment at the time of evaluation are mentioned for descriptive purposes only and were not included in the final analysis.

All pulpectomy treatments were carried out following a standard operative protocol as follows: after administering local anesthesia, caries affected dental tissues were removed and the occlusal surface was reduced by about 1.5 mm for the stainless-steel crown (SSC). After that an access cavity was achieved and

the root canals were identified. The infected pulp tissue was removed, using Hedstrom files to a length of 12 mm and to a minimum size of ISO35, along with the use of sodium hypochlorite (0.6%) as an irrigant. After cleaning and shaping, the root canals were dried using sterile paper points. A calcium-hydroxide/iodoform paste was injected into the canals and the pulp chamber was sealed with zinc phosphate cement. As a final step, the SSC was used as a definitive restoration.

Pulpectomized primary anterior teeth along with patients who did not return for the follow-up period were excluded. Success of primary tooth pulpectomy at the department is judged mainly based on clinical assessment; routine posttreatment radiologic assessment following pulpectomy is not the standard due to radiation protection. Posttreatment radiologic examination following a pulpectomy is carried out only with the presence of clinical signs of failure. Therefore, clinical success of the treatment was determined when:

- no clinical signs of abscess and/or fistula were documented, and
- there was absence of pain and complaints by the patients, and
- further treatments after pulpectomy were not necessary, or
- the tooth exfoliated at the average chronologic age, or
- the tooth had to be extracted as a result of severe mobility associated with normal physiologic exfoliation at the appropriate chronologic age with the absence of pathology.[9,12]

Clinical failure of the treatment was determined when:
- clinical and/or radiologic signs and symptoms of pathology were documented, or
- the tooth had to be extracted as a result of abscess or sinus tract, or
- the tooth had to be extracted as a result of extreme mobility related to nonphysiologic root resorption at an age earlier than the appropriate chronologic age.

Data collection and statistical analysis

To evaluate the outcome of pulpectomy and the possible impact of behavior management modality on success up to 4 years follow-up, the 92 identified patients' records were screened and resulted in the recognition of 117 pulpectomized primary teeth, 12 of which were anterior teeth and, therefore, were excluded leaving 105 pulpectomized primary molars at baseline. Of these, 65 out of 105 had adequate documentation regarding follow-up visits and thus were included in the final analysis. The subsequent factors related to the individual pa-

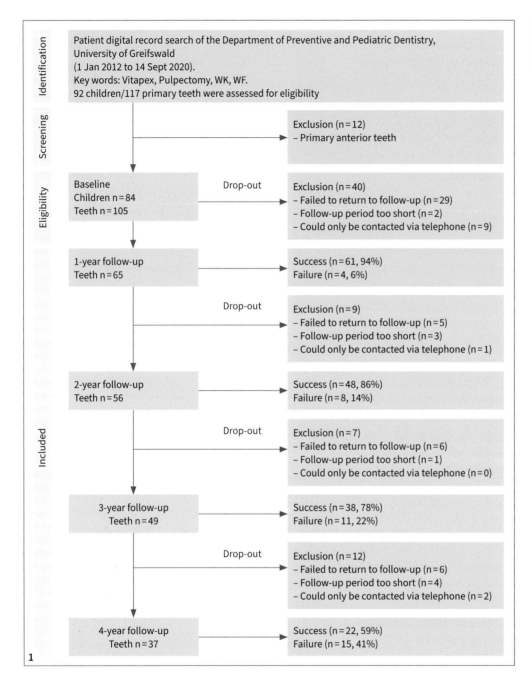

tients, teeth, and treatments that might have affected the success of the pulpectomy were also analyzed:

- patient-related factors:
  - sex
  - age at day of treatment
  - caries experience (dmft) at day of treatment
  - general health status
  - travel distance to clinic (in km)

- tooth-related factors:
  - tooth type
  - arch
  - pulpal and periapical condition prior to treatment
- treatment-related factors:
  - treatment indication
  - setting of treatment (GA, sedation, LA alone)
  - academic qualification of the operator
  - number of visits
  - posttreatment restoration.

After transferring the identified data from patients' digital records into a Microsoft Excel data sheet, data had to be coded for descriptive and analytical purposes. Regarding the indication of the treatment as reported in the documentation, the cases were coded as follows:

- primary molars with a history of spontaneous pain or deep caries with/without pulpal involvement or primary molars with pulpal necrosis with no signs of apical radiolucency
- necrotic primary molars with signs of apical radiolucency without clinical signs of abscess or fistula
- primary molars with clinical signs of fistula
- primary molars with clinical signs of an abscess
- previously pulpotomized primary molars with clinical and/or radiographic signs of failure
- primary molars with unknown diagnosis due to insufficient documentation and absence of a radiograph.

As this study was a retrospective analysis of real-life treatment in highly selected patients, radiographs were not available in all cases and were used on individual, case-based needs, classified as follows:

- radiograph was no older than 6 months from the date of treatment
- radiograph was older than 6 months from the date of treatment
- no radiograph was taken at all.

After that, a native speaker pediatric specialist audited the extracted data to ensure high data quality and to avoid misunderstanding of the clinical documentation. Where there was unclear documentation or diagnosis, the issue was discussed with a second clinical expert to settle any disagreements.

The descriptive analyses comprised ranges, distributions, mean values for numerical data with a normal distribution (age, caries prevalence), and standard deviations. Chi-square tests were used to investigate the possible impact that various factors might have on the success of the pulpectomy treatment.

In an attempt to enhance the follow-up numbers, efforts to contact the patients' parents via telephone were undertaken for those who failed to attend recall visits. At baseline only nine parents could be interviewed through the telephone and were asked about the status of the treated primary molar (Fig 1). Nevertheless, these teeth were pooled together and were not included in the final analysis of the success and failure rates of the pulpectomy treatment in the light of the inferior level of scientific evidence acquired through telephone contact, solely. These nine teeth are mentioned for informative purposes.

In order to evaluate the positive effect of the secondary factors a multivariate regression analysis was conducted. The data set was analyzed with the statistical Excel plugin. Due to the multitude of different variables the adjusted squared multiple R was used to avoid overfitting of the regression.

Results

General characteristics of the study sample

Data were retrieved from 92 patients' records during 2012 to 2020. The total number of patients included in this study was 84; nearly half of them (n = 41; 48.8%) were females (Table 1). The vast majority (n = 79; 94%) were healthy and many of them (n = 61; 72.7%) had to travel a minimum of 11 km to reach the University clinic (Table 1). Over the years, the total number of patients attending regular recall visits dropped to 30 at 4 years posttreatment. This drop, however, did not seem to affect the proportion of patients who had to travel greater distances to reach the University clinic, as it remained constant (Table 1).

Characteristics at tooth level

The study sample largely comprised young children (mean 5.0 ± 1.4 years, Table 2) with high caries risk (mean 8.0 ± 3.8 dmft, Table 2). Roughly half of the pulpectomy treatments (42.9%) were completed under GA (Table 2). The distribution of the different treatment modalities (LA, N_2O sedation, and GA) differed between the mandibular and maxillary arch, and over time regarding the different follow-up periods. At baseline there were more cases of LA treatments in the maxillary arch (43.6%) compared to the mandibular arch (33.3%), whereas a lower percentage of pulpectomies were conducted under GA in the maxillary arch (38.5% vs 45.5% mandibular). The proportion of pulpectomies under N_2O sedation was almost the same (17.9% maxillary vs 21.2% mandibular).

The patient profile showed that usually as a part of the first visit these children were subjected to panoramic radiographs for complex treatment planning due to multiple caries lesions affecting mostly all quadrants. The absence of radiograph in some patients (3.8%, Table 2) was due to the need to adjust the treatment plan from pulpotomy to pulpectomy, as a result of persistent bleeding. Placement of SSCs after pulp therapy of primary molars is the standard procedure at the department, reflected in the present study, as this was the posttreatment restoration of choice in 98.1% of the cases (Table 2).

Table 1 General characteristics of the study sample (data based on number of patients)

Category	Factor	Baseline, n = 84	1-y follow-up, n = 52	2-y follow-up, n = 45	3-y follow-up, n = 39	4-y follow-up, n = 30
Sex	Male	43 (51.2%)	21 (40.4%)	19 (42.2%)	16 (41.0%)	12 (40.0%)
	Female	41 (48.8%)	31 (59.6%)	26 (57.8%)	23 (59.0%)	18 (60.0%)
Health status	Healthy	79 (94.0%)	50 (96.2%)	43 (95.6%)	37 (94.9%)	28 (93.3%)
	Chronic disease	5 (6.0%)	2 (3.8%)	2 (4.4%)	2 (5.1%)	2 (6.7%)
Location	Radius < 10 km	23 (27.4%)	16 (30.8%)	14 (31.1%)	11 (28.2%)	11 (36.7%)
	Radius 11 – 40 km	35 (41.7%)	22 (42.3%)	19 (42.2%)	17 (43.6%)	14 (46.7%)
	Radius 41 – 70 km	15 (17.9%)	9 (17.3%)	9 (20.0%)	8 (20.5%)	2 (6.7%)
	Radius > 70 km	11 (13.1%)	5 (9.6%)	3 (6.7%)	3 (7.7%)	3 (10.0%)

Outcome of primary molar pulpectomy up to 4 years posttreatment

The overall success and failure rates over the years are presented in Table 3. Clinical criteria of success were the absence of clinical signs and symptoms of abscess, fistula, or pathologic mobility, absence of periapical pathology, and without premature extraction. At the 1-year follow-up examination 93.8% of the pulpectomy treatments were successful. After 4 years the success dropped to 59.5%, with an average follow-up time of 3.2 years (based on the 65 teeth with a minimum follow-up period of 1 year). The success of the pulpectomy treatment slightly increased upon adding primary molars that were followed up through telephone contact only at 1 and 4 years posttreatment to 94.6% and 65.1%, respectively.

Behavior management technique

Treatment modality had a decisive role in the outcome of the pulpectomy treatment, as treatments performed under GA had the lowest failure rates through the years rising to only 21.4% after 4 years (Table 3). This was followed by treatments carried out under N$_2$O sedation combined with a LA agent. Apparently, treatments were the least successful under LA alone, with a success rate of 43.8% four years following treatment.

Similarly, arch type appeared to have an impact on the outcome of the treatment. The success of the treatment carried out in primary molars in the maxillary arch decreased significantly with every follow-up year to reach 38.5% after 4 years (Table 3). This impact was most evident at both the 1- and 2-year follow-up examinations.

Multivariate regression analysis

The multivariate regression analysis showed a low squared multiple R (0.22) as well as a low adjusted squared multiple R (0.09) and therefore no good fit of the regression analysis. The P value of each variable was above .05 and, therefore, not statistically significant besides the variables "dmft" (.017), "number of visits" (.020), and coronal lesion (.026, Table 4).

Discussion

To the best of the present authors' knowledge, this is one of the few studies in the literature to investigate the possible influence of different treatment settings on the success of pulpectomy treatment in primary molars, which in turn could help clinicians in decision making when planning treatments.

The treatment setting of the study was found to have an impact on the outcome of primary molar pulpectomy. Treatments carried out under GA had the highest success rate at all follow-up periods and was considerably high 4 years posttreatment (78.6%). This finding came as no surprise given the rather strict indications and the nonconservative nature of dental treatment under sedation or especially GA. Treatments carried out under GA are planned carefully, and only teeth with predictable and good prognosis (free of radiologic and clinical signs of abscess or fistula) are usually treated and maintained to avoid possible posttreatment complications and the necessity of a second intervention. In addition, the cooperation of the child does not affect the result under GA, and therefore, quality of treatment is also easier to assure. In addition, oral rehabilitation under GA of young uncooperative children suffer-

Table 2 General characteristics of the study sample (data based on number of primary molars)

Category	Factor	Baseline, N = 105, n (%)	1-y follow-up, n = 65, n (%)	2-y follow-up, n = 56, n (%)	3-y follow-up, n = 49, n (%)	4-y follow-up, n = 37, n (%)
Treatment modality, n (%)	Local anesthesia	39 (37.1%)	23 (35.4%)	21 (37.5%)	19 (38.8%)	16 (43.2%)
	Nitrous oxide sedation	21 (20.0%)	14 (21.5%)	11 (19.6%)	11 (22.4%)	7 (18.9%)
	General anesthesia	45 (42.9%)	28 (43.1%)	24 (42.9%)	19 (38.8%)	14 (37.8%)
Arch, n (%)	Maxillary	39 (37.1%)	26 (40.0%)	20 (35.7%)	17 (34.7%)	13 (35.1%)
	Mandibular	66 (62.9%)	39 (60.0%)	36 (64.3%)	32 (65.3%)	24 (64.9%)
Age (y), n (%)	3	6 (5.7%)	5 (7.7%)	3 (5.4%)	3 (6.1%)	3 (8.1%)
	4	29 (27.6%)	20 (30.8%)	19 (33.9%)	16 (32.7%)	11 (29.7%)
	5	30 (28.6%)	13 (20.0%)	12 (21.4%)	12 (24.5%)	8 (21.6%)
	6	21 (20.0%)	15 (23.1%)	12 (21.4%)	9 (18.4%)	6 (16.2%)
	7	10 (9.5%)	7 (10.8%)	5 (8.9%)	5 (10.2%)	5 (13.5%)
	8	6 (5.7%)	5 (7.7%)	5 (8.9%)	4 (8.2%)	4 (10.8%)
	9	2 (1.9%)	0 (0.0%)	0 (0.0%)	0 (0.0%)	0 (0.0%)
	10	1 (1.0%)	0 (0.0%)	0 (0.0%)	0 (0.0%)	0 (0.0%)
Mean baseline age (±SD), y		5.0±1.4				NA
Mean baseline dmft (±SD)		8.0±3.8				
Treatment indication, n (%)	Irreversible pulpitis/ Necrosis	71 (67.6%)	44 (67.7%)	37 (66.1%)	30 (61.2%)	23 (62.2%)
	Apical radiolucency	18 (17.1%)	11 (16.9%)	10 (17.9%)	10 (20.4%)	9 (24.3%)
	Fistula	4 (3.8%)	3 (4.6%)	3 (5.4%)	3 (6.1%)	1 (2.7%)
	Abscess	3 (2.9%)	1 (1.5%)	1 (1.8%)	1 (2.0%)	1 (2.7%)
	Failed pulpotomy	4 (3.8%)	4 (6.2%)	3 (5.4%)	3 (6.1%)	2 (5.4%)
	Unknown	5 (4.8%)	2 (3.1%)	2 (3.6%)	2 (4.1%)	1 (2.7%)
Operator, n (%)	Master student	38 (36.2%)	26 (40.0%)	24 (42.9%)	22 (44.9%)	17 (45.9%)
	Pedodontist/Professor	21 (20.0%)	11 (16.9%)	9 (16.1%)	8 (16.3%)	5 (13.5%)
	General dentist	46 (43.8%)	28 (43.1%)	23 (41.1%)	19 (38.8%)	15 (40.5%)
Number of visits, n (%)	One visit	99 (94.3%)	60 (92.3%)	52 (92.9%)	46 (93.9%)	36 (97.3%)
	Two visits	6 (5.7%)	5 (7.7%)	4 (7.1%)	3 (6.1%)	1 (2.7%)
Posttreatment restoration, n (%)	Preformed metal crown	103 (98.1%)	64 (98.5%)	55 (98.2%)	48 (98.0%)	36 (97.3%)
	Composite filling	2 (1.9%)	1 (1.5%)	2 (3.6%)	2 (4.1%)	2 (5.4%)
Tooth type, n (%)	2nd primary molar	86 (81.9%)	52 (80.0%)	45 (80.4%)	38 (77.6%)	29 (78.4%)
	1st primary molar	19 (18.1%)	13 (20.0%)	11 (19.6%)	11 (22.4%)	8 (21.6%)
Radiograph, n (%)	Yes	90 (85.7%)	57 (87.7%)	49 (87.5%)	42 (85.7%)	34 (91.9%)
	No	4 (3.8%)	1 (1.5%)	1 (1.8%)	1 (2.0%)	0 (0.0%)
	Radiograph older than 6 months	11 (10.5%)	7 (10.8%)	6 (10.7%)	6 (12.2%)	3 (8.1%)
Type of radiograph, n (%)	Periapical radiograph	40 (38.1%)	25 (38.5%)	21 (37.5%)	17 (34.7%)	12 (32.4%)
	Panoramic radiograph	59 (56.2%)	37 (56.9%)	32 (57.1%)	29 (59.2%)	23 (62.2%)
	Panoramic radiograph half side	2 (1.9%)	2 (3.1%)	2 (3.6%)	2 (4.1%)	2 (5.4%)
	No radiograph	4 (3.8%)	1 (1.5%)	1 (1.8%)	1 (2.0%)	0 (0.0%)
Type of caries lesion, n (%)	Occlusal	12 (11.4%)	9 (13.8%)	8 (14.3%)	8 (16.3%)	8 (21.6%)
	Approximal 2 or 3 surfaces	93 (88.6%)	56 (86.2%)	48 (85.7%)	41 (83.7%)	29 (78.4%)

NA, not applicable.

ing from ECC is the most efficient way to achieve sustainable results and enhance the overall OHRQoL.[14,15]

Treatments under N_2O sedation in conjunction with LA had slightly lower success than GA, showing that N_2O is a powerful tool in reducing or eliminating a child's fear and anxiety, which in turn elevates pain reaction threshold and reduces fatigue.[16] Another favorable effect of N_2O sedation is that it makes children relax and sudden movements are eliminated, facilitating lengthy and optimal procedures.[16] Not surprisingly, treatments performed under LA alone had the highest failure rates; this

Table 3 Retrospective outcome of pulpectomy in primary molars in relation to the main important variables (data based on number of primary molars) up to 4 years in bivariate analysis

Variable		1-y follow-up		2-y follow-up		3-y follow-up		4-y follow-up	
		Success, n (%)	Failure, n (%)	Success, n (%)	Failure, n (%)	Success, n (%)	Failure, n (%)	Success, n (%)	Failure, n (%)
Treatment modality	Chi-square test	$X^2=0.02$		$X^2=0.06$		$X^2=0.02$		$X^2=0.15$	
	LA	19 (82.6%)	4 (17.4%)	15 (71.4%)	6 (28.6%)	11 (57.9%)	8 (42.1%)	7 (43.8%)	9 (56.3%)
	N_2O	14 (100.0%)	0 (0.0%)	10 (90.9%)	1 (9.1%)	9 (81.8%)	2 (18.2%)	4 (57.1%)	3 (42.9%)
	GA	28 (100.0%)	0 (0.0%)	23 (95.8%)	1 (4.2%)	18 (94.7%)	1 (5.3%)	11 (78.6%)	3 (21.4%)
Arch	X^2	$X^2=0.01$		$X^2=0.01$		$X^2=0.12$		$X^2=0.00$	
	Maxillary	22 (84.6%)	4 (15.4%)	14 (70.0%)	6 (30.0%)	11 (64.7%)	6 (35.3%)	5 (38.5%)	8 (61.5%)
	Mandibular	39 (100.0%)	0 (0.0%)	34 (94.4%)	2 (5.6%)	27 (84.4%)	5 (15.6%)	17 (70.8%)	7 (29.2%)
Treatment indication	Chi-square test	$X^2=0.61$		$X^2=0.16$		$X^2=0.19$		$X^2=0.18$	
	Irreversible pulpitis/ necrosis	41 (93.2%)	3 (6.8%)	32 (86.5%)	5 (13.5%)	25 (83.3%)	5 (16.7%)	16 (69.6%)	7 (30.4%)
	Apical radiolucency	11 (100.0%)	0 (0.0%)	9 (90.0%)	1 (10.0%)	6 (60.0%)	4 (40.0%)	4 (44.4%)	5 (55.6%)
	Fistula	3 (100.0%)	0 (0.0%)	3 (100.0%)	0 (0.0%)	3 (100.0%)	0 (0.0%)	1 (100.0%)	0 (0.0%)
	Abscess	1 (100.0%)	0 (0.0%)	1 (100.0%)	0 (0.0%)	1 (100.0%)	0 (0.0%)	0 (0.0%)	1 (100.0%)
	Failed pulpotomy	3 (75.0%)	1 (25.0%)	1 (33.3%)	2 (66.7%)	1 (33.3%)	2 (66.7%)	0 (0.0%)	2 (100.0%)
	Unknown	2 (100.0%)	0 (0.0%)	2 (100.0%)	0 (0.0%)	2 (100.0%)	0 (0.0%)	1 (100.0%)	0 (0.0%)
Coronal lesion	Chi-square test	$X^2=0.95$		$X^2=0.82$		$X^2=0.60$		$X^2=0.38$	
	Occlusal	9 (100.0%)	0 (0.0%)	8 (100.0%)	0 (0.0%)	8 (100.0%)	0 (0.0%)	7 (87.5%)	1 (12.5%)
	Approximal two or three surfaces)	52 (92.9%)	4 (7.1%)	40 (83.3%)	8 (16.7%)	30 (73.2%)	11 (26.8%)	15 (51.7%)	14 (48.3%)
Age (y)	Chi-square test	$X^2=0.00$		$X^2=0.00$		$X^2=0.07$		$X^2=0.07$	
	3	5 (100.0%)	0 (0.0%)	3 (100.0%)	0 (0.0%)	3 (100.0%)	0 (0.0%)	3 (100.0%)	0 (0.0%)
	4	20 (100.0%)	0 (0.0%)	18 (94.7%)	1 (5.3%)	15 (93.8%)	1 (6.3%)	9 (81.8%)	2 (18.2%)
	5	12 (92.3%)	1 (7.7%)	11 (91.7%)	1 (8.3%)	10 (83.3%)	2 (16.7%)	4 (50.0%)	4 (50.0%)
	6	15 (100.0%)	0 (0.0%)	10 (83.3%)	2 (16.7%)	5 (55.6%)	4 (44.4%)	1 (16.7%)	5 (83.3%)
	7	4 (57.1%)	3 (42.9%)	2 (40.0%)	3 (60.0%)	2 (40.0%)	3 (60.0%)	2 (40.0%)	3 (60.0%)
	8	5 (100.0%)	0 (0.0%)	4 (80.0%)	1 (20.0%)	3 (75.0%)	1 (25.0%)	3 (75.0%)	1 (25.0%)
Operator	Chi-square test	$X^2=0.74$		$X^2=0.47$		$X^2=0.97$		$X^2=0.33$	
	Master student	24 (92.3%)	2 (7.7%)	19 (79.2%)	5 (20.8%)	17 (77.3%)	5 (22.7%)	10 (58.8%)	7 (41.2%)
	Pedodontist/Professor	10 (90.9%)	1 (9.1%)	8 (88.9%)	1 (11.1%)	6 (75.0%)	2 (25.0%)	2 (40.0%)	3 (60.0%)
	General dentist working in a pediatric dental clinic	27 (96.4%)	1 (3.6%)	21 (91.3%)	2 (8.7%)	15 (78.9%)	4 (21.1%)	10 (66.7%)	5 (33.3%)
Number of visits	Chi-square test	$X^2=0.55$		$X^2=0.40$		$X^2=0.34$		$X^2=0.22$	
	One visit	56 (93.3%)	4 (6.7%)	44 (84.6%)	8 (15.4%)	35 (76.1%)	11 (23.9%)	22 (61.1%)	14 (38.9%)
	Two visits	5 (100.0%)	0 (0.0%)	4 (100.0%)	0 (0.0%)	3 (100.0%)	0 (0.0%)	0 (0.0%)	1 (100.0%)
Posttreatment restoration	Chi-square test	$X^2=1.00$		$X^2=1.00$		$X^2=0.99$		$X^2=0.95$	
	SSC	60 (93.8%)	4 (6.3%)	47 (85.5%)	8 (14.5%)	37 (77.1%)	11 (22.9%)	21 (58.3%)	15 (41.7%)
	Filling	1 (100.0%)	0 (0.0%)	1 (100.0%)	0 (0.0%)	1 (100.0%)	0 (0.0%)	1 (100.0%)	0 (0.0%)
Tooth type	Chi-square test	$X^2=0.12$		$X^2=0.68$		$X^2=0.66$		$X^2=0.54$	
	2nd primary molar	50 (96.2%)	2 (3.8%)	39 (86.7%)	6 (13.3%)	30 (78.9%)	8 (21.1%)	18 (62.1%)	11 (37.9%)
	1st primary molar	11 (84.6%)	2 (15.4%)	9 (81.8%)	2 (18.2%)	8 (72.7%)	3 (27.3%)	4 (50.0%)	4 (50.0%)

might be due to the preference to retain these primary molars especially in cooperative children, as in case of failure only a second treatment for extraction is needed and not a second GA or N_2O sedation.

Behavior management technique and the resulting setting for dental treatment was found to be statistically significant not only for 1 year, but also 3 years posttreatment in bivariate analysis. Even though treatment modality was no longer statis-

Table 4 Results of the multivariate regression analysis of the outcome after 4 years

Variable	Coefficients	Standard deviation	t-statistic value	P value
Intersection	−0.1059	1.6181	−0.0654	.9480
Sex	−0.1041	0.2369	−0.4395	.6614
Overall health condition of the patient	−0.9017	0.5246	−1.7188	.0891
Treatment modality	0.0384	0.1785	0.2152	.8301
Arch type	−0.1941	0.2644	−0.7342	.4647
Age at day of treatment	0.0192	0.0996	0.1931	.8473
dmft at day of treatment	0.0910	0.0375	2.4252	.0173
Indication of treatment	−0.0497	0.1089	−0.4565	.6491
Operator	0.2148	0.1446	1.4860	.1408
Number of visits	1.2852	0.5423	2.3699	.0199
Posttreatment restoration	−0.1163	0.4368	−0.2663	.7906
Tooth type	−0.0864	0.3242	−0.2664	.7905
Radiograph available	0.0529	0.2239	0.2362	.8138
Type of radiograph	0.1741	0.2402	0.7248	.4705
Coronal lesion	0.8694	0.3852	2.2570	.0264

tically significant 4 years posttreatment, probably due to the decreased remaining sample, a clinically relevant difference was found. This may also be the reason for the low fit in the multivariate analysis leading to a statistically nonsignificant correlation.

Possible further reasons for the clinical effect of the modality are likely not the treatment itself, but a combination of GA and a certain expected prognosis. For pulpectomy with LA alone the risk of retreatment due to failure is also considered, but it is not viewed as a clear contraindication as the child will manage the extraction in case of a failure.

In contrast to the present results, a recent study found no significant difference in the survival rate of pulpectomized primary teeth performed under GA and LA after 5 years posttreatment.[17] Even though the study was also a retrospective analysis, in that study both anterior and posterior primary teeth were included, and only those with irreversible pulpitis or pulp necrosis with or without apical/interradicular radiolucency.[17] The inability to completely eliminate all pathogens from the dental pulp and root canals of the severely infected teeth was believed to be the primary source of failure. In the present study, all primary molars that underwent pulpectomy treatment were included regardless of the pretreatment status of the pulp and/or periapical/radicular area. Moreover, different root canal filling materials were used. Therefore, the previous results are not fully comparable with the present study as these factors might have influenced the outcome as a confounder.

In the bivariate analysis, the dental arch was also found to be statistically significant 4 years following treatment; this is in agreement with a previous study,[13] probably related to the wide anatomical variations of primary maxillary molars, such as a double canal system in the mesiobuccal root[18] and great divergence of the distobuccal root.[19] Moreover, the ease of manipulation of primary molars in the mandibular arch and the possibility of direct vision might have contributed to the greater success. Most likely a confounding of the factor "arch" on the behavior management modality can be excluded as, in general, the distribution between the three different behavior management modalities stays more or less constant.

One of the important aspects that contribute to the success of the pulpectomy treatment is the choice of a posttreatment restoration that provides a tight coronal seal. SSCs are durable, can be easily fitted, and provide long-term clinical success.[20] Furthermore, SSCs are more likely to reduce the risk of major failures than fillings;[21] they have a survival probability of 98% four years following placement on second primary molars under general anesthesia,[22] making them the ideal restoration to be used in primary molars following a pulpotomy or pulpectomy.[23,24] In a similar manner, as only one tooth received a composite filling following the pulpectomy treatment, the remaining teeth restored with a SSC reflect the overall success rate of the pulpectomy treatment.

One of the strengths of the present study was the diversity of the operators who carried out the pulpectomy treatment. All treatments had similar success rates with no statistically signif-icant difference among the different groups, perhaps owing to the antimicrobial properties of the calcium-hydroxide/iodo-form paste and ease of application. This in turns excludes an allocation bias of the complex cases to the more specialized and experienced operators. This is important as in real life not only specialized pediatric dental practitioners treat children but also general dental practitioners and dental students.

Another strength of the present study was the inclusion of all primary molars that underwent pulpectomy treatment to avoid influencing the outcome; this contrasts with other studies that used much stricter inclusion criteria excluding teeth, eg, with clinical abscess or fistula.[11,12] Though the majority of the pulpec-tomized primary molars in the present study were second pri-mary molars, tooth type did not show an effect on the success of the treatment. This finding is in accordance with a study in which tooth type did not seem to have any effect on the outcome 18 months posttreatment.[25] Nevertheless, the importance of sec-ond primary molars in guiding the eruption of first permanent molars to prevent mesial shifting followed by arch length loss and finally crowding is well-known.[26] Alternatively, fixed space maintainers with a distal shoe may be applied when extraction of a second primary molar before eruption of the first permanent molar is performed. Nonetheless, the survival rate of fixed space maintainers in the same clinic as the present study was unsatis-factory, especially for fixed appliances with distal shoe (~60%).[27] For this reason it is of utmost importance to preserve primary second molars, ideally until their natural exfoliation to act as nat-ural space maintainers and maintain arch integrity.

The retrospective nature of the present study comes with some limitations such as the inability to control external factors, as well as missing important data and incomplete documenta-tion in some cases. This can influence the outcome and impact of variables on the success of the treatment. Another weakness is the limited sample size, since retrospective studies often re-quire a large number of patients especially when trying to find a correlation between various factors and their influence on the outcome. Moreover, success of primary tooth pulpectomy in the literature is based on clinical and radiographic assessment,[28] whereas the present study relied mainly on clinical assessment alone.

In children between 4 and 5 years of age, maintaining pri-mary molars through root canal treatment should always be considered even with the prognosis of a modest 4-year success of the treatment. When the first permanent molar erupts, it will be easier to place a space maintainer after the extraction, or this may no longer be necessary as the space would be natu-rally retained if the opposing first permanent molars are locked in a stable relationship.[29] ⠿

Conclusion

Primary molar pulpectomy performed under GA showed a high success rate several years following treatment and should be considered during treatment planning in complex oral rehabil-itation. Even in general practice this easily applicable tech-nique should be considered in order to prevent space loss in the molar area.

Disclosure

The authors declare there are no conflicts of interest.

References

1. Tinanoff N, Baez RJ, Diaz Guillory C, et al. Early childhood caries epidemiology, aetiology, risk assessment, societal burden, management, education, and policy: Global perspective. Int J Paediatr Dent 2019;29: 238–248.

2. Kher MS, Rao A. Pulp therapy in primary teeth. Clin Dent Rev 2020;4:340.

3. Chen KJ, Gao SS, Duangthip D, Lo ECM, Chu CH. Prevalence of early childhood caries among 5-year-old children: A systematic review. J Investig Clin Dent 2019;10:e12376.

4. Monte-Santo AS, Viana SVC, Moreira KMS, Imparato JCP, Mendes FM, Bonini GAVC. Prevalence of early loss of primary molar and its impact in schoolchildren's quality of life. Int J Paediatr Dent 2018;28: 595–601.

5. Ahmed HMA. Pulpectomy procedures in primary molar teeth. Eur J Gen Dent 2014;3:3–10.

6. Wagner Y, Knaup I, Knaup TJ, Jacobs C, Wolf M. Influence of a programme for pre-vention of early childhood caries on early orthodontic treatment needs. Clin Oral Investig 2020;24:4313–4324.

7. Rewal N, Thakur AS, Sachdev V, Mahajan N. Comparison of endoflas and zinc oxide eugenol as root canal filling materials in primary dentition. J Indian Soc Pedod Prev Dent 2014;32:317–321.

8. Lokade A, Thakur S, Singhal P, Chauhan D, Jayam C. Comparative evaluation of clinical and radiographic success of three different lesion sterilization and tissue repair techniques as treatment options in primary molars requiring pulpectomy: An in vivo study. J Indian Soc Pedod Prev Dent 2019;37: 185–191.

9. Chen X, Liu X, Zhong J. Clinical and radiographic evaluation of pulpectomy in primary teeth: an 18-months clinical randomized controlled trial. Head Face Med 2017;13:12.

10. American Academy of Pediatric Dentistry. Behavior guidance for the pediatric dental patient. The Reference Manual of Pediatric Dentistry. American Academy of Pediatric Dentistry, 2021:306–324.

11. Pramila R, Muthu MS, Deepa G, Farzan JM, Rodrigues SJL. Pulpectomies in primary mandibular molars: a comparison of outcomes using three root filling materials. Int Endod J 2016;49:413–421.

12. Al-Ostwani AO, Al-Monaqel BM, Al-Tinawi MK. A clinical and radiographic study of four different root canal fillings in primary molars. J Indian Soc Pedod Prev Dent 2016;34:55–59.

13. Al-Attiya H, Schmoeckel J, Mourad MS, Splieth CH. One year clinical success of pulpectomy in primary molars with iodoform-calcium hydroxide paste. Quintessence Int 2021;52:528–537.

14. Boukhobza S, Stamm T, Glatthor J, Meißner N, Bekes K. Changes in oral health-related quality of life among Austrian pre-school children following dental treatment under general anaesthesia. Clin Oral Investig 2021;25:2821–2826.

15. Jiang H-F, Qin D, He S-L, Wang J-H. OHRQoL changes among Chinese preschool children following dental treatment under general anesthesia. Clin Oral Investig 2020;24:1997–2004.

16. Wright GZ. Behavior management in dentistry for children. Ames: John Wiley & Sons, 2014.

17. Songvejkasem M, Auychai P, Chankanka O, Songsiripradubboon S. Survival rate and associated factors affecting pulpectomy treatment outcome in primary teeth. Clin Exp Dent Res 2021;7:978–986.

18. Fumes AC, Sousa-Neto MD, Leoni GB, et al. Root canal morphology of primary molars: a micro-computed tomography study. Eur Arch Paediatr Dent 2014;15:317–326.

19. Gaurav V, Srivastava N, Rana V, Adlakha VK. A study of root canal morphology of human primary incisors and molars using cone beam computerized tomography: an in vitro study. J Indian Soc Pedod Prev Dent 2013;31:254–259.

20. Dimitrov E, Georgieva M, Dimova-Gabrovska M, Andreeva R, Belcheva-Krivorova A. Preformed metal crowns as a prosthetic restorations in pediatric dentistry. J IMAB 2017;23:1627–1632.

21. Innes NPT, Ricketts D, Chong LY, Keightley AJ, Lamont T, Santamaria RM. Preformed crowns for decayed primary molar teeth. Cochrane Database Syst Rev 2015;12:CD005512.

22. Azadani EN, Peng J, Kumar A, et al. A survival analysis of primary second molars in children treated under general anesthesia. J Am Dent Assoc 2020;151:568–575.

23. Lin GSS, Hisham ARB, Cher CIY, Cheah KK, Ghani NRNA, Noorani TY. Success rates of coronal and partial pulpotomies in mature permanent molars: a systematic review and single-arm meta-analysis. Quintessence Int 2021;3:196–208.

24. Aksoy B, Güngör HC, Uysal S, Gonzales CD, Ölmez S. Ferric sulfate pulpotomy in primary teeth with different base materials: a 2-year randomized controlled trial. Quintessence Int 2022;53:782–789.

25. Mendoza-Mendoza A, Caleza-Jiménez C, Solano-Mendoza B, Iglesias-Linares A. Are there any differences between first and second primary molar pulpectomy prognoses? A retrospective clinical study. Eur J Peadiatr Dent 2017;18:41–44.

26. Law CS. Management of premature primary tooth loss in the child patient. J Calif Dent Assoc 2013;41:612–618.

27. Abdin M. Survival and failure of fixed space maintainers placed in different clinical settings: a 5-year retrospective analysis: Master thesis. University of Greifswald, 2021.

28. Boutsiouki C, Frankenberger R, Krämer N. Clinical and radiographic success of (partial) pulpotomy and pulpectomy in primary teeth: a systematic review. Eur J Peadiatr Dent 2021;22:273–285.

29. Albati M, Showlag R, Akili A, et al. Space maintainers application, indication and complications. Int J Community Med Public Health 2018;5:4970.

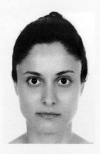

Haneen Al-Attiya

Haneen Al-Attiya Specialist Pediatric Dentist, Department of Preventive and Pediatric Dentistry, University of Greifswald, Greifswald, Germany

Mhd Said Mourad Specialist Pediatric Dentist and Postgraduate Supervisor, Department of Preventive and Pediatric Dentistry, University of Greifswald, Greifswald, Germany; and Department of Orthodontics, University of Greifswald, Greifswald, Germany

Christian H. Splieth Professor and Head of Department of Preventive and Pediatric Dentistry, University of Greifswald, Greifswald, Germany

Julian Schmoeckel Assistant Professor, Department of Preventive and Pediatric Dentistry, University of Greifswald, Greifswald, Germany

Correspondence: Prof Dr Christian Splieth, Department of Preventive and Pediatric Dentistry, University of Greifswald, Fleischmann-straße 42-44, 17475 Greifswald, Germany. Email: splieth@uni-greifswald.de

First submission: 29 Jul 2022
Acceptance: 13 Aug 2022
Online publication: 15 Nov 2022

UNDERSTANDING THE LANGUAGE OF CELLS

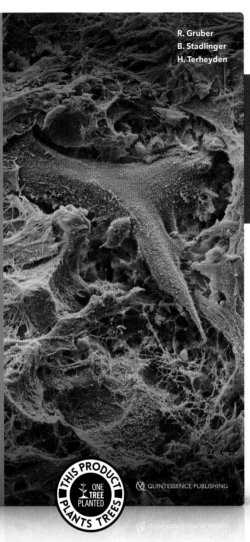

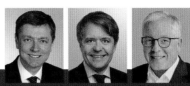

Reinhard Gruber | Bernd Stadlinger | Hendrik Terheyden (Eds.)

CELL-TO-CELL COMMUNICATION
CELL-ATLAS – VISUAL BIOLOGY IN ORAL MEDICINE
Volume 7

Hardcover, 244 pages, 298 illus.
ISBN 978-1-78698-107-3, €86

The deepest understanding of the cells of the oral system will be found in decoding their communication and seeing how it is regulated. Once we have understood their language, clinicians migh be able to talk to cells and control their action.

This book by 47 world-renowned experts – for each chapter at leas one clinician and one basic scientist – highlights a reliable and actu state of research regarding this topic that quickly moves forward. Beyond the classic cell types addressed in the first part of the book and visualized by colored scanning electron microscopic (SEM) images, organ systems or model systems of cell-to-cell communication of a more generic type are presented in four additional chapters in the second part.

This book – accompanied by an augmented reality (AR) app that allows you to experience the process of bone resorption virtually – should help to open the vision of how we can regenerate tissues ar heal diseases by controlling the language of the cells, and shows u the direction in which research and therapy will go in the future.

OUTLINE

Part 1: Cell Atlas of the Oral System "A to Z"
Ameloblasts (R. J. Miron, A. Lussi)
B-Cells / T-Cells (J. Konkel, I. Chapple)
Cementoblasts & Cementocytes (B. L. Foster, M. Sanz)
Chondrocytes and Fibrochondrocytes
(D. S. Nedrelow, M. S. Detamore, M. E. Wong)
Dental Stem Cells: Developmental Aspects (J. Krivanek, K. Fried)
Epithelial Cells (V.-J. Uitto, U. K. Gursoy)
Fibroblasts (G. Pompermaier Garlet, D. S. Thoma)
Macrophages (J. CW. Wang, W. V. Giannobile)
Microvascular Cells: Endothelium and Pericytes (A. Banfi, S. Kühl)
Myocytes (S. W. Herring, S. Kiliaridis)
Nerve Cells (S. Bae Oh, Pa Reum Lee, D. A. Ettlin)
Odontoblasts (D. D. Bosshardt, P. R. Schmidlin)
Osteoblasts (F. E. Weber, B. Lethaus)

Osteoclasts / Odontoclasts (R. Nishimura, H. Terheyden)
Osteocytes (R. Gruber, B. Stadlinger)
Polymorphonuclear Cells (Neutrophils) (J. Deschner, S. Jepsen)
Salivary Acinar Cells (G. B. Procter, A. Vissink)

Part 2: Cellular Interactions – Insights and Outlooks
Oral Microbiota, Biofilms and Their Environment
(N. Bostanci, G. N. Belibasakis)
Mesenchymal Stromal Cells: Therapeutic Aspects
(Q. Vallmajo-Martin, J. S. Marschall, E. Avilla-Royo, M. Ehrbar)
Model Systems for Investigation of Cell-to-Cell Communication
(P. Korn, M. Gelinsky)
Linking Molecular Function with Tissue Structure in the Oral Cavity
(C. Porcheri, C. T. Meisel, T. A. Mitsiades)

Supported by

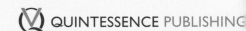 QUINTESSENCE PUBLISHING

▦ COMMUNITY DENTISTRY

Racial and oral health disparity associated with perinatal oral health care utilization among underserved US pregnant women

Nisreen Al Jallad, DDS*/Shruti Vasani, BDS, MPH*/Tong Tong Wu, PhD/Rita Cacciato, RDH, MS/
Marie Thomas/Nour Lababede/Ayah Lababede/Jin Xiao, DDS, MS, PhD

Objective: The study aims to identify specific determinants of dental care utilization during the perinatal period (prenatal and 1-year postnatal) among underserved US women residing in Upstate New York. **Method and materials:** The prospective cohort study included 186 low-income US pregnant women. Demographic-socioeconomic parameters and medical-dental conditions were obtained from questionnaires, electronic medical-dental records, and dental examinations. Multivariate regression analyses were used to assess factors associated with perinatal dental care utilization. As an exploratory effort, a separate logistic model assessed factors associated with adverse birth outcomes. **Results:** The results demonstrated unmet oral health needs among the underserved US pregnant women residing in Upstate New York. Despite an average of 2.7 ± 3.6 untreated decayed teeth per person during pregnancy, only 39.3% and 19.9% utilized prenatal and 1-year postnatal dental care, respectively. Previous dental care utilization was a notable factor contributing to a higher uptake of perinatal dental care at a subsequent period. Prenatal dental care utilization was significantly lower among African American women (odds ratio 0.43 [95% CI 0.19, 0.98], $P = .04$) and positively associated with dental caries severity (OR 2.40 [1.09, 5.12], $P = .03$). Post-

natal utilization was associated with caries severity (OR 4.70 [1.73, 12.74], $P = .002$) and prevalent medical conditions (hypertension, diabetes mellitus, and emotional conditions). Pregnant women who achieved prenatal caries-free status had a lower odds of experiencing adverse birth outcomes; however, this was an insignificant finding due to limited adverse birth cases. **Conclusion:** Racial and oral health disparity is associated with perinatal oral health care utilization among underserved US pregnant women in New York. While both prenatal and postnatal dental care utilization was positively associated with oral health status, specifically, postnatal utilization was driven by existing medical conditions such as emotional condition, hypertension, and diabetes mellitus. The results add to existing information on inherent barriers and postulated needs to improve access to perinatal oral care, thereby informing statewide recommendations to maximize utilization. Considering this is a geographically restricted population, the findings are particularly true to this cohort of underserved pregnant women. However, future more robust studies are warranted to assess effective strategies to further improve perinatal dental care utilization among underserved pregnant women.
(Quintessence Int 2022;53:892–902; doi: 10.3290/j.qi.b3095001)

Key words: birth outcomes, caries, dental care utilization, pregnancy, prenatal oral health

Inter-relationships between systemic and oral diseases have led to the recognition of oral health as an integral component of overall total health.[1] The oral cavity may be susceptible to physiologic hormonal imbalances and pathologic changes during pregnancy. Some commonly reported pregnancy-associated oral manifestations include pregnancy-related gingivitis, pregnancy periodontal tumor, xerostomia, and resultant dental caries and periodontal infection.[2] Maternal periodontal health has been linked to adverse birth outcomes such as preterm birth, low-birth-weight babies, and preeclampsia.[3] Moreover, the mother's oral health is considered strongly related to their offspring's oral health. Various studies demonstrated that improved oral health during pregnancy significantly reduced the incidence of early childhood caries (ECC) among children.[4] Furthermore, poor periodontal health during pregnancy may also be correlated to significantly compromised quality of life in terms of increased pain and discomfort, restricted function, and psychologic stress.[5]

Despite the importance and benefits of maintaining desirable oral health care during pregnancy,[6,7] prenatal dental care utilization remains low, especially among the low-income and socioeconomically underserved population. Therefore, understanding the determinants of oral health care utilization during pregnancy is essential to implementing effective strategies to improve care utilization. A 2018 systematic review study reported that psychosocial stigma, fear and anxiety, lack of adequate knowledge, and financial and time constraints were among the most common predictors of the utilization of oral health care during pregnancy.[8] A retrospective study on factors that influence access to prenatal care among pregnant women who were provided care by the University of North Carolina (UNC) prenatal oral care program and community health clinics detected significant underutilization of oral care as compared to the need for treatment (42% versus 87% respectively).[9] Medicaid insurance coverage was significantly positively associated with the number of dental visits ($P = .001$), highlighting the need for improved coverage during pregnancy.[9] Adeniyi et al[10] identified interprofessional collaborative practices, including in-service training and education, as a critical approach to successfully integrated prenatal oral care.

Although previous studies have assessed determinants of prenatal oral health care behavior among pregnant women,[11-13] there is limited literature attempting to evaluate specific determinants of prenatal oral care utilization at the community level focusing on underprivileged women residing within New York. In addition to assessing sociodemographic and lifestyle determinants, limited studies have considered the impact of medical and oral health conditions on dental care utilization during pregnancy. Furthermore, most previous reports utilized a cross-sectional dataset without longitudinal assessment of dental utilization during pregnancy and after the child is born. The objective of this study was to assess the association between demographic-sociotechnical-behavior factors, medical-dental conditions, and perinatal (prenatal and 1-year postnatal) dental care utilization among 186 underserved pregnant women. It was hypothesized that perinatal oral care utilization is associated with racial and oral health disparities among underserved pregnant women residing in Upstate New York.

Method and materials

Study population and design

The study was a prospective cohort study including 186 pregnant women who were sampled from the patient population of socioeconomically disadvantaged women visiting the University of Rochester Medical Center (URMC) Highland Family Medicine (HFM), and Eastman Institute for Oral Health (EIOH) from 2017 to 2020. The study participants were mothers in a birth cohort study (186 mother-infant dyads) that examined factors associated with early childhood caries (ECC) onset in early life.[14] The URMC clinics provide care to a large patient population from low-income communities. The New-York state-supported Medicaid type insurance status (eg, Medicaid, Blue Choice, MVP Option, Fidelis Care – Medicaid) was used to determine the socioeconomic status of the study participants. Accordingly, pregnant women with NY state supported medical insurance determined by income levels (ie, ≤138% of federal poverty line) were eligible to participate. The study protocol was approved by the University of Rochester Research Subject Review Board (#1248).

Inclusion and exclusion criteria

All study subjects who met the inclusion and exclusion criteria were enrolled in the study. The inclusion criteria were as follows:
- >18 years
- over 28 weeks of gestation
- pregnant with a single fetus.

The exclusion criteria were as follows:
- having a severe systemic disease such as acquired immunodeficiency syndrome (AIDS) that rendered them susceptible to infections
- diagnosed with oral cancer
- with maxillofacial deformity (eg, cleft lip/palate).

Data collection and examination

The sociodemographic information was acquired through a self-reported questionnaire that the study participants filled out. Parameters on the questionnaire included sociodemographic information, including age, race, ethnicity, marital status, level of education, number of other children, and employment status. Information on medical conditions was obtained from URMC electronic health records (eRecord). The medical information included physician-diagnosed medical conditions (eg, diabetes, asthma, hypertension, emotional condition such as anxiety, depression), a list of current medications, long-term use of antibiotic therapy for more than 3 months, anti-fungal therapy in the past 3 months, and any history of recent yeast infection, and birth outcomes (term of the pregnancy and infant birth weight). In addition, the subjects self-reported information of oral health behavior such as smoking status and brushing habits. A comprehensive oral examination was conducted using standard examination equipment and protocol to obtain oral health conditions. Oral health status, as well as dental caries, was reported using Decayed, Missing, and Filled teeth (DMFT) index per the World Health Organization (WHO) recommendations and International Caries Detection and Assessment System (ICDAS).[15,16] Plaque Index (PI) was recorded as described by Löe and Sillnes.[17] Information on perinatal (prior to pregnancy, during pregnancy, 1-year postnatal) dental care utilization was obtained from URMC Axium dental electronic system. Accordingly, information on type of dental care received (eg, urgent care or routine care) was obtained at each of the specified time periods. For instance, routine dental care included a wide range of dental procedures such as examination and diagnosis, prophylaxis, scaling and root planing, amalgam and composite restorations, endodontic treatment, post and core, fixed prosthesis as well as extractions. In contrast, emergency care involved all kinds of palliative treatment for dental pain including prescription medications. At the prenatal and postnatal examination visit, all those women who completed total oral health rehabilitation were characterized to achieve caries-free status (Y/N).

Sample size consideration

The sample size was calculated based on the assumption that the possibility of approximately 72% of pregnant women who had dental visits prior to pregnancy would utilize prenatal dental care. Moreover, approximately 35% of pregnant women who did not have prior-to-pregnancy dental care would utilize prenatal dental care.[12,18,19] Thus, a total sample size of 142 study participants was required to detect the proposed difference, assuming that the exposure rate to nonexposure is 1:9, to achieve 80% power with a two-tailed test of significance at 5%.[18,19]

Statistical analysis

Baseline characteristics of the two groups (pregnant women who received dental care vs pregnant women who did not receive dental care) were compared at all the three time-periods

(eg, prior pregnancy, prenatal, and 1-year postnatal periods) using the Pearson chi-square test or Fisher exact test for categorical independent variables including sociodemographic factors (eg, age group, race, ethnicity, education level, marital status, number of other children and employment status), medical conditions (eg, asthma, diabetes mellitus, hypertension, emotional condition, antibiotic use > 3 months, anti-fungal therapy in the last 3 months, and history of yeast infection), oral health behavior (eg, smoking, brushing frequency) as well as adverse birth outcomes (eg, preterm birth and low birth weight). For continuous variables including oral health status (eg, PI, DMFT index, and ICDAS scores) pairwise mean comparison test or Kruskal-Wallis nonparametric test was used depending on normality distribution. Spearman rank test was used to assess correlation among each of the independent covariates mentioned earlier.

At prenatal and 1-year postnatal periods, two types of outcome variables were used:

- Binary outcome routine dental care (exam and hygiene) utilization (Y/N)
- Ordinal outcome: the type of dental services (no care, urgent care, and routine care).

Multivariate and ordinal logistic regression analyses were conducted for the binary and ordinal outcomes, respectively. Subsequently, exploratory analysis was conducted, and a separate multivariate logistic regression model was established using adverse birth outcome (preterm birth/low birthweight) as a dichotomous dependent variable to assess association with the above-mentioned independent covariates. The independent variables were included in the regression model in multiple steps. First, all pertinent independent variables to be included in the initial model were selected based on the results of exploratory univariate analysis and biologic plausibility. According to previous studies, some independent variables (eg, age group, race, level of education, brushing habits) considered essential and relevant were retained in the model even with high insignificant P values. Pre-pregnancy care (Y/N) and prenatal dental care (Y/N) were used as predictor variables in the regression model with prenatal and postnatal utilization as the outcome of interest to assess utilization patterns at a subsequent time-period. All statistical analysis was performed using STATA software (version 12, STATA).

Results

A total of 186 low-income pregnant women participated in the study. Demographic-socioeconomic and medical conditions of

Table 1 Demographic-socioeconomic-behavior-medical-dental conditions

Parameter		Pre-pregnancy dental exam Y (n = 22)	N (n = 164)	P value	Prenatal dental exam Y (n = 73)	N (n = 113)	P value	Postnatal dental exam Y (n = 37)	N (n = 149)	P value
Age group (y)	18–30	77.27%	68.29%	.39	67.12%	70.80%	.60	64.86%	70.47%	.51
	>30	22.73%	31.71%		32.88%	29.20%		35.14%	29.53%	
Ethnicity	White	13.64%	31.71%	.12	32.88%	27.43%	.70	32.43%	28.86%	.53
	African-American	72.73%	50.00%		49.32%	54.87%		56.76%	51.68%	
	Others	13.64%	18.29%		17.81%	17.70%		10.81%	19.46%	
Hispanic (Y)		4.55%	14.02%	.21	10.96%	14.16%	.53	10.81%	13.42%	.79
History of yeast infection (Y)		18.18%	20.12%	.83	17.81%	21.24%	.57	18.92%	20.13%	.87
Antibiotics usage >3 mo (Y)		0.00%	3.05%	.41	3.54%	1.37%	.65	2.70%	2.68%	.68
Anti-fungal therapy in past 3 mo (Y)		18.18%	4.88%	.02*	4.42%	9.59%	.16	2.70%	7.38%	.47
Tooth-brushing	1. Twice daily	77.27%	64.63%	.35	72.60%	61.95%	.26	67.57%	65.77%	.98
	2. Once daily	22.73%	29.27%		24.66%	30.97%		27.03%	28.86%	
	3. Not everyday	0.00%	6.10%		2.74%	7.08%		5.41%	5.37%	
Diabetes (Y)		9.09%	6.10%	.59	4.11%	7.96%	.37	10.81%	5.37%	.26
Asthma (Y)		4.55%	14.02%	.21	10.96%	14.16%	.53	13.51%	12.75%	.90
Emotional condition (Y)		27.27%	35.37%	.45	31.51%	36.28%	.50	45.95%	31.54%	.10
High blood pressure (Y)		9.09%	15.85%	.41	13.70%	15.93%	.68	8.11%	16.78%	.30
Smoking (Y)		4.55%	17.07%	.13	15.07%	15.93%	.87	18.92%	14.77%	.53
Employed (Y)		63.64%	48.17%	.17	47.95%	51.33%	.65	51.35%	49.66%	.85
Education	Middle school	9.09%	8.54%	.35	8.22%	8.85%	.05	8.11%	8.72%	.73
	High school	45.45%	51.22%		53.42%	48.67%		43.24%	52.35%	
	Associate	4.55%	14.63%		5.48%	18.58%		16.22%	12.75%	
	College or higher	40.91%	25.61%		32.88%	23.89%		32.43%	26.17%	
Marital status	Married	27.27%	21.34%	.53	17.81%	24.78%	.26	21.62%	22.15%	.95
	Single and other	72.73%	78.66%		82.19%	75.22%		78.38%	77.85%	
Number of other children	0	40.91%	33.54%	.78	35.62%	33.63%	.67	27.03%	36.24%	.57
	1	22.73%	27.44%		23.29%	29.20%		29.73%	26.17%	
	≥2	36.36%	39.02%		41.10%	37.17%		43.24%	37.58%	
Adverse birth outcome (Y)		9.09%	5.49%	.50	8.22%	4.42%	.28	0.00%	7.38%	.13
Plaque Index (mean ± SD)		1.5±0.6	1.7±0.6	.34	1.6±0.6	1.7±0.6	.15	1.6±0.6	1.7±0.6	.77

*Statistically significant, $P<.05$.

the study participants are summarized in Table 1. The two groups (eg, pregnant women who utilized dental care and those who did not) were similar at all three time-periods (ie, pre-pregnancy, prenatal, and 1-year postnatal) in terms of demographic factors such as age group, race, ethnicity, education level, employment status, marital status, number of other children, medical background, oral health behaviors such as smoking, brushing habits, and eventual adverse birth outcome experience ($P>.05$) except those who received antifungal therapy in

the past 3 months significantly differed during pre-pregnancy period ($P=.02$). Table 2 presents the oral health condition of the women during pregnancy. Women who used or did not use prenatal dental care differed significantly in oral health condition reflected by DMFT and DMFS scores ($P<.05$). The correlation between demographic, health behaviors, and medical parameters is illustrated in Fig 1. The results demonstrated unmet oral health needs among the underserved US pregnant women. Despite an average of 2.7 ± 3.6 untreated decayed teeth per person

Table 2 Oral health condition of pregnant women

	Prenatal dental care + (n = 73)	Prenatal dental care − (n = 113)	P value
Decayed teeth	2.9±4.2	2.6±3.2	.95
Missing teeth	1.2±1.7	1.0±3.0	.04*
Filled teeth	3.8±3.5	2.5±3.2	.001*
DMFT	7.8±5.8	6.1±4.7	.04*
Decayed surface	5.0±9.0	3.6±6.0	.31
Missing surface	5.7±7.7	4.9±14.1	.04*
Filled surface	7.3±8.6	3.6±5.4	.0001*
DMFS	17.9±16.6	12.1±15.3	.002*
ICDAS	3.7±2.6	3.3±2.3	.20

*Statistically significant, $P<.05$.
DMFS, decayed, missing, and filled surface; DMFT, decayed, missing, and filled teeth; ICDAS, International Caries Detection and Assessment System

during pregnancy, only 39.3% and 19.9% utilize prenatal and 1-year postnatal dental care, respectively. In addition, 41% of the pregnant women had a DMFT scores over 7, and 55% of them had caries severity score (ICDAS) over 3.

Factors associated with utilization of dental services during pregnancy

During the prenatal phase, approximately 39.3% of subjects utilized routine dental care. The factors significantly associated with dental visits during pregnancy are presented in Fig 2a. Of particular interest, significant differences were observed in the cohort's oral care utilization by race. For example, African American women displayed significantly lower odds (odds ratio [OR] 0.43 [95% confidence interval (CI) 0.19, 0.98]) of utilizing prenatal dental care when compared to White women ($P<.05$). In addition, among the other determinants of dental services utilization, the severity of oral disease as measured by the ICDAS scoring system was significantly associated with increased dental visits during pregnancy. Specifically, pregnant women with ICDAS scores>3 were 2.4 (1.09, 5.12) times more likely to utilize prenatal dental visits when compared to those with ICDAS scores≤3 ($P<.05$). Furthermore, a remarkable positive oral health care utilization pattern was observed among the study participants. Pregnant women who had dental visits prior to pregnancy had 7.8 (2.28, 22.66) times higher odds of seeking prenatal dental visits than those who did not utilize dental care prior to pregnancy ($P<.05$).

Factors associated with the type of dental services used during pregnancy

The type of dental services used during pregnancy was categorized into three ordinal levels: level 1 represented women who had no dental care during pregnancy, level 2 included women who used only emergency dental care, and level 3 included women who used both emergency and routine dental care during pregnancy. It was noted that only 9% of women utilized urgent dental care and 29% subjects utilized both urgent and routine dental care during pregnancy. Racial differences were observed, which indicated that African American women were less likely (OR 0.30 [0.14, 0.67]) to use higher-level dental services, including emergency and routine care, compared to White women (Fig 2b) ($P<.05$). Likewise, those who had dental services prior to pregnancy had a greater likelihood (OR 10.5 [3.45, 32.31]) of higher-level dental care usage in the prenatal period than those who did not use dental services prior to pregnancy (Fig 2b) ($P<.05$).

Factors associated with utilization of dental services during the 1-year postpartum

At 1-year postpartum, approximately 19.9% of women in the study utilized routine dental care. It was observed that dental care use during the postnatal phase was particularly driven by prevailing medical conditions as well as oral disease severity (Fig 3a). Higher odds of utilizing postnatal dental care were seen among pregnant women with an existing emotional condition

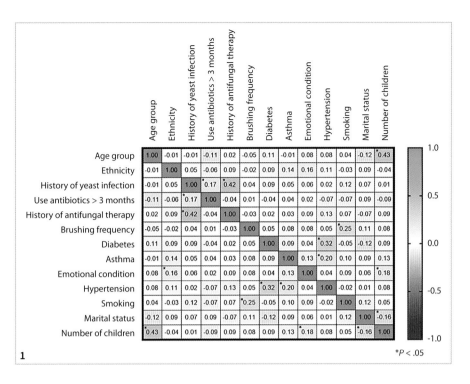

Fig 1 Correlation between demographic-socioeconomic-behavior-medical-dental conditions. Blue indicates positive correlation, whereas red indicates negative correlation, with brighter color indicating stronger correlation (*P < .05).

such as anxiety or depression (OR 2.80 [1.16, 6.57]), or diabetes mellitus (OR 8.10 [1.36, 47.70]) (*P* < .05). In contrast, women with hypertension had lower odds (OR 0.18 [0.03, 0.99]) when compared to women without this medical condition (*P* < .05). In addition, women with ICDAS scores >3 measured during pregnancy had a greater likelihood (OR 4.70 [1.73, 12.74]) of having more dental visits postnatally than those with ICDAS scores ≤3 (*P* < .05). A striking observation was that the unique positive oral health behavior pattern seen during the prenatal phase was exhibited postnatally. Pregnant women with prenatal dental visits had increased odds (OR 3.60 [1.50, 8.60]) of having 1-year postnatal dental care (*P* < .05).

Factors associated with type of dental service used during the 1-year postpartum

The postnatal dental service utilization was characterized similarly as described in the prenatal phase. Approximately, 10% of subjects used urgent dental services and 12% used both routine and urgent dental services during the postnatal phase. The care utilization pattern from no dental care to increased use of emergency plus routine dental care was also determined by the presence of severe dental caries and prevalent medical conditions as described previously (Fig 3b). Greater likelihood of use of both emergency and routine care was seen in women with

emotional condition (OR 4.6 [1.92, 11.07]), diabetes mellitus (OR 10.5 [1.98, 55.98]), and ICDAS scores >3 (OR 6.0 [2.16, 16.44]) when compared to women without these conditions and those with ICDAS scores ≤3, respectively (*P* < .05). Hypertensive women had lower odds (OR 0.17 [0.04, 0.86]) of using increased dental services (*P* < .05). Analogous to the prenatal phase, increased odds (OR 8.72 [3.32, 22.91]) of postnatal utilization of dental services were seen among those who had previously utilized increased dental services in the prenatal period (*P* < .05).

Factors associated with adverse birth outcomes

Exploratory analysis was conducted of factors associated with adverse birth outcomes characterized as preterm and low-birth-weight delivery. A total of 11 women (5.9%) experienced adverse birth outcomes including preterm and low-birth weight delivery. Pregnancy-related hypertension was associated with higher odds (OR 9.28 [1.94, 44.48]), whereas having one or more other children was associated with lower odds (OR 0.10 [0.02, 0.58]) of experiencing an adverse birth outcome (*P* < .05). In addition, higher odds were observed among women with age >30 years, African American women, pregnancy-associated diabetes mellitus, and past antifungal therapy, but it failed to reach statistical significance. Interestingly, those women who achieved prenatal caries-free status after the pregnancy total oral rehabilitation

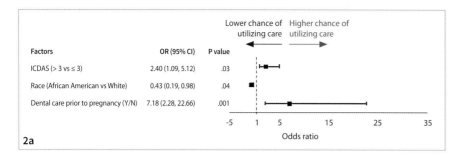

2a

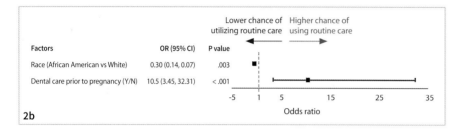

2b

Figs 2a and 2b *(a)* Forest plot for factors that were significantly associated with routine dental care (exam and hygiene) utilized during pregnancy. *(b)* Forest plot for factors that were significantly associated with type of dental care (no care, urgent care, routine care) utilized during pregnancy. African American women had significantly lower odds of utilizing increased dental services during pregnancy, whereas women with severe dental disease (ICDAS > 3) and women who utilized dental care prior to pregnancy had significantly higher odds of seeking prenatal dental care (*P* < .05). Factors adjusted in the model included sociodemographics (eg, age, race, ethnicity, employment status, education level, marital status), medical (eg, recent antifungal therapy, diabetes mellitus, hypertension, emotional condition), oral behaviors and status (eg, brushing frequency, smoking, Plaque Index, ICDAS scores, decayed teeth number) and prior-to-pregnancy dental care utilization.

(PTOR) therapy also had lower odds of experiencing adverse birth outcomes (OR 0.85 [0.17, 4.25], *P* > .05). However, it did not reach statistical significance, possibly due to a small number of cases of an adverse birth outcome experience.

Discussion

The results from this study identified specific determinants of oral health care utilization during critical perinatal periods, including during pregnancy and the 1-year postpartum within this cohort of pregnant women. Numerous studies have detected determinants of dental service utilization; however, there is limited evidence on prenatal oral care utilization among the underserved population residing in New York. Since most of the previous studies have been cross-sectional analyses, the strength of the present study is that study participants were prospectively followed up to determine the factors that influence dental services usage at each period. Also, unlike cross-sectional analysis, a follow-up prospective cohort study allows the establishment of temporality. Understanding the impacts of unmet prenatal oral health needs among the vulnerable populations from a geographically limited sample such as the one used in this study will help address inherent barriers that led to unequal access within the population.

According to Healthy People 2030, approximately 4.6% of the US population nationwide lacked complete access to dental care or had untimely delayed care.[20] The 2019 PRAMS data report that in New York State alone, approximately 8.5% of pregnant women were uninsured 1 month before pregnancy compared to the overall 13.8% of the combined participating states.[21] This highlights the increasing need to improve coverage among pregnant women, especially in New York State. In the past, dental insurance coverage has been recognized as one of the strongest predictors of oral health care utility during pregnancy.[22] The current study used NY state-supported insurance coverage status as determined by income levels to classify low socioeconomic status. The 2011–2016 NHANES survey data analysis describes sociodemographic predictors of dental use among a nationally representative sample of US women. Racial disparities, as well as ethnic minorities such as Mexican American women, less than high school education, younger age group, and uninsured, were among those who were least likely to use dental care (*P* < .025).[23] Racial disparities and financial constraints have also been attributed to suboptimal oral hygiene practices during pregnancy.[12]

In the current analysis, racial disparities were observed among African American pregnant women, who displayed significant underutilization of prenatal oral care (OR 0.43 [0.19, 0.98], *P* = .04). This is consistent with findings from a 2004–2006 population-based survey analysis that reported significantly lower utilization rates during pregnancy along with the substantially increased prevalence of oral diseases among Black

Figs 3a and 3b *(a)* Forest plot for significantly associated with routine 1-year postnatal dental care utilization (exam and hygiene). *(b)* Forest plot for significantly associated with types of 1-year postnatal dental care utilized (no care, urgent care, routine care). Prevailing medical conditions such as emotional condition (anxiety, depression), diabetes mellitus, and severity of dental disease (ICDAS scores > 3) were significantly associated with higher odds of utilizing dental care (*P* < .05). Those who utilized dental care prenatally had a greater likelihood of seeking dental care postnatally as well suggestive of a positive oral health behavior pattern. Factors adjusted in the model included sociodemographics (eg, age, race, ethnicity, employment status, education level, marital status), medical (eg, recent antifungal therapy, diabetes mellitus, hypertension, emotional condition), oral behaviors and status (eg, brushing frequency, smoking, plaque index, ICDAS scores, decayed teeth number) and prenatal dental care utilization.

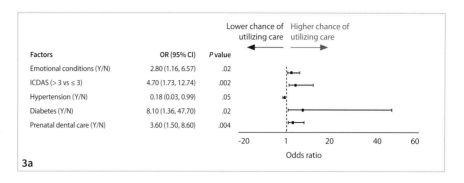

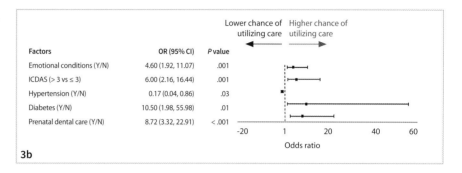

non-Hispanic women when compared to White non-Hispanic women (OR 0.87 [0.77, 0.98] and OR 1.19 [1.05,1.35], respectively).[24] Furthermore, dental caries severity, particularly ICDAS score > 3, was found to be associated with higher odds of seeking increased dental service utilization during pregnancy (OR 2.4 [1.09, 5.12], *P* = .03). Comparably, preliminary analysis from a cross-sectional study correlated the oral health status during pregnancy and the corresponding disease burden with the socioeconomic characteristics of the study subjects.[25] Again, this can be related to findings from the present study, where the increased oral disease burden driven by socioeconomic status was correlated with dental care usage.

In addition, the present study revealed that prior dental care utilization as an impact factor that contributed to higher care utilization rates at a subsequent time point. To the best of the authors' knowledge, this is one of the first prospective studies that assessed existing behavior patterns in oral health care utilization among pregnant women. A distinctively positive oral health behavior pattern was uniquely demonstrated by participating subjects in this study at each time-period. Accordingly, those who previously utilized oral care had the highest odds of seeking dental care at subsequent periods. It can be advantageous to track such behavior patterns and incorporate them

into a program intervention that encourages positive health behaviors such as theory of planned behavior (TPB) based interventions. TPB is one of the most widely used health education models.[26] A qualitative cross-sectional analysis including academic student participants demonstrated that current oral health behavior attitudes strongly predicted intentions to improve oral health compared to perceived oral health behaviors.[26] Therefore, future interventional studies can assess the efficacy of current oral health behavior patterns like the one identified in this study to improve prenatal oral care access.

At the 1-year postpartum period, prevalent medical conditions such as diabetes mellitus and emotional conditions (eg, anxiety, depression) during pregnancy were strong predictors of dental care use. Previous research has reported a seven-fold increase in the risk of developing subsequent type II diabetes mellitus for women with gestational diabetes mellitus (GDM) during pregnancy.[27] Likewise, pregnant women with GDM and subsequent type II diabetes mellitus have a higher risk of increased dental caries and periodontal diseases.[28] Self-perceived poor oral health has also been positively correlated with postpartum depression along with concomitant increased dental caries disease burden.[29] The present findings also indicate that resultant higher untreated dental caries associated with persistent moderate to severe depressive symptoms postnatally significantly predicted dental care usage (OR 2.8 [1.16, 6.57], *P* = .022). This may explain the increased use of dental services postnatally among pregnant women with these existing medical conditions.

Interestingly, postnatal dental care was also significantly determined by higher ICDAS scores, ie scores > 3 (OR 4.7 [1.73, 12.74], *P* = .002). ICDAS assessment is a more robust criterion than DMFT. It incorporates noncavitated early caries lesions and therefore denotes a continuing disease progression state.[30] This indicates that both prenatal and postnatal dental care utilization was dependent upon the severity of dental diseases. Consistent with previously reported inconclusive results, pregnant women's education level was not one of the strongest predictors of both pre- and postnatal dental care usage with this cohort.[31,32] Further, it can be implied that factors other than women's education level such as lack of awareness and knowledge gaps regarding associated risks of poor oral health in pregnancy can serve as a barrier to access to care.[33]

In the present study, as an exploratory effort, factors impacting the eventual adverse birth outcome experience on follow-up were further assessed. A total of 11 women reported an adverse birth outcome (preterm birth or low birth weight). Extensive literature establishes a link between poor oral health and periodontal infection during pregnancy and a subsequent adverse birth outcome experience.[3,34,35] Exclusive to this study, a preliminary analysis of factors that can be attributed to adverse pregnancy outcomes pertinent to this cohort was conducted. The results from the study identified pregnancy-related hypertension was associated with an increased risk of a consequent adverse birth outcome. This was consistent with previous research demonstrating that it was a clinically apparent hypertensive state that correlated with an adverse birth outcome experience. However, a dose-response relationship is also demonstrated between critical blood pressure levels at different trimesters, which can be positively correlated to an adverse birth outcome experience.[36,37] Also, having one or more other children was associated with reduced odds of an adverse birth outcome (OR 0.10 [0.02, 0.68], *P* = .018). An earlier case-control study attempted to determine the association between the number of previous live births and an adverse birth outcome experience.[38] No significant correlation could be established, but the majority of cases in that study had less than three live births, which is consistent with the present results.[38] Furthermore, increasingly higher odds for adverse birth outcomes were seen among age > 30 years, African American women, non-Hispanics, and existing type II diabetes mellitus; however,

this failed to reach statistical significance. Interestingly, women who achieved prenatal caries-free status after PTOR therapy also had lower odds of experiencing an adverse birth outcome. Again, however, it did not reach statistical significance, possibly due to limited adverse birth cases, which is one of the limitations of the study. Furthermore, more robust future studies are required to further explore the impacts of PTOR therapy on an adverse birth outcome experience.

An unmet oral health need is where maximum disease burden exists. It is important that the clinician is aware of inherent barriers within the population to be able to implement strategies that counteract unequal access and reduce disease burden. Although dental care usage was predominantly reliant upon dental disease severity, the present results indicated significant underutilization. This highlights the crucial role of general dental practitioners in addressing community-level barriers by promoting oral health screenings and preventive dental services during pregnancy, which can significantly alleviate risks. In addition, interprofessional collaborative practices with prenatal medical providers and meaningful engagement with policymakers can enable a comprehensive approach to oral care during pregnancy.

There were other potential limitations of the present study. The study subjects were sampled from a birth cohort of an existing study and included a geographically restricted population. Therefore, the study's findings lack external validity and generalizability. Also, certain information, such as oral hygiene habits, was self-reported by the study participants and could be prone to bias or inaccuracies. Moreover, dental care utilization was obtained from electronic dental records. Although the URMC-EIOH is one of the primary dental care facilities that accommodate dental needs and provide dental care to the majority of the underserved pregnant women residing in Rochester, New York, information on dental care occurred outside of URMC-EIOH was not obtained. Therefore, the present results could underestimate and overestimate the impact of identified factors associated with perinatal dental care utilization. ⊞

Conclusion

Racial and oral health disparity is associated with perinatal oral healthcare utilization within this cohort of underserved pregnant women. The results indicate unmet oral health needs among underserved pregnant women residing in Upstate New York. Both prenatal and postnatal dental care utilization was positively associated with dental caries severity, especially postnatal care which was dependent upon existing medical conditions (eg, hypertension, diabetes mellitus, and emotional condition). Further, pregnancy-associated hypertension was associated with significant risk, whereas having more than one other child alleviated risk of an adverse birth outcome experience, as per exploratory analysis. Although an insignificant finding, post oral rehabilitation, caries-free pregnant women had lower odds of experiencing an adverse birth outcome. As this was a geographically limited sample, the results are particularly true for this cohort. Besides, these findings add to existing information on oral care determinants among low-income populations that can guide statewide efforts to maximize dental care usage in pregnancy. Future robust studies are warranted to assess effective strategies further to improve perinatal dental care utilization among underserved pregnant women and demonstrate health benefits, including birth outcomes from receiving prenatal dental care.

Acknowledgment

This study was supported by the National Institute of Dental and Craniofacial Research grant K23DE027412 and R01 DE031025. Dr Wu's work is also supported by grant from the National Science Foundation NSF-CCF-1934962. The authors report there are no conflicts of interest.

References

1. Nazir MA, Izhar F, Akhtar K, Almas K. Dentists' awareness about the link between oral and systemic health. J Family Community Med 2019;26:206–212.

2. Steinberg BJ, Hilton IV, Iida H, Samelson R. Oral health and dental care during pregnancy. Dent Clin North Am 2013;57:195–210.

3. Puertas A, Magan-Fernandez A, Blanc V, et al, Association of periodontitis with preterm birth and low birth weight: a comprehensive review. J Matern Fetal Neonatal Med 2018;31:597–602.

4. Xiao J, Alkhers N, Kopycka-Kedzierawski DT, et al. Prenatal oral health care and early childhood caries prevention: a systematic review and meta-analysis. Caries Res 2019; 53:411–421.

5. Geevarghese A, Baskaradoss JK, Sarma PS. Oral health-related quality of life and periodontal status of pregnant women. Matern Child Health J 2017;21:1634–1642.

6. Jang H, Al Jallad N, Wu TT, et al. Changes in Candida albicans, Streptococcus mutans and oral health conditions following prenatal total oral rehabilitation among underserved pregnant women. Heliyon 2021;7:e07871.

7. Jang H, Patoine A, Wu TT, Castillo DA, Xiao J. Oral microflora and pregnancy: a systematic review and meta-analysis. Sci Rep 2021;11:16870.

8. Rocha JS, Arima L, Chibinski AC, Werneck RI, Moysés SJ, Baldani MH. Barriers and facilitators to dental care during pregnancy: a systematic review and meta-synthesis of qualitative studies. Cad Saude Publica 2018;34:e00130817.

9. Byrd MG, Quinonez RB, Lipp K, Chuang A, Phillips C, Weintraub JA. Translating prenatal oral health clinical standards into dental education: results and policy implications. J Public Health Dent 2019;79:25–33.

10. Adeniyi A, Donnelly L, Janssen P, Jevitt C, von Bergman H, Brondani M. A qualitative study of health care providers' views on integrating oral health into prenatal care. JDR Clin Trans Res 2021;6:409–419.

11. Naavaal S, Brickhouse TH, Hafidh S, Smith K. Factors associated with preventive dental visits before and during pregnancy. J Womens Health (Larchmt) 2019;28:1670–1678.

12. Boggess KA, Urlaub DM, Massey KE, Moos MK, Matheson MB, Lorenz C. Oral hygiene practices and dental service utilization among pregnant women. J Am Dent Assoc 2010;141:553–561.

13. Gadson A, Akpovi E, Mehta PK. Exploring the social determinants of racial/ethnic disparities in prenatal care utilization and maternal outcome. Semin Perinatol 2017; 41:308–317.

14. Alkhars N, Zeng Y, Alomeir N, et al. Oral Candida predicts Streptococcus mutans emergence in underserved US infants. J Dent Res 2022;101:54–62.

15. Shivakumar K, Prasad S, Chandu G. International Caries Detection and Assessment System: A new paradigm in detection of dental caries. J Conserv Dent 2009;12:10–16.

16. Petersen PE, Baez RJ, World Health Organization. Oral health surveys: basic methods. 5th ed. Geneva: World Health Organization, 2013.

17. Löe H. The Gingival Index, the Plaque Index and the Retention Index Systems. J Periodontol 1967;38(Suppl):610–616.

18. Hulley SB, Cummings SR, Browner WS, Grady DG, Newman TB. Designing Clinical Research. Philadelphia: Wolters Kluwer, 2013.

19. Fleiss JL, Tytun A, Ury HK. A simple approximation for calculating sample sizes for comparing independent proportions. Biometrics 1980;36:343–346.

20. Reduce the proportion of people who can't get the dental care they need when they need it — AHS-05. Healthy People 2030, Objectives and Data, Health Care Access and Quality. https://health.gov/healthypeople/objectives-and-data/browse-objectives/health-care-access-and-quality/reduce-proportion-people-who-cant-get-dental-care-they-need-when-they-need-it-ahs-05. Accessed 10 January 2022.

21. Prevalence of Selected Maternal and Child Health Indicators for New York City, Pregnancy Risk Assessment Monitoring System (PRAMS), 2016–2019. https://www.cdc.gov/prams/prams-data/mch-indicators/states/pdf/2019/New-York-City_PRAMS_Prevalence-of-Selected-Indicators_ 2016-2019_508.pdf. Accessed 10 January 2022.

22. Lee H, Marsteller JA, Wenzel J. Dental care utilization during pregnancy by Medicaid dental coverage in 26 states: Pregnancy risk assessment monitoring system 2014–2015. J Public Health Dent 2022;82:61–71.

23. Gupta A, Feldman S, Perkins RB, Stokes A, Sankar V, Villa A. Predictors of dental care use, unmet dental care need, and barriers to unmet need among women: results from NHANES, 2011 to 2016. J Public Health Dent 2019;79:324–333.

24. Hwang SS, Smith VC, McCormick MC, Barfield WD. Racial/ethnic disparities in maternal oral health experiences in 10 states, pregnancy risk assessment monitoring system, 2004–2006. Matern Child Health J 2011;15:722–729.

25. Chung LH, Gregorich SE, Armitage GC, Gonzalez-Vargas J, Adams SH. Sociodemographic disparities and behavioral factors in clinical oral health status during pregnancy. Community Dent Oral Epidemiol 2014;42:151–159.

26. Dumitrescu AL, Wagle M, Dogaru BC, Manolescu B. Modeling the theory of planned behavior for intention to improve oral health behaviors: the impact of attitudes, knowledge, and current behavior. J Oral Sci 2011;53:369–377.

27. Bellamy L, Casas JP, Hingorani AD, Williams D. Type 2 diabetes mellitus after gestational diabetes: a systematic review and meta-analysis. Lancet 2009;373(9677):1773–1779.

28. Friedlander AH, Chaudhuri G, Altman L. A past medical history of gestational diabetes: its medical significance and its dental implications. Oral Surg Oral Med Oral Pathol Oral Radiol Endod 2007;103:157–163.

29. Cademartori MG, Demarco FF, Freitas da Silveira M, Barros FC, Corrêa MB. Dental caries and depression in pregnant women: The role of oral health self-perception as mediator (Epub ahead of print, 2 Feb 2021). Oral Dis doi: 10.1111/odi.13789.

30. Gugnani N, Pandit IK, Srivastava N, Gupta M, Sharma M. International Caries Detection and Assessment System (ICDAS): A new concept. Int J Clin Pediatr Dent 2011;4:93–100.

31. Timothé P, Eke PI, Presson SM, Malvitz DM. Dental care use among pregnant women in the United States reported in 1999 and 2002. Prev Chronic Dis 2005;2:A10.

32. Amin M, ElSalhy M. Factors affecting utilization of dental services during pregnancy. J Periodontol 2014;85:1712–1721.

33. Swathi K, Koothati RK, Motor RR, Priyadarshini, RajaShekar CH, Vallakonda S. Knowledge and experience of women about dental services utilization during pregnancy: a cross-sectional questionnaire study. J Pharm Bioallied Sci 2021;13(Suppl 2):S1042–S1046.

34. Cobb CM, Kelly PJ, Williams KB, Babbar S, Angolkar M, Derman RJ. The oral microbiome and adverse pregnancy outcomes. Int J Womens Health 2017;9:551–559.

35. Cho GJ, Kim SY, Lee HC, et al. Association between dental caries and adverse pregnancy outcomes. Sci Rep 2020;10:5309.

36. Bakker R, Steegers EA, Hofman A, Jaddoe VW. Blood pressure in different gestational trimesters, fetal growth, and the risk of adverse birth outcomes: the generation R study. Am J Epidemiol 2011;174:797–806.

37. Zhu B, Huang K, Bao W, et al. Dose-response relationship between maternal blood pressure in pregnancy and risk of adverse birth outcomes: Ma'anshan birth cohort study. Pregnancy Hypertens 2019;15:16–22.

38. Abadiga M, Mosisa G, Tsegaye R, Oluma A, Abdisa E, Bekele T. Determinants of adverse birth outcomes among women delivered in public hospitals of Ethiopia, 2020. Arch Public Health 2022;80:12.

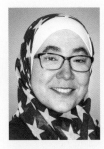

Nisreen Al Jallad

Nisreen Al Jallad* Research Fellow, Eastman Institute for Oral Health, University of Rochester Medical Center, Rochester, NY, USA

Shruti Vasani* Research Fellow, Eastman Institute for Oral Health, University of Rochester Medical Center, Rochester, NY, USA

Tong Tong Wu Associate Professor, Department of Biostatistics and computational biology, University of Rochester Medical Center, Rochester, NY, USA

Rita Cacciato Human Subject Research Coordinator II, Eastman Institute for Oral Health, University of Rochester Medical Center, Rochester, NY, USA

Marie Thomas Health Project Coordinator, Department of Family Medicine, University of Rochester Medical Center, Rochester, NY, USA

Nour Lababede 4th year Undergraduate Student, Case Western University, Cleveland, OH, USA

Ayah Lababede 2nd year Undergraduate Student, Case Western University, Cleveland, OH, USA

Jin Xiao Associate Professor, Director for Perinatal Oral Health, Eastman Institute for Oral Health, University of Rochester Medical Center, Rochester, NY, USA

*Equal contribution.

Correspondence: Associate Professor Jin Xiao, Director, Perinatal Oral Health, Eastman Institute of Oral Health, University of Rochester, 625 Elmwood Ave, Rochester, NY 14620, USA. Email: jin_xiao@urmc.rochester.edu

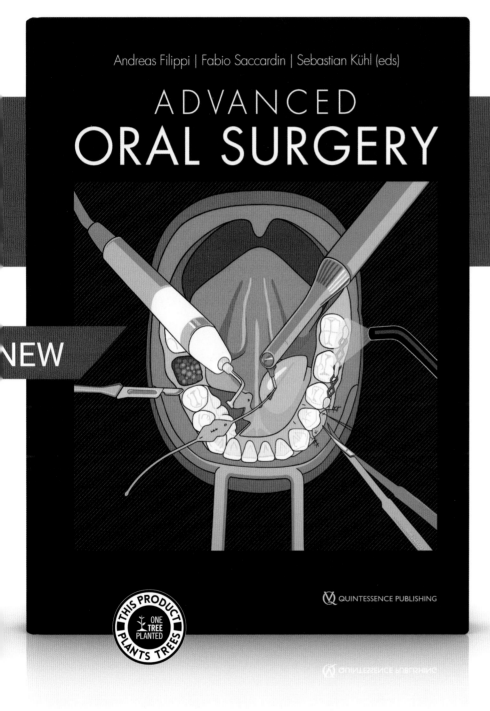
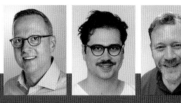

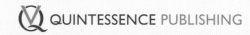

Oral health disparities among the 65+ age group

Ayelet Berg-Warman, PhD/Ile Kermel-Schiffman, PhD/Shlomo Paul Zusman, DMD, MSc(DPH), MPA, DDPH.RCS/
Lena Natapov, DMD, MPH, MPA

Objective: Oral and dental health significantly impacts the quality of life and nutrition of the older population. While government action has been taken in Israel to reduce barriers to using dental care services by welfare recipients among older adults, there are still disparities associated with socioeconomic status in the older adult population. In 2019, a dental care reform for the older adults was implemented in Israel assuring dental Universal Health Coverage (UCH) for them. This has improved accessibility to dental services and reduced cost barriers. The aim of the present article was to explore the oral health disparities among the 65+ age group by their socioeconomic situation, and their additional barriers to using dental services at the start of the reform. **Method and materials:** Telephone interviews were conducted with a representative sample of 512 older adults aged 65+ from February to April 2020. **Results:** The self-perceived oral health status was rated as better in the higher socioeconomic group (73.4% perceived their oral health status as good or very good), compared with the lower socioeconomic group (52.5%). In the lower socioeconomic group, 38.5% were edentulous, compared with 18.1% of the higher socioeconomic group. The latter group had four more natural teeth, on average, than the former. Regarding the prevalence of dental problems, double and triple gaps were also found, as well as loose, sore, and sensitive teeth, and difficulty chewing. Oral health behavior, as reflected in tooth brushing patterns and routine preventive check-ups, was found to be better in the higher socioeconomic group than in the lower socioeconomic group. Dental care costs were found to be a barrier to dental care, primarily in the lower socioeconomic group (18.2%, compared with 4.8% of the higher socioeconomic group, were faced with a financial barrier). At the same time, 66.7% of the higher socioeconomic group were aware of the inclusion of dental care services for the older adult population in the basket of health services provided by the health plans, compared with 27.8% of the lower socioeconomic group. **Conclusions:** Lack of awareness to proper oral health behavior and to their legal rights were the main barriers to dental care in the lower socioeconomic groups. Dental practitioners play a vital role and have an opportunity to lower these barriers. Existing disparities and barriers should be monitored as a vital part of including dental care in Universal Health Coverage. *(Quintessence Int 2023;54:344–352; doi: 10.3290/j.qi.b3819531)*

Key words: dental health policy, dental service utilization, elderly, oral health, oral health disparities, Universal Health Coverage

As stated in the draft Global Oral Health Action Plan (2023 to 2030), "The vision of the global strategy on oral health is UHC [Universal Health Coverage] for oral health for all individuals and communities by 2030, enabling them to enjoy the highest attainable state of oral health and contributing to healthy and productive lives."[1] Rightly so, since aging is correlated with deterioration of oral and dental health, both of which have a significant negative impact on the ability to chew, swallow, and speak. Those limitations negatively impact nutrition and thus overall physical health and quality of life during later life. They also affect the social engagement and self-esteem of older adults.[2]

Accessibility to dental care is vital for the maintenance of oral health. Low-income and low-education groups as well as minority and immigrant groups, home-bound older adults, and institution residents are at a high risk of dental morbidity.[3-8]

The oral health status of older adults is affected in part by their barriers to using dental care services. Barriers include cohort and age, race, income and education, availability of dental services and medical insurance, and functional health.[9] In the US, Hispanic and non-Hispanic black aged 65 years and over were more likely to have unmet needs for dental care due to cost.[10]

A nationwide study conducted in Israel about 22 years ago[11] indicated dental morbidity differences between socioeconomic groups: about 70% of older adults aged 65+ in the lowest-income third were edentulous, compared with 45% of older adults aged 65+ in the highest-income third. Study also showed that about 88% of low-income older adults aged 65+ reported having maxillary and/or mandibular dentures, compared with 63% of high-income older adults aged 65+.

A study by Adut et al[12] indicated that 54.4% of older adults aged 65+ living in the community were edentulous, whereas others had 10.4 teeth on average. The highest percentage of edentulous older adults aged 65+ was found in the Arab population in Israel (67.2%).

A study by Natapov et al[13] investigated the effect of oral health on nutritional status among older people and found lower energy intake among people with complete dentures compared to those who had natural teeth.

Studies conducted in Israel[8,9,14] emphasized the economic barriers and the importance of including preventive, restorative, and reconstructive treatments in the basket of services of the National Health Insurance Law (NHIL).

This long-needed UHC reform for older people was implemented in 2019 with the aim of improving the older adults' access and reducing their barriers to the use of these services. Since February 2019, preventive and restorative treatments (procedures to repair and restore damaged teeth) have been included in the basket of services guaranteed by NHIL for those 75+, and since October 2019 reconstructive treatments (procedures to replace missing teeth, and repair damaged teeth and faulty bites) have been included for 80+ years old. The reform was widened in 2022 and the entitlement age was lowered to 72 years of age.

Is the UHC the panacea? Including preventive and restorative treatments in the basket of services guaranteed by NHIL for older adults was the second step after starting UHC in Israel for children in 2010.[15] Report of the benefits of the UHC for children has been published.[16]

In a former article,[12] the oral health of the 65+ age group in Israel was presented. One of the conclusions was that one of "The main barriers [is] … the cost of care for people with financial difficulty."

For deeper scrutiny of this issue, the present study explored oral health disparities and oral health behavior patterns among older adults immediately after the start of the UHC reform by their socioeconomic status (SES).

The information provided will enable the examination and identification of oral health disparities between different socio-economic groups and help policy makers to further improve the provision of dental care services to the older adult population, as part of UHC.

Method and materials

The study population consisted of all older adults aged 65+ living in the community in Israel (1,056 million people). Older adults in institutions were excluded from the study.

The sampling method has been described elsewhere.[14] A random sample of 1,250 people aged 65+ was drawn from computerized telephone books. From the random sample of 1,250 people 65+ years old, 64 had died, in 174 cases the telephone numbers were wrong, and 258 subjects could not be reached by phone over several weeks. The remaining 754 older adults aged 65+ with validated phone numbers were included in the study.

The interview questionnaire included validated questions from international comparative surveys – the first[17] and second[18] International Collaborative Study (ICS I and ICS II) – conducted by the World Health Organization; and by the National Institute of Dental Research.[19] The questionnaire dealt with the following issues: older adults' self-perceived oral health status, their awareness of the vital importance of oral and dental health, and their knowledge of proper oral health behavior. In order to accommodate two large non-Hebrew speaking groups, the questionnaire was translated into Arabic and Russian (questionnaire available upon request). The questionnaire was pretested on 15 interviewees. Since only minor changes were needed, subsequently those interviews were added to the study.

The interviews were conducted by experienced interviewers who received specific guidelines from the researchers. An interview took 30 minutes on average.

Data analysis

Weighting was done to improve the representativeness of the sample. Weights were calculated according to percentages of age groups, ethnic groups, and socioeconomic status (SES), in accordance with the Central Bureau of Statistics data.[20]

The distribution of the characteristics examined was calculated, and comparative analyses were conducted according to SES, which was measured by the ability to cover monthly household expenses:

- covering expenses without difficulty (high SES)
- managing to cover expenses (middle SES)
- finding it difficult or failing to cover expenses (low SES).

Table 1 Background characteristics classified by socioeconomic status (N = 512)

Characteristic		Total[†]	Socioeconomic status		
			Low	Middle	High
Participants	Number	512	121	258	103
	%	100.0	25.1	53.5	21.4
Sex* (%)	Men	48.0	39.0	48.8	65.2
	Women	52.0	61.0	51.2	34.8
Age group (%)	65–74 y	59.2	52.0	62.4	63.8
	75–84y	28.6	35.0	24.5	31.9
	85+ y	12.2	13.0	13.1	4.3
Marital status* (%)	Married	71.2	61.5	71.6	89.5
	Widowed	20.8	30.3	19.5	7.4
	Divorced/single/separated	8.0	8.2	8.8	3.2
Education*** (%)	Primary	18.6	39.1	14.4	5.4
	Secondary	33.9	34.5	34.9	22.5
	Post-secondary	15.1	10.0	16.2	15.1
	Academic	32.4	16.4	34.5	57.0
Religion* (%)	Jewish	89.1	79.8	91.0	96.8
	Muslim	6.6	15.6	4.3	3.2
	Other	4.4	4.6	4.7	0.0
Working* (%)		24.5	19.3	23.2	46.8

*P<.05; ***P<.001.
[†]Including 30 interviewees who failed to answer the question regarding the ability to cover monthly household expenses.

Comparative analyses of some of the characteristics examined were conducted according to sex and population group. The comparative analyses were conducted using chi-square tests, and independent samples *t* tests were used to compare the average number of natural teeth by age, sex, and population group. A linear regression was used to explain oral health status, using background and oral health behavior as independent variables. Statistical significance was indicated at P<.05.

Ethics

The study was approved by the Helsinki Committee at the Ministry of Health (No. 16/2019; 11 July 2019) and by the Ethics Committee of the Myers-JDC-Brookdale Institute (23 July 2019). The prospective interviewees in the sample were informed of the study background and goals and subsequently asked to give their explicit consent to take part in the study. Interviews were conducted only with those who agreed to be interviewed.

Results

From the 754 participants in the study, 168 declined to take part, and 74 were not interviewed for other reasons (language barrier, communication problems, or completion of the study). Telephone interviews were conducted with 512 participants (response rate of 67.9%). The interviews were conducted from February to April 2020. In those cases where the interviewee could not respond due to declining health or cognitive status, a close family member was interviewed. Altogether, 34 family members were interviewed and asked to provide information on the oral health status of the older adult, for instance, the number of natural teeth retained and the frequency of visits to a dental care clinic.

The average age of the interviewees was 75.6 years (standard deviation [SD] 6.4). Table 1 presents the interviewees' characteristics classified by their SES. As shown in Table 1, 52.0% of the interviewees were women, and 71.2% were married. Differences between the SES groups were found in the proportion of women (61.0% of the low SES group compared with 34.8% of the high SES group); in the marital status (61.5% of the low SES group

Table 2 Oral health status and characteristics by socioeconomic status (%) (n = 512).

Status and characteristics		Total[†]	Socioeconomic status		
			Low	Middle	High
Self-perceived oral health status* (%)	Very good	15.4	9.2	16.5	18.1
	Good	50.1	43.1	50.6	55.3
	Not so good	25.0	29.4	26.0	16.0
	Not good	9.5	18.3	6.9	10.6
Retained natural teeth	None retained*** (%)	23.9	38.5	18.6	18.1
	All retained (%)	9.9	3.7	12.1	9.4
	No. of teeth (partially and completely dentulous) (mean ± SD) (n)	19.1 ± 10.5	18.2 ± 10.4	18.7 ± 10.8	22.2 ± 9.6
	No. of teeth (65+ age group) (mean ± SD) (n)	14.0 ± 12.3	10.3 ± 12.0	14.8 ± 12.3	18.2 ± 12.2
	Sore or sensitive gums*** (%)	20.0	28.4	17.6	13.8
	Bleeding gums (%)	14.3	16.4	13.2	20.0
Dental and periodontal problems (%)	Loose teeth***	11.7	26.5	8.5	7.8
	Swollen gums*	10.4	15.6	9.0	10.6
	Difficulty chewing***	19.6	33.9	17.4	9.5
	Suffering from bad breath (often or occasionally)	17.2	18.1	17.9	8.0

*$P<.05$; ***$P<.001$.
[†]Including 30 interviewees who failed to answer the question regarding the ability to cover monthly household expenses.

were married, compared with 89.5% of the high SES group); in the education level (16.4% of the low SES group had academic education, compared with 57.0% of the high SES group); and in the work force participation rate (19.3% of the low SES group, compared with 46.8% of the high SES group).

Oral health status and characteristics

The interviewees' responses regarding their oral, dental, and periodontal health status are presented in Table 2. As shown, 65.5% of the interviewees perceived their oral health status as very good or good; 25.0% rated it as not so good; and 9.5% rated it as not good. As further shown, 23.9% were edentulous while 9.9% retained all their natural teeth.

Analysis of the interviewees' oral health characteristics classified by their SES indicated a positive correlation between the self-perceived oral health status and the SES. This positive correlation was further corroborated by the proportion of edentulous, partially dentulous, and completely dentulous participants in the different SES groups: 18.1% of the high SES group

were edentulous and the rest had 22.2 teeth on the average; in contrast, 38.5% of the low SES group were edentulous and the rest had 18.2 teeth on the average. Of the 65+ age group, 63.0% (70.4% of the low SES group and 45.9% of the high SES group) reported having 20 teeth or less (not shown in the table); 20 is the minimum number of teeth required for adequate oral function, according to the World Health Organization.[20]

Likewise, the prevalence of dental and periodontal problems was higher in the low SES group compared with the high SES group, as specifically reflected in the percentage of those reporting having loose teeth (26.5% compared with 7.8%, respectively), sore and sensitive teeth (28.4% compared with 13.8%, respectively), or difficulty chewing (33.9% compared with 9.5%, respectively).

Virtually no differences were found between men and women with respect to the number of retained natural teeth: 23.9% of women reported being edentulous, compared with 26.8% of men ($P=.720$); similarly, the number of retained natural teeth reported by women was 19.7 and that reported by men was 18.4 ($P=.279$). Significant differences were found between Jews and non-Jews: 22.4% of Jews reported being edentulous, compared with 50.0% of

Table 3 Use patterns of dentures classified by socioeconomic status (%) (N = 512)

Characteristic		Total[†]	Socioeconomic status		
			Low	Middle	High
Having dentures		43.8	49.0	43.3	32.6
Frequency of use of the dentures*	All the time	48.0	43.6	44.7	73.5
	Only during waking hours	42.7	40.0	46.6	26.5
	Just for eating	3.5	3.6	3.9	0.0
	Only in social settings	0.9	0.0	1.9	0.0
	Not using	4.8	10.9	2.9	0.0

*$P < .05$.
[†]Including 30 interviewees who failed to answer the question regarding the ability to cover monthly house-hold expenses.

non-Jews ($P < .001$). The data analysis also indicated a higher prevalence of periodontal problems among women: 23.9% of the women reported having sore or sensitive gums, compared with 17.2% of the men ($P = .045$). Similarly, 14.5% of the women reported having swollen gums, compared with 7.5% of the men ($P = .011$).

Table 3 presents the use patterns of dentures by SES. As shown, 43.8% of the interviewees reported having dentures, and a higher percentage was reported by the low SES group (49.0%) compared with 32.6% of the high SES group ($P = .177$). Of the low SES group, 10.9% reported that they had never used dentures, while none of the high SES group reported this.

As for the problems associated with the use of dentures, about 10% reported that they suffered pain or sores using the dentures and about 20% reported that they had difficulty eating while wearing their dentures. In this respect, no differences at a significance level of 5% were found between men and women. For dental implants, 39% of all participants had implants; 28.4% of the low SES group compared with 46.8% of the high SES group ($P < .05$). Of the latter, 47% were satisfied with their implants, compared with 78% in low SES (not significant, results not shown).

Oral health awareness, knowledge, and behavior patterns

Oral health behavior patterns, which may affect oral health status, were examined with reference to three indicators: tooth brushing, oral care by a dental hygienist, and visits to the dental practitioner for routine preventive check-ups (Table 4). In total, 69.4% of the interviewees reported that they regularly brush their teeth at least twice a day; 23.2% regularly brush their teeth once a day; a lower frequency of tooth brushing was reported by 4.0% of the interviewees; and 3.4% reported that they never

brush their teeth (6.4% of the low SES group, compared with 3.2% of the high SES group). Furthermore, the percentage of interviewees who reportedly had never received oral care by a dental hygienist is 3.1 times higher in the low SES group than in the high SES group (52.7% and 17.2%, respectively).

About 40% of the interviewees regularly visit a dental practitioner for preventive check-ups to identify and take care of oral health problems before they become more acute and cause pain. In total, 31.0% of the interviewees reported that they visit a dental practitioner for preventive check-ups at least once a year, and a lower frequency was reported by 8.9%. Interviewees who reportedly never visit a dental practitioner for routine preventive check-ups were asked to explain the reasons for their failure to do so. The two main reasons cited were lack of awareness of the importance of routine preventive check-ups (63.6%) and the costs involved (6.7%). It was also found that oral health behavior patterns differ by SES: 27.5% of the low SES group regularly visit a dental practitioner for routine preventive check-ups, compared with 50.6% of the high SES group. In total, 18.2% of the low SES group attributed their failure to visit a dental practitioner for routine preventive check-ups to the costs involved, compared with 4.8% of the high SES group (Table 4). In total, 66.7% of the high SES group were aware of the dental care reform for older adults, compared with 27.8% of the low SES group and 43.9% of the middle SES group.

Knowledge of proper oral health behavior and attitudes towards it were also examined. In total, 44.8% of the interviewees noted that the consumption of sweets is very harmful for dental health; 17.2% believe that it is moderately harmful for dental health; 9.8% believe that it is not so harmful; and 28.2% stated that it is not at all harmful or that they do not know whether it is harmful for dental health.

Table 4 Oral health behavior patterns classified by socioeconomic status (%) (N = 512)

Oral health behavior		Total†	Socioeconomic status		
			Low	Middle	High
Tooth brushing	At least twice a day	69.4	68.8	68.8	75.5
	Less than twice a day	27.2	24.7	29.1	21.3
	Never	3.4	6.4	2.1	3.2
Oral care by a dental hygienist	Visited a dental hygienist in the last year	35.5	31.0	57.4	45.3
	Never visited a dental hygienist	44.5	52.7	45.5	17.2
Frequency of routine preventive check-ups*	At least once a year	31.0	26.4	31.9	42.5
	At a lower frequency	8.9	1.1	10.2	8.1
	Never	60.1	72.4	58.0	49.4
Reasons for failure to visit the dentist for routine preventive check-ups or for infrequent visits*	Lack of time	3.6	4.5	2.5	14.3
	The costs involved	6.7	18.2	3.4	4.8
	Waiting times/distance from the dental practitioner's clinic	2.8	3.0	2.5	7.1
	Lack of awareness of the importance of routine preventive check-ups	63.6	54.5	66.4	50.0
	Forgetfulness/laziness	6.3	8.3	6.7	4.8
	Other	17.0	12.1	17.6	19.0

*$P < .05$.
†Including 30 interviewees who failed to answer the question regarding the ability to cover monthly household expenses.

To examine the unique effect of different variables on oral health, a multivariate analysis was used. The number of natural teeth was a proxy for oral health status (see Table 5). A multivariate linear regression was used to determine the effect of the following variables:

- age group (1, ≥ 85 years; 0, < 85 years)
- sex (1, women; 0, men)
- SES (1, covering monthly household expenses; 0, finding it difficult or failing to cover expenses)
- population group/religion (1, Jews; 0, non-Jews)
- oral health behavior patterns (1, regularly visits a dental practitioner for routine preventive check-ups; 0, never visits)
- frequency of tooth brushing (1, at least twice a day; 0, less than twice a day)
- knowledge of proper oral health behavior (1, sweets are harmful for dental health; 0, sweets are not harmful for dental health).

It was found that background characteristics and oral health behavior patterns have an impact on oral health status. The variables with the greatest impact were:

- age – a negative correlation was found between age and number of natural teeth (as age increases fewer teeth are retained)

- frequency of visits to the dental practitioner for routine preventive check-ups – a positive correlation was found between the frequency of visits and the number of retained natural teeth
- SES – those in the high and middle SES groups retained more natural teeth
- population group/religion – Jews retained more natural teeth
- tooth brushing frequency – the higher the frequency the higher the number of natural teeth retained.

The multivariate linear regression model accounted for 15% of the variance of the dependent variable ($R^2 = 0.151$; F = 8.44).

Discussion

This paper presents study findings regarding oral health inequalities and oral health behavior differences among older adults aged 65+ in Israel at the beginning of inclusion of oral health for elderly in UHC by their socioeconomic situation. The proportion of edentulousness was 2.2 times higher in the lower SES group (38.5%) than in the higher SES group (18.1%). Similarly, the average number of retained natural teeth was low (18.2) in the lower SES group, compared with 22.2 in the higher SES group. Furthermore, the prevalence of reported periodon-

Table 5 Linear regression coefficients accounting for the number of natural teeth retained (N = 512)

Parameter	B	Standard deviation	Beta	t	P
Age (85+ years)	−8.314	2.007	−2.214	−4.142	<.001
Regularly visiting a dental practitioner for routine preventive check-ups vs not visiting regularly for routine check-ups	4.708	1.277	0.190	3.688	<.001
Economic status (high and middle vs low SES)	4.429	1.575	0.147	2.812	.005
Population group/religion (Jewish vs non-Jewish)	5.239	2.292	0.119	2.286	.023
Tooth brushing frequency (twice a day vs less)	2.562	1.375	0.096	1.864	.063
Sex (women vs men)	1.588	1.271	0.065	1.250	.212
Knowledge (sweets are harmful for dental health vs not harmful)	0.125	1.262	0.005	0.099	.921
Constant	5.354	2.788		0.615	.539

tal problems and cases of loose teeth, which cause chewing difficulties, was higher in the lower SES group, compared with the higher SES group.

According to the World Health Organization,[21] the number of teeth required for adequate oral function is 20. With fewer teeth, there is a brusque drop in comfortable eating and social engagement. The current study presents a gloomy picture of the oral health status of older adults in Israel by SES: 63.0% of the 65+ age group (70.4% of the lower SES group and 45.9% of the higher SES group) reported having 20 teeth or less.

However, virtually no differences in oral health status were found between men and women in the present study or in other studies.[4,8] While the present study shows that the oral health status (as expressed by number of teeth) of women is somewhat better than that of men, no sex-related statistically significant differences were indicated.

Also, in line with a previous study by Adut et al,[10] the present study shows that the oral health status of the 65+ age group has improved and that the Jewish population in Israel has better oral health than that of the non-Jewish population.

The differences in oral health status may be attributed, inter alia, to differences in oral health behavior patterns, eg, tooth brushing, visits to the dental practitioner for routine preventive check-ups, and oral care by a dental hygienist. The main reasons for the failure to maintain a proper oral health routine were lack of awareness of its importance, and dental care costs, which are the major barriers to dental care, primarily in the lower SES group, as shown by the present study as well as by previous studies conducted in Israel and in other countries.[6,9,22,23] As all these

studies further show, SES and advanced age are key predictors of oral health.

The present study also shows that the majority of older adults fail to visit a dental practitioner for routine preventive check-ups and that most of them are unaware of the importance of routine preventive check-ups. The percentage of older adults aged 65+ of lower SES status who visit a dental practitioner for routine preventive check-ups is lower than that of their age group peers who are of higher SES. Still, considering the situation about 22 years ago,[8] the present study indicates a certain improvement in oral health behavior patterns, as reflected in the higher percentage of older adults visiting a dental practitioner for routine preventive check-ups as well as in the reported higher tooth brushing frequency. Thus, the percentage of older adults brushing their teeth at least twice a day increased from 61% in 1998 to 69% in 2020 and the percentage of older adults visiting a dental practitioner for routine preventive check-ups increased from 20% to 40%.[8]

The disparities regarding oral health and oral health behavior may result from dental care costs and or lack of awareness of the importance of routine dental care, and lack of knowledge to entitlement to dental care services by law, especially in the lower SES group and the non-Jewish population.

Balaji wrote that with "inclusion of oral health in UHC, impending changes in outlook of dental health care would provide an ample opportunity for the policymakers and dental researchers to recalibrate their priorities."[24] To his list we can add dental practitioners.

UHC is a crucial first step to reduce dental health disparities. The WHO is correct to propagate UHC, but in view of these barriers, action should be taken to ensure the accessibility of the services, first and foremost, for older adults aged 65+ of lower SES and those in minority populations. In addition, information campaigns should be conducted to raise awareness of the legal rights to dental services and to the importance of routine dental care in the 65+ age group.

It is expected that UHC for older patients will bring more of them to the dental clinics, especially those patients who did not visit before, as happened when UHC for children was implemented in Israel.[25] The dental profession has a responsibility and a unique opportunity to actively contribute to achieving all benefits from UHC.

This study may help to inform policy and serve as a basis for decision-making on the provision of dental care services at the national level, the nationwide deployment of the services, and the reduction of barriers to the use of dental care services as part of UHC.

Conclusion

There has been an improvement in the oral health status and oral health behavior of older adults aged 65+ in Israel during the last two decades.

Disparities regarding oral health and oral health behavior may be the result of dental care costs, due to lack of awareness of the importance of proper oral health behavior, routine dental care, and lack of knowledge of entitlement to dental care services, especially in the lower SES group and the minority population.

As part of UHC, action should be taken to ensure the accessibility of the services for older adults of lower SES and those in the minority population. Information campaigns are needed to raise awareness to the legal rights to dental services and to the importance of routine dental care in the 65+ age group.

The dental profession should make sure to provide comprehensive dental health education to all elderly patients who come to the dental clinics as a result of the UHC lowering the cost barrier.

Study limitations

The study has two main limitations: the subjective reporting of the self-perceived oral health status and the self-reporting of the use of dental care services, which may be biased due to aging-associated memory decline. Another limitation concerns the interviews conducted with 34 family members that might have influenced the findings. ▦

Acknowledgment

The study was funded with the assistance of the Research Fund of the Chief Scientist at the Ministry of Health, Israel.

Disclosure

The authors have no conflicts of interest to disclose.

References

1. World Health Organization Discussion Paper. Draft Global Oral Health Action Plan (2022–2030). https://cdn.who.int/media/docs/default-source/ncds/mnd/eb152-draft-global-oral-health-action-plan.pdf?sfvrsn=ecce482e_4. Accessed 15 Oct 2022.

2. Aarabi G, Reissmann DR, Seedorf U, Becher H, Heydecke G, Kofahl C. Oral health and access to dental care – a comparison of elderly migrants and non-migrants in Germany. Ethnicity Health 2017;23:703–717.

3. Fleming E, Afful J, Frenk, SM. Prevalence of edentualism in adults aged >65 years, by age group and race/Hispanic origin – National Health and Nutrition Examination Survey, 2011–2014. MMWR Morb Mortal Wkly Rep 2017;66:94.

4. Griffin, SO, Griffin PM, Li C, Bailey WD, Bruson D, Jones JA. Changes in older adults' health and disparities: 1999 to 2004 and 2011 to 2016. J Am Geriatr Soc 2019;67:1152–1157.

5. Raphael C. Oral health and aging. Am J Public Health 2017;107:S44–S45.

6. Masood M, Newton T, Bakri NN, Khalid T. The relationship between oral health and oral health related quality of life among elderly people in United Kingdom. J Dent 2017;56:78–83.

7. Shariff JA, Burkett S, Watson CW, Cheng B, Noble JM, Papapanou PN. Periodontal status among elderly inhabitants of northern Manhattan: The WHICAP ancillary study of oral health. J Clin Periodontol 2018;45:909–919.

8. Berg A, Zusman SP, Horev T. Social and economic aspects of dental care in Israel in the era of national health insurance [Hebrew]. Jerusalem: The Myers-JDC-Brookdale Institute, 2001, RR 359-01.

9. Kiyak HA, Reichmuth M. Barriers to and enablers of older adults' use of dental services. J Dent Educ 2005;69:975–986.

10. Kramarow EA. Dental care among adults aged 65 and over, 2017. NCHS Data Brief 2019;337:1–8.

11. Berg-Warman A, Horev T, Zusman SP. Oral health status of older adults in Israel and their use patterns of dental care services [Hebrew]. Gerontol Geriatr 2004;31:43–54.

12. Adut R, Mann J, Sgan-Cohen HD. Past and present geographic location as oral health markers among older adults. J Public Health Dent 2004;64:240–243.

13. Natapov L, Kushnir D, Goldsmith R, Dichtiar R, Zusman SP. Dental status, visits, and functional ability and dietary intake of elderly in Israel. Isr J Health Policy Res 2018; 7:58.

14. Berg-Warman A, Kermel Schiffman I, Zusman SP, Natapov L. Oral health of the 65+ age group in Israel-2020. Isr J Health Policy Res 2021;10:58.

15. Zusman SP. Dental care as part of universal health coverage. Quintessence Int 2018;49:779–780.

16. Natapov L, Sasson A, Zusman SP. Does dental health of 6-year-olds reflect the reform of the Israeli dental care system? Isr J Health Policy Res 2016;5:26.

17. Barmes DE, Cohen LK. International collaborative study of dental manpower systems: Interim report. Albany: World Health Organizations Publications, 1981.

18. Chen MS, Andersen RM, Barmes DE, Leclerq MH, Lyttle CS. Comparing oral health care systems: a second international collaborative study. (No. WHO/ORH/ICSII/97.1). Geneva: World Health Organization, 1997.

19. National Institute of Dental Research (US). Epidemiology, & Oral Disease Prevention Program. Oral Health of United States Adults: The National Survey of Oral Health in US Employed Adults and Seniors, 1985–1986: Regional Findings (No. 88). Epidemiology and Oral Disease Prevention Program, National Institute of Dental Research, US Department of Health and Human Services, Public Health Service, National Institutes of Health, 1988.

20. Central Bureau of Statistics. The Social Survey, 2013, #1594. Jerusalem: CBS, 2015.

21. World Health Organization. Recent Advances in Oral Health. WHO Technical Report Series N. 826. Geneva: World Health Organization, 1992:16–17.

22. Friedman PK, Kaufman LB, Karpas SL. Oral health disparity in older adults: dental decay and tooth loss. Dent Clin North Am 2014;58:757–770.

23. Müller F, Naharro M, Carlsson GE. What are the prevalence and incidence of tooth loss in the adult and elderly population in Europe? Clin Oral Implants Res 2007;18:2–14.

24. Balaji SM. Oral health, universal health coverage, and dental research. Indian J Dent Res 2019;30:486.

25. Ashkenazi Y, Yankellevich A, Zusman SP, Natapov L. Patterns of utilization and experiences of children in dental care following the reform of dental care in Israel. Jerusalem: Myers-JDC-Brookdale Institute, 2016. English Executive summary: https://brookdale-web.s3.amazonaws.com/uploads/2018/01/710-16_English_Summary-updated.pdf. Accessed 15 Oct 2022.

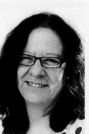

Ayelet Berg-Warman

Ayelet Berg-Warman Senior Researcher, The Myers-JDC-Brookdale Institute, Jerusalem, Israel

Ile Kermel Schiffman Researcher, The Myers-JDC-Brookdale Institute, Jerusalem, Israel

Shlomo Paul Zusman Retired, Former Director of Dental Health, The Ministry of Health, Division of Dental Health, Tel Aviv, Israel

Lena Natapov Director of Dental Health, The Ministry of Health, Division of Dental Health, Tel Aviv, Israel

Correspondence: Prof Shlomo Zusman, 42/19 Pinkas Street, Tel Aviv, Israel. Email: zusmans@gmail.com

First submission: 15 Oct 2022
Acceptance: 14 Jan 2023
Online publication: 18 Jan 2023

■ ORAL MEDICINE AND OROFACIAL PAIN

Temporomandibular disorders: current status of research, education, policies, and its impact on clinicians in the United States of America

Gary D. Klasser, DMD, Cert.Orofacial Pain/Elliot Abt, DDS, MS, MSc/Robert J. Weyant, DMD, DrPH/
Charles S. Greene, DDS

Temporomandibular disorders (TMDs) encompass a number of different musculoskeletal disorders often accompanied by pain and dysfunction. Most TMDs are acute, but can become chronic leading to disability and quality of life issues. There is wide variation in treatment of TMDs, including both conservative/reversible therapies as well as invasive/irreversible treatments, which present difficulties for clinicians, patients, and third-party payers as to what constitutes appropriate care. **Data sources:** A recent report by the National Academies of Sciences, Engineering, and Medicine highlighted a number of deficiencies, most notably in the education of TMDs within United States of America dental schools at both the predoctoral and postdoctoral (dental) levels as well as addressing the historic inconsistencies in both diagnosis and treatment. New areas for research and interprofessional collaboration should assist in the understanding of TMDs, and updated clinical practice guidelines should help reduce variation in the delivery of evidence-based care. Recently, the American Dental Association recognized orofacial pain as a specialty, which should increase the level and availability of expertise in treating these issues. **Summary:** Based on the current best evidence, this report is an attempt to alert the profession to discontinue irreversible and invasive therapies for the vast majority of TMDs and recognize that the majority of these disorders are amenable to conservative, reversible interventions. *(Quintessence Int 2023;54:328–334; doi: 10.3290/j.qi.b3999673)*

Key words: American Dental Association, Commission on Dental Accreditation, dental education and research, National Academies of Sciences, Engineering, and Medicine, temporomandibular disorders

The American Academy of Orofacial Pain (AAOP) defines temporomandibular disorders (TMDs) as a group of musculoskeletal and neuromuscular conditions that involve the temporomandibular joints (TMJs), the masticatory muscles, and all associated tissues.[1] Furthermore, TMDs have been identified as a major cause of nondental pain in the orofacial region[2,3] often associated with pain and/or dysfunction. Many TMDs are acute and transitory in nature, but can become long-lasting and chronic, leading to significant morbidity and quality of life issues.[4,5] Individuals suffering from TMDs often feel stigmatized and invalidated by family members, friends, and the health community as a whole, resulting in significant psychosocial issues.[6,7] TMDs can also co-occur or be comorbid with other health conditions such as fibromyalgia, back pain, irritable bowel syndrome, and headache.[8]

While variation in treatment modalities may be present in many areas of health care, perhaps nowhere in dentistry is there greater diversity of therapies than in treating TMDs. These interventions include reversible therapies such as passive oral appliances, physical therapy, and analgesics, and irreversible ones such as active (purposefully designed to alter maxillomandibular relationships) oral appliances, occlusal adjustments, orthodontics, dental reconstructions, and surgery. Accurate diagnosis is the key to providing appropriate care, which can become complicated due to the complexity and sheer number of TMDs. However, despite these issues, clinical practice guidelines exist for TMDs[1] and reinforce the need for evidence-based, conservative care for the majority of cases.

There have been several positive developments recently in the TMD field. In 2019, the National Academies of Sciences, Engineering, and Medicine (NASEM) initiated a 15-month study on the current status of research, education, and care in the field of TMD. Their 400-page report entitled "Temporomandibular Disorders: Priorities for Research and Care"[9] was published in 2020 and followed by a guest editorial in this journal.[10] This project highlighted the many advancements in the field of TMD, along with deficiencies, such as the need for better education at the predoctoral (undergraduate) level and the need for more programs with unified curricula at the postdoctoral (graduate) level at dental schools in the USA. The report also calls for dental practitioners to reject old mechanistic models such as those related to occlusal and jaw relationship factors being the primary etiological factors for TMDs. Instead, it encourages the profession to move into modern application of the biopsychosocial model, based on the current understanding that TMDs are multifactorial conditions with overlapping comorbidities often associated with central nervous system dysregulation.[11] Additionally, in March 2020, the American Dental Association (ADA) made orofacial pain a recognized specialty, a significant development in terms of recognizing those with advanced training in the field.

This narrative report highlights the many changes in the TMD field and is a call for various stakeholders involved in TMD research, education, and clinical practice in the USA to conform to an evidence-based approach to improve outcomes of care.

Dental education in TMD

Historically, dental education in the USA related to orofacial pain (including TMDs) for predoctoral students has somewhat improved and progressed in both qualitative and quantitative standards over the last several decades.[12,13] However, until recently there was a lack of specific TMD curriculum guidelines regarding the teaching of this topic in predoctoral dental education. A major change to remedy this situation occurred in August 2020, when the Commission on Dental Accreditation (CODA), nationally recognized by the United States Department of Education (USDE) as the sole agency to accredit USA dental and dental-related education programs conducted at the post-secondary level, approved a revision to Standard 2-24k contained within the Accreditation Standards for Dental Education Programs.[14] The revision mandated the teaching of TMDs in the predoctoral curriculums of all USA dental schools by July 2022.[14] The mission of CODA is to serve the public and dental professions by developing and implementing accreditation standards that promote and monitor the continuous quality and improvement of dental education programs.[14] However, the function of CODA does not include authority to determine how these standards are defined, implemented, or assessed. Therefore, each dental school is responsible for setting their requirements regarding each standard. This created a need for development of a national TMD educational guideline to ensure that evidence-based content, with consistent quality and depth, is being taught at all dental schools throughout the USA. This prompted the AAOP to form an expert task force to develop a core curriculum framework for implementation of CODA Standard 2-24k. This framework is based on the 2020 NASEM report,[9] previous recommendations, and a consensus on present and future educational needs in TMD education.[15] This competency-based core curriculum envisions that all graduates of accredited dental schools in the USA will understand the basic mechanisms, etiology, evaluation, diagnosis, treatment, and prevention of TMDs. Moreover, it is expected that graduates will apply contemporary evidence-based knowledge and collaborate with orofacial pain specialists and pertinent health professionals in caring for and preventing TMDs.[16]

There are five domains which frame this predoctoral curriculum with each having their own specific objectives and learning outcomes.[16] The included domains are:

- knowledge base of TMDs and orofacial pain
- screening, evaluation, diagnosis, and risk assessment
- health promotion and prevention of TMDs
- clinical decision making, treatment planning, evidence-based TMD management, communication, and interdisciplinary collaboration in clinical practice
- practice management and informatics.

Ideally, this didactic curriculum should be supplemented by actual clinical exposure to symptomatic TMD patients within the dental colleges. This would aid in the development of real-life competencies in screening and triage of such patients. If the students can be educated to recognize more complex patients, they could avoid doing wasteful and often harmful primary care in those cases, and instead learn how to refer to more expert practitioners for appropriate management. Ultimately, this will result in better educated dental practitioners and improved access to care for those with TMDs, and assist in preventing the development of chronic pain and disability.

This situation is somewhat different for postdoctoral dental education. Over the past 40 to 50 years, a number of orofacial pain postdoctoral residency training programs were developed and expanded in the USA. Those programs have produced a number of knowledgeable clinicians, but overall they are limited in size and cannot produce enough practitioners for managing large numbers of patients with complex pain problems. CODA oversees and sanctions the educational guidelines for evaluating and accrediting these postdoctoral residency programs through the lens of the Advanced General Dentistry Education Programs in Orofacial Pain.[17] The goals set forth by CODA for Advanced Dental Education Programs in Orofacial Pain are to provide education in orofacial pain at a level beyond predoctoral education, using applied basic and behavioral sciences. The programs are designed to expand the scope and depth of the graduates' knowledge and skills to enable them to provide care for individuals with orofacial pain.[17] Monitoring of these programs has been under the scrutiny of CODA for a number of years.

Current and future research in TMD

The history of research related overall to TMDs and specifically to the TMJ goes back many years. Basic science research has been conducted at universities on a global basis since the last half of the 20th century, and clinical research has been encouraged and supported by government health agencies in several countries. However, there has been little collaboration between researchers working in various locations, despite the sharing of findings via the many journals that publish these scientific peer-reviewed articles as well as congregating together at the various conferences where expert speakers present their data and concepts. However, this merely represents a "siloed" approach to a field that needs much more interdisciplinary and collaborative research in order to advance understanding of these complex disorders. Furthermore, the discovery that there are several other medical conditions that are comorbid with TMDs increases both the complexity of the situation and the need for an expanded research agenda.

In recent years, the only notable effort to accomplish some of these collaborative goals has been the Orofacial Pain Prospective Evaluation and Risk Assessment (OPPERA) studies, which for a period of over 12 years focused on the etiopathogenesis of TMDs in a population of over 3,000 subjects.[18,19] Using a longitudinal prospective research design, the project emphasized the genomic and epigenetic factors that contributed to TMD onset cases, while also testing the patients for biologic sensitivity factors as well as psychologic and other environmental factors that were associated with the various phenotypes of clinical symptomatology.

Another organization interested in advancing TMD research is the Medical Device Epidemiology Network (MDEpiNet). This organization is a global public-private partnership that brings together leadership, expertise, and resources from various stakeholders to advance a national patient-centered medical device evaluation and surveillance system. In 2018, there was a meeting at which proposals for future research were presented by the MDEpiNet TMJ Patient Led RoundTable, an interagency, multi-stakeholder initiative.[20] The research priorities in this plan were established through two initiatives of the RoundTable. First, those research priorities identified as most important to patients and other stakeholder groups at an 11 May 2018 meeting of the RoundTable were included and second, additional research priorities were extracted from a Briefing Report prepared by the four Working Groups of the RoundTable. The proposed research will focus on two aspects of TMDs:

1. Studies gathering information to assess the quality, safety, and reliability of TMJ replacement implants, and studies to predict those subjects at greatest risk of harm from TMJ implant devices (mechanical failures, tissue reactions, etc)
2. Studies collecting data on TMD subjects without implanted devices to determine the progression of pain, dysfunction, changes in quality of life, and the development of other comorbidities stratified as:

- those with no invasive or noninvasive procedures to the joints
- those with nonsurgical procedures to manipulate or realign the joints (eg, stabilization splints, bite guards), often followed by various dental procedures to permanently change jaw relationships
- those with invasive procedures such as arthrocentesis, arthroscopy, condylotomy arthroplasty, reconstructive surgery, Botox injections, steroid treatments, etc.

As the NASEM report emphasizes, there is a need for major improvement in collaborative research, with special emphasis on delivering better care for TMD patients. Therefore, following the release of the NASEM report, The National Advisory Dental & Craniofacial Research Council met on 25 January 2022 to receive state-of-the-Institute reports from the National Institute of Dental and Craniofacial Research (NIDCR) Director, other staff, and guest scientists to learn about proposed new policies, activities, and research concepts. One proposal was to establish a TMD Collaborative for Improving Patient-Centered Translational Research (TMD IMPACT).

What followed was an outline of research goals and projects to: "advance Temporomandibular Disorders (TMD) basic and clinical research, research training and translation to evidence-based treatment and improved clinical care – through the establishment of a national, interdisciplinary, trans-NIH, patient-centered research Collaborative." This proposed Collaborative would include relevant research areas from tissue engineering and regeneration, TMD pain, and disease prevention, building the evidence base for existing treatments, and developing scientifically based new treatments, emphasizing the multidisciplinary nature of the Collaborative as well as the multidisciplinary composition of the teams that would carry out the research. Implicit in that statement is the Institute's recognition that TMDs are complex multifactorial disorders, not dental conditions mainly treated by dentists. A systemic and collaborative interdisciplinary approach to research in TMDs will clearly improve the evidence base, leading to improved clinical practice guidelines (CPGs) and more appropriate care.

Clinical practice guidelines in TMD

There is a hierarchy of evidence that assigns systematic reviews and CPGs at the highest level primarily due to reduced bias and confounding inherent in their methodologic designs. CPGs are at the highest level of scientific evidence as they employ an expert panel to conduct a systematic review of the literature to answer a clinical question.[21] Guidelines are needed in health care to improve the quality and outcomes of care, reduce inappropriate variation in clinical practice, promote efficient use of resources, and inform public policy. Perhaps no other discipline in dentistry has greater breadth of treatment modalities, while at the same time having a dearth of evidence based on high-quality science, than TMDs. Interventions have ranged from conservative, reversible therapies, to irreversible treatments such as dental reconstructions, orthodontics, and surgery.

CPGs summarize the evidence in a particular field and provide a recommendation for (sealants) or against (antibiotics to prevent prosthetic joint infection) a specific clinical practice. While CPGs aid health care professions to improve patient care and inform public policy, challenges exist in the creation, dissemination, and implementation arenas. The three main issues are lack of quality evidence, the ability to get evidence into clinical practice, and financial constraints.

High-quality randomized controlled trials abound in primary care medicine due to the ease and relatively low cost of drug trials on surrogate markers. However, due to funding and methodologic issues, there are fewer randomized trials in dentistry, leaving an evidence base dominated by observational studies. Thus, CPGs related to TMDs are dependent on the quality/quantity of the existing evidence.

There are several significant barriers to getting research evidence into practice. It is well documented that publication of a study, including CPGs, even in widely read journals, does not guarantee that clinicians will be aware of its existence, have read or understand its implications, and will implement results into practice.[22-26] Thus, sponsoring organizations need other vehicles to ensure dissemination and implementation of findings from CPGs including methods to update and transmit findings as evidence evolves.

Despite these issues and concerns, AAOP has undertaken the task of publishing guidelines for orofacial pain including TMDs since 1990. To date, AAOP has published six editions, with the most current being published in 2018.[1] A seventh edition is scheduled for release in 2023. The proposed guidelines, which have changed over the years due to new scientific discoveries, adhere to an evidence-based approach, when available. The reader of this CPG is provided with scientifically sound and effective diagnostic and management options, often recommending conservative and reversible therapies for the majority of TMDs based upon current peer-reviewed literature. Incorporating this CPG into clinical practice will enable clinicians to provide better chairside patient care, based on a sound scientific approach.

NASEM report summary

In 2020, NASEM released a consensus study report titled: "Temporomandibular Disorders: Priorities for Research and Care."[9] This study was sponsored by the Office of the Director of the National Institutes of Health and the NIDCR. This report was the output of an 18-member ad hoc committee convened by NASEM and charged with examining "the current state of knowledge regarding TMD research, education, and training, safety and efficacy of clinical treatment of TMDs, and burden and costs associated with TMDs."[9] The purpose of the review was to provide recommendations that would lead to improved health and well-being of individuals with TMDs. The committee approached its work through literature reviews along with interviews of TMD patients and their families, clinicians, researchers, policy makers, and research funders.[9] Based on their findings, the committee provided 11 recommendations aimed at identifying the need for expanded research in several areas as well as strategies for improving clinical care for TMD patients:[9]

- Create and sustain a national collaborative research consortium for TMDs.
- Strengthen basic research and translational efforts.
- Strengthen population-based research on the public health burden of TMDs.
- Bolster clinical research efforts to build the evidence base for patient-centered care and public health interventions for TMDs.

- Improve the assessment and risk stratification of TMDs to advance patient care.
- Develop and disseminate evidence-based clinical practice guidelines and quality metrics for care of TMDs.
- Improve reimbursements and access to high-quality assessment, treatment, and management of TMDs.
- Develop centers of excellence for TMDs and orofacial pain.
- Improve education and training on TMDs for health care professionals.
- Establish and strengthen advanced/specialized training in care of orofacial pain and TMDs.
- Raise awareness, improve education, and reduce stigma.

The report highlights research needs in several areas. First, it was clear that additional epidemiologic research must be done to document the extent that TMDs lead to individual and societal harms. These harms include major impacts on quality of life and economic well-being of families and communities. The committee also stressed the need for additional basic and clinical research that could lead to the identification of risk factors and elucidate pathophysiologic mechanisms involved in the various TMDs. Additional research efforts should be directed toward evaluation of outcomes of current clinical interventions, and those results could be used to support development of new approaches to clinical care that could be developed into clinical guidelines.

Current approaches to care for those suffering from both acute and chronic TMDs were reviewed. The committee found that many approaches to care featured siloed or isolated treatment approaches within various health care disciplines, often using treatments that lacked evidence of effectiveness. As a result, the committee stressed the need for guideline development aimed at improving diagnostic and treatment approaches based on documentation of effectiveness. With appropriate guidelines in place, it would become possible to develop and implement an evidence-based curriculum across all disciplines involved in TMD care that includes interdisciplinary training. The committee strongly supported adopting a biopsychosocial model of TMD care, which necessitates an interdisciplinary and coordinated approach to TMD diagnosis and treatment among the various health care disciplines that engage in TMD treatment. The committee also emphasized the need for adopting a conservative and graduated approach to TMD treatment, noting that much of the current care being delivered to TMD patients is often irreversible and lacks evidence of effectiveness, leading in many cases to more harms than benefits.

Orofacial pain recognized as a specialty in dentistry

AAOP, founded in 1975, is the professional membership organization representing the field of orofacial pain and is an organization of dentists and other health professionals that is dedicated to alleviating pain and suffering through the promotion of excellence in education, research, and patient care. Over the years, this organization has attempted to have the field of orofacial pain recognized as a specialty in the USA. This situation changed in March 2020, when AAOP's request to recognize orofacial pain as a dental specialty was granted by the National Commission on Recognition of Dental Specialties and Certifying Boards (NCRDSCB) based on compliance with the Requirements for Recognition of Dental Specialties as determined by the ADA.

The ADA states that, "Dental specialties are recognized by the National Commission on Recognition of Dental Specialties and Certifying Boards to protect the public, nurture the art and science of dentistry, and improve the quality of care. Specialties are recognized in those areas where advanced knowledge and skills are essential to maintain or restore oral health (Association policies are contained in the ADA Principles of Ethics and Code of Professional Conduct)."[27]

Adopted by NCRDSCB as of September 2020, orofacial pain is now considered a specialty of dentistry in the USA that encompasses the diagnosis, management, and treatment of pain disorders of the jaw, mouth, face, head, and neck. The specialty is dedicated to the evidence-based understanding of the underlying pathophysiology, etiology, prevention, and treatment of these disorders and improving access to interdisciplinary patient care.

Overall, recognition of this specialty solidifies another link between dentistry and medicine, acknowledging that the orofacial region, oral cavity, and masticatory system are an integral part of total patient care.[28] The benefits of these past events are numerous and include: improved access to care by providing a resource for referral of patients not responding to basic therapy; the maintaining of educational standards for postgraduate orofacial pain training programs thereby educating and providing a supply of properly trained clinicians and faculty; the ability to emphasize the importance of orofacial pain in predoctoral dental education resulting in enhanced patient care through orofacial pain training for newly graduating dental practitioners; allowing for the protection and ability to serve the public by identifying qualified dental practitioners treating TMDs and orofacial pain; and to insure a standard of care through a certified credentialing process administered by a recognized board.

Summary

This report summarizes the current status and future proposed actions for five important aspects of the TMD field. Beginning with the issue of education, the deficiencies of current dental school curricula as well as the prospects for great improvement under new CODA guidelines were discussed as it relates to USA dental schools. The need for a broader multidisciplinary approach to TMD research as well as more focus on related comorbid pain conditions was explained in detail. The value of CPGs was emphasized, because practicing dental practitioners need to have authoritative guidance in order to avoid reproducing the errors of past treatments and to recognize what treatment approaches are required following the current biopsychosocial model. A brief summary of the massive NASEM Report[9] was presented, and the reader is encouraged to obtain and read that important document. Finally, with the recognition of orofacial pain as a specialty in the USA, the management of complex TMDs has become identified as a special set of challenges requiring postgraduate training in diagnosis and treatment at the tertiary care level. This combination of topics presents the reader with a broad overview of the current and future status of the TMD field.

Acknowledgments

The authors thank Ms Terrie Cowley, President of the TMJ Association, and her colleagues for their valuable contributions to the "Current and future research in TMD" section. Some parts of this have appeared previously in their organizational newsletter, while others have appeared in the Research Plan prepared by the MDEpiNet TMJ Patient Led RoundTable. The authors declare no conflicts of interest.

References

1. De Leeuw R, Klasser GD. Orofacial Pain: Guidelines for Assessment, Diagnosis, and Management. 6th edition. Chicago: Quintessence, 2018.

2. Greene CS. Managing the care of patients with temporomandibular disorders: a new guideline for care. J Am Dent Assoc 2010; 141:1086–1088.

3. Okeson JP. Bell's Oral and Facial Pain. 7th edition. Hanover Park: Quintessence Publishing, 2014.

4. Dahlstrom L, Carlsson GE. Temporomandibular disorders and oral health-related quality of life. A systematic review. Acta Odontol Scand 2010;68:80–85.

5. Cao Y, Yap AU, Lei J, Zhang MJ, Fu KY. Oral health-related quality of life of patients with acute and chronic temporomandibular disorder diagnostic subtypes. J Am Dent Assoc 2022;153:50–58.

6. Fillingim RB, Ohrbach R, Greenspan JD, et al. Psychological factors associated with development of TMD: the OPPERA prospective cohort study. J Pain 2013;14(12 Suppl): T75–T90.

7. Cole HA, Carlson CR. Mind-body considerations in orofacial pain. Dent Clin North Am 2018;62:683–694.

8. Klasser GD, Bassiur J, de Leeuw R. Differences in reported medical conditions between myogenous and arthrogenous TMD patients and its relevance to the general practitioner. Quintessence Int 2014;45:157–167.

9. National Academies of Sciences, Engineering, and Medicine. Temporomandibular Disorders: Priorities for Research and Care. Washington, DC: The National Academies Press, 2020.

10. Greene CS, Ohrbach R. Guest Editorial: Major US scientific academy proposes significant changes in understanding and managing TMDs. Quintessence Int 2021;52:657–658.

11. List T, Jensen RH. Temporomandibular disorders: Old ideas and new concepts. Cephalalgia 2017;37:692–704.

12. Greene CS. Teaching undergraduate dental students about TMJ disorders: survey and proposal. J Dent Educ 1973;37:16–19.

13. Klasser GD, Greene CS. Predoctoral teaching of temporomandibular disorders: a survey of U.S. and Canadian dental schools. J Am Dent Assoc 2007;138:231–237.

14. Commission on Dental Accreditation. Accreditation standards for dental education programs. Chicago: American Dental Association, 2022. https://coda.ada.org/~/media/CODA/Files/predoc_standards.pdf?la=en. Accessed 29 July 2022.

15. Fricton J, Chen H, Shaefer JR, et al. New curriculum standards for teaching temporomandibular disorders in dental schools: A commentary. J Am Dent Assoc 2022;153:395–398.

16. AAOP Committee on TMD Predoctoral Education, Chen H, Fricton J, et al. Temporomandibular disorders core curriculum for predoctoral dental education: recommendations from the American Academy of Orofacial Pain. J Oral Facial Pain Headache 2021;35: 271–277.

17. Commission on Dental Accreditation. Accreditation standards for advanced general dentistry education programs in orofacial pain. Chicago: American Dental Association, 2022. https://coda.ada.org/~/media/CODA/Files/Orofacial_Pain_Standards.pdf?la=en. Accessed 29 July 2022.

18. Fillingim RB, Slade GD, Diatchenko L, et al. Summary of findings from the OPPERA baseline case-control study: implications and future directions. J Pain 2011;12(11 Suppl): T102–T107.

19. Slade GD, Fillingim RB, Sanders AE, et al. Summary of findings from the OPPERA prospective cohort study of incidence of first-onset temporomandibular disorder: implications and future directions. J Pain 2013;14(12 Suppl):T116–T124.

20. TMJ RoundTable Working Groups. The TMJ Patient-Led RoundTable: A history and summary of work. The Medical Device Epidemiology Network (MDEpiNet), 2018. https://www.mdepinet.net/tmj. Accessed 18 September 2022.

21. Sutherland SE, Matthews DC. Conducting systematic reviews and creating clinical practice guidelines in dentistry: lessons learned. J Am Dent Assoc 2004;135:747–753.

22. Haynes B, Haines A. Barriers and bridges to evidence based clinical practice. BMJ 1998;317:273–276.

23. Clarkson JE. Getting research into clinical practice: barriers and solutions. Caries Res 2004;38:321–324.

24. Andermann A, Pang T, Newton JN, Davis A, Panisset U. Evidence for Health II: Overcoming barriers to using evidence in policy and practice. Health Res Policy Syst 2016;14:17.

25. Bero LA, Grilli R, Grimshaw JM, Harvey E, Oxman AD, Thomson MA. Closing the gap between research and practice: an overview of systematic reviews of interventions to promote the implementation of research findings. The Cochrane Effective Practice and Organization of Care Review Group. BMJ 1998;317:465–468.

26. Grimshaw JM, Eccles MP, Lavis JN, Hill SJ, Squires JE. Knowledge translation of research findings. Implement Sci 2012;7:50.

27. Council on Ethics, Bylaws and Judicial Affairs. Principles of Ethics and Code of Professional Conduct. American Dental Association Chicago; 2021. https://www.ada.org/about/principles/code-of-ethics. Accessed 18 September 2022.

28. Heir GM. Orofacial pain, the 12th specialty: The necessity. J Am Dent Assoc 2020; 151:469–471.

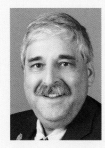

Gary D. Klasser

Gary D. Klasser   Professor, Louisiana State University Health Sciences Center, School of Dentistry, Department of Diagnostic Sciences, New Orleans, LA, USA

Elliot Abt   Adjunct Associate Professor, University of Illinois at Chicago, College of Dentistry, Department of Oral Medicine, Chicago, IL, USA

Robert J. Weyant   Professor and Chair, University of Pittsburgh, Department of Dental Public Health, Pittsburgh, PA, USA

Charles S. Greene, DDS   Clinical Professor Emeritus, University of Illinois at Chicago, College of Dentistry, Department of Orthodontics, Chicago, IL, USA

Correspondence: Professor Gary D. Klasser, Louisiana State University Health Sciences Center, School of Dentistry, Department of Diagnostic Sciences, 1100 Florida Avenue, Box #8, New Orleans, LA 70119, USA. Email: gklass@lsuhsc.edu

First submission: 15 Nov 2022
Acceptance: 17 Dec 2022
Online publication: 22 Dec 2022

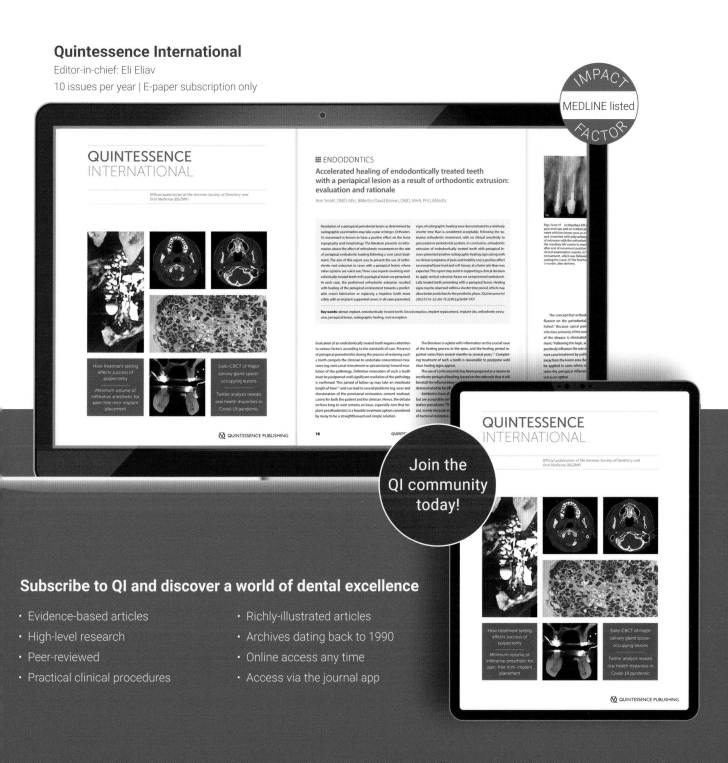

QUINTESSENCE INTERNATIONAL
SERVING THE NEEDS OF THE GENERAL DENTAL PRACTITIONER

Quintessence International
Editor-in-chief: Eli Eliav
10 issues per year | E-paper subscription only

IMPACT FACTOR — MEDLINE listed

Join the QI community today!

Subscribe to QI and discover a world of dental excellence

- Evidence-based articles
- High-level research
- Peer-reviewed
- Practical clinical procedures

- Richly-illustrated articles
- Archives dating back to 1990
- Online access any time
- Access via the journal app

Europe
www.quint.link/qi

North and South America
www.quint.link/qi-us

Rest of the world
www.quint-link/qi-uk

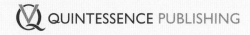

Oral health status in patients with inherited epidermolysis bullosa: a comparative multicenter study

Clara Joseph, DDS, PhD/Mathieu Marty, DDS, PhD/Sophie-Myriam Dridi, DDS, PhD/Veroniek Verhaeghe, DDS/
Isabelle Bailleul-Forestier, DDS, PhD/Christine Chiaverini, MD, PhD/Thomas Hubiche, MD/
Juliette Mazereeuw-Hautier, MD, PhD/Olivier Deny, DDS/Dominique Declerck, DDS, PhD/Philippe Kémoun, DDS, PhD

Objective: Epidermolysis bullosa (EB) is a rare genetic mucocutaneous disorder characterized by epithelial fragility leading to blister formation on skin and mucous membranes with even minor mechanical trauma. Most EB oral health publications give fragmented information, focusing on only one oral health aspect or one EB type. The aim of this study was to expand the knowledge of the overall oral health status of individuals with dystrophic, junctional, and simplex EB. **Method and materials:** A comparative multicenter study, including a control group, and based on questionnaires and clinical examinations, was undertaken in three EB expert centers. **Results:** Most EB (90.2%) participants brushed their teeth at least once a day despite the pain. The prevalence of enamel defects and caries experience did not differ between the 42 EB participants and the 42 age-/sex-matched healthy controls. Gingival inflammation unrelated to dental plaque accumulation was found in EB participants. Blisters, erythema, and erosion/ulceration mainly involved gingiva, buccal mucosa, lips, and palate, with different topographic patterns according to EB type. EB patients whatever the age showed a similar lesion distribution. Simplex and dystrophic EB patients under 12 years old displayed higher lesion severity than junctional EB ones. Only dystrophic type exhibited microstomia and ankyloglossia. **Conclusion:** Oral health status seemed to benefit from a close collaboration between dental practitioner and dermatologist, and from regular dental examination, starting at a young age and with a focus on prevention. The new appreciation of oral health involvement highlighted by this study is essential for EB patients care, regarding comorbidities and quality of life. *(Quintessence Int 2023;54:34–43; doi: 10.3290/j.qi.b3479975)*

Key words: dystrophic epidermolysis bullosa, gingival inflammation, inherited epidermolysis bullosa, junctional epidermolysis bullosa, oral health, oral lesion, simplex epidermolysis bullosa

Inherited epidermolysis bullosa (EB) is a group of rare genodermatoses characterized by mechanical fragility of skin/mucous membranes as a result of cleavage within dermal-epidermal layers leading to blistering. Bullous lesions can severely handicap individuals because of their local and systemic consequences (Fig 1).[1] People with EB have general complications such as digestive, respiratory, ocular, and urogenital manifestations and possible malignant degeneration. In the most severe cases, the condition is life-threatening, and life expectancy is shortened (by about 30 years).[1] Moreover, this disease has a significant impact on quality of life.[2] Four major types of EB are described, based on the localization of the split at the epidermal ultrastructural level: simplex EB (SEB; intra-epidermal cleavage); junctional EB (JEB; dermal-epidermal split); dystrophic EB (DEB; intradermal cleavage); and Kindler syndrome (multifocal).[3] No acquired forms of EB were considered in this study.

The oral cavity is especially affected because of constant exposure to oral functions from an early age. Oral lesions are characterized by erythema, blistering, and their aftermath (eg, erosions, ulcerations, crusts, and atrophic scarring).[4] Number, frequency, and severity of the lesions hinge on the type of EB (Figs 2 and 3).[5] Except for reports by Wright et al[6-9] in the 1990s (including a cohort of 292 patients) and Fortuna et al[5] (92 patients), most studies bring fragmented information focusing on only one aspect of oral health (oral soft-tissue lesions, oral hygiene, caries, or enamel defects),[4,5,10-12] or only one type of EB.[13-16] Recently, the present authors' group reported that the distribution of oral mucosal lesions depends on the type of disease and

Figs 1a and 1b Two-year-old patient with severe DEB, presenting hemorrhagic blisters, crust, and erythema: preparation for dental treatment under general anesthesia.

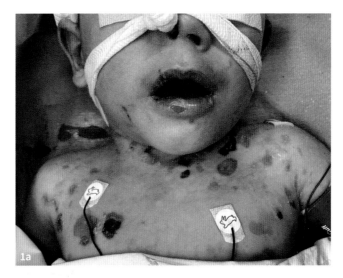
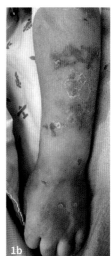

that gingival inflammation might be a specific feature reflecting the intrinsic fragility of the gingival tissues.[17] However, many questions remain regarding EB oral health status, such as the prevalence of functional sequelae (in particular ankyloglossia and microstomia),[15] caries experience, enamel defects, oral hygiene, and dietary habits. This information is especially relevant in the pediatric population, requiring special attention.

The aim of the present study was to report global oral health (prevalence and distribution of oral lesions at the level of mucosa, periodontal tissues, and dental structures) and oral health-related habits (hygiene and diet) in a cohort of individuals with DEB, JEB, and SEB as compared with age and sex-matched controls.

Method and materials

Study design

This comparative multicenter study including a control group was conducted in three EB expert centers, in Belgium (Leuven) and France (Nice, Toulouse) between September 2017 and December 2019. The protocol received institutional approval (Commission Nationale de l'Informatique et des Libertés: CNIL, identifier no. R0172003095), and the study was registered at ClinicalTrials.gov (NCT04217538).

Participants

EB group

All EB patients, regardless of sex, age, and type of inherited EB, in any of the three expert centers were invited to participate during the dental consultation, part of their regular care. To be eligible, patients and/or guardians needed to understand French (Nice and Toulouse) or Dutch (Leuven) in order to capture all information and to provide their consent. If oral clinical examination could not be performed, mostly because of a lack of cooperation, the patient was excluded.

Control group

For each individual enrolled in the EB group, an age- and sex-matched healthy patient consulting (for regular treatment or check-up only) was included in the same timeframe at the Toulouse Hospital dentistry department.

Questionnaire and clinical procedures

All seven dental practitioners involved in the clinical examinations were specialists in oral medicine and/or pediatric dentistry, and perform their clinic in pediatric dentistry, periodontology, or special care. Before the beginning of the study, all examiners met several times to discuss different representative clinical controls and EB cases to calibrate themselves for the diagnosis, until reaching a full agreement. The oral clinical examination was performed following World Health Organization recommendations.[18] The reference indices chosen to describe the oral health condition of the participants were the Decayed, Missing, Filled Teeth index (DMFT) to summarize dental caries experience (cavitated lesions), the Plaque Index (PI) to describe the presence of dental plaque accumulation reflecting the level of oral hygiene, and the Gingival Index (GI) to describe the extent of gingival inflammation. Presence of enamel hypoplasia

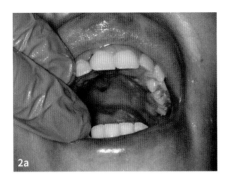

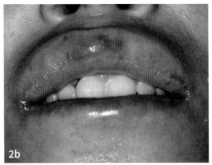

Figs 2a to 2d Thirteen-year-old patient with DEB exhibiting microstomia, ulcerations, and blisters (lips, oral commissures, gingiva, vestibule, tongue) typical of the disease. The entire gingival area shows inflammation unrelated to dental plaque accumulation that is characterized by redness, fading of mucogingival line, papillary hypertrophy, and spontaneous bleeding.

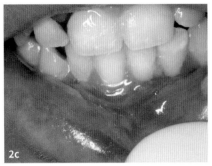

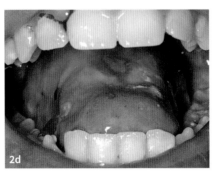

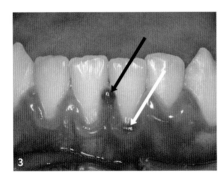

Fig 3 Intraoral photograph of a 12-year-old JEB patient, showing light dental plaque deposit with a wide gingival inflammation, with erythema and edema. Note the small gingival blister (black arrow) and the erosion (white arrow).

was reported. The epidermolysis bullosa oropharyngeal severity (EBOS)[19] score (range 0 to 60) was used to assess the severity of oral mucosal involvement.

Examinations took place in a dental setting with use of a dental probe, mirror, and light source. Data collection was completed with information obtained by simple questioning on dietary habits, oral hygiene routine, and dental care (Table 1).

All data were entered in an anonymized file that was designed by all expert dental practitioners involved in the study. In some cases, when indicated, radiography was performed for diagnostic purposes but was not part of data collection within the framework of the study.

Statistical analyses

Frequencies (percentages) are given for categorical variables and mean ± standard deviation (SD) or range for continuous variables. As patients under 12 years old undergo periodontal changes with regular local inflammation caused by physiologic dentition changes, a subdivision of the sample at 12 years old was decided as a cutoff for comparison in each EB and control groups in order to improve the relevance of the results for oral examination, by making sure that these physiologic changes were not the cause of any oral lesion, as all permanent teeth (except the third molars) are erupted.[20]

Table 1 Questionnaire on dietary habits, oral hygiene routine, and dental care that was asked of each participant/parents

Dietary habits	Hygiene practices	Dental care
Are you able to feed yourself or do you need a feeding tube?	How many times a day do you brush your teeth? Once? twice? or three times a day?	Do you have a dentist?
Do you eat hard or soft food, or both?	Do you brush your teeth on your own or are you assisted by your parents? Do they watch over you when you do it?	Have you ever had some cavity treated or some tooth removed?
How many times a day do you eat?	Which kind of toothbrush do you use? Soft? Hard? Manual or electric?	Was the treatment performed in general practice or under general anesthesia?
Do you eat soft and sticky food?	Do you have difficulty brushing your teeth? Because of lack of dexterity, limitation of mouth opening, or because of the pain and/or bleeding of your gum?	When was the last time you saw your dentist? Was it for a checkup, a treatment, or an emergency?
Do you eat candy? Or drink sugary drinks? Everyday? Once or more a day? A few times a week? Sometimes for special occasions?	Which kind of toothpaste do you use? Does it contain fluoride? How much?	
Do you eat in between meals?	Do you use any of other oral hygiene products, ie mouth wash, dental floss, interdental brushes?	
Do you eat at school facility? Or at home?	Did you take any fluoride supplement?	

The Wilcoxon test was used for comparing groups. Stata software (StataCorp) was used for analysis. If one of the groups had missing data, the associated unpaired data were excluded from analyses. $P < .05$ was considered statistically significant.

Results

Participants characteristics

Among the 42 individuals with EB included in the study, 25 (59.5%) had a diagnosis of DEB (4 dominant and 21 recessive forms), 5 (11.9%) JEB, and 12 (28.6%) SEB. The mean age of the EB group was 13 ± 15.1 years (range 2 to 78), with a female:male ratio of 19:23. In the < 12-year-old subgroup, the mean age was 7 ± 2.9 years (range 2 to 12), with a female:male ratio of 11:18. In total, 42 age- and sex-matched controls were included.

Dental attendance, hygiene, and dietary habits

Both EB participants and controls had regular follow-up and prophylaxis consultations with the dental practitioner (Table 2). Most EB (90.2%) and control (97.6%) participants brushed their teeth at least once every day. These results were similar for patients < 12 years old. Nevertheless, less than half of EB participants (43.9%) reported brushing only once a day, whereas most controls (73.8%) brushed twice a day. More than half of EB participants (predominantly those with DEB) reported difficulties with toothbrushing. The main issues mentioned by all EB pa-

tients were "pain" and "limitation of mouth opening" (42.9% and 16.7%, respectively), more frequently in DEB than in other participants (52.0% and 20.0%). In addition, DEB and JEB participants reported difficulties with chewing and swallowing; one-third of them consumed only soft food. For patients < 12 years old, brushing was generally performed by the parents, especially for those with JEB (100.0%) or DEB (94.1%) as compared with the control group (66.6%). The frequency of "gingival bleeding when brushing" was higher for EB participants than controls (32.5% vs 17.5%), regardless of age. The frequency of sugar consumption did not differ between EB participants and controls.

Oral mucosa examination

EB participants exhibited mainly oral mucosal erythema, blisters, and erosions/ulcerations (Table 3 and Fig 4). Ten (23.8%) EB participants (predominantly SEB) did not show any oral mucosal lesions on clinical examination.

The mean EBOS score was 3.3 ± 3.0. DEB participants had the highest mean score (4.4 ± 2.9) and SEB participants the lowest (1.4 ± 2.1). Microstomia and ankyloglossia were found only in DEB (40.0% and 48.0% of total DEB, respectively). Oral lesions showed a wide distribution over the mucosal surfaces, in all types of EB, with the exception of the oral cavity floor, which was never affected in SEB. Gingiva (81% of total EB), oral mucosa on the cheeks (73.8% of total EB), lips (64.3% of total EB), and palate (61.9% of total EB) were the most affected areas. Despite the overall similar oral mucosa lesion distribution within each EB

Table 2 Oral hygiene, dietary habits, and function in participants with epidermolysis bullosa (EB) and controls, for the total sample and for participants aged under 12 years old

			Control group (n = 42)	Total EB group (n = 42)	DEB (n = 25)	JEB (n = 5)	SEB (n = 12)
Total sample, all ages							
Patient characteristics							
Oral hygiene	Toothbrushing frequency	Less than once a day	1 (2.4%)	4 (9.5%)	4 (16.7%)	0 (0.0%)	0 (0.0%)
		Once a day	10 (23.8%)	18 (43.9%)	12 (48.0%)	2 (40.0%)	5 (41.7%)
		Twice a day or more	31 (73.8%)	19 (46.3%)	9 (37.5%)	3 (60.0%)	7 (58.3%)
	Difficulties brushing (y/n)	All difficulties included	NR	23 (54.7%)	16 (64.0%)	2 (40.0%)	5 (41.7%)
		Pain*	NR	18 (42.9%)	13 (52.0%)	1 (20.0%)	4 (33.3%)
		Limitation of mouth opening*	NR	7 (16.7%)	5 (20.0%)	0 (0.0%)	2 (16.7%)
		Presence of enamel hypoplasia	5 (11.9%)	7 (16.6%)	3 (12.0%)	3 (60.0%)	1 (8.3%)
		Gingival bleeding when brushing	7 (17.5%)	13 (32.5%)	10 (47.8%)	2 (40.0%)	1 (8.3%)
Diet/function	Food consistency*	Soft	NR	13 (31.0%)	11 (44.0%)	1 (20.0%)	1 (8.3%)
		Mixed	NR	29 (69.0%)	14 (56.0%)	4 (80.0%)	11 (91.7%)
	Sugar consumption	Once a day	8 (19.1%)	24 (57.1%)	15 (60.0%)	3 (60.0%)	6 (50.0%)
		Several times a day	15 (35.7%)	18 (42.9%)	10 (40.0%)	2 (40.0%)	6 (50.0%)
	Functional difficulties (y/n)*	Chewing	NR	19 (45.2%)	13 (52.0%)	4 (80.0%)	2 (16.7%)
		Swallowing	NR	14 (33.3%)	9 (36.0%)	3 (60.0%)	2 (16.7%)
			Control group (n = 29)	Total EB group (n = 29)	DEB (n = 17)	JEB (n = 4)	SEB (n = 8)
Subgroup, children under 12 years of age							
Patient characteristics							
Oral hygiene and health	Toothbrushing frequency	Less than once a day	1 (0.0%)	4 (13.8%)	3 (18.7%)	0 (0.0%)	0 (0.0%)
		Once a day	6 (20.7%)	12 (42.9%)	7 (43.8%)	2 (50.0%)	3 (37.5%)
		Twice a day or more	22 (75.9%)	13 (46.4%)	6 (37.5%)	2 (50.0%)	5 (62.5%)
	Difficulties to brush (y/n)	All difficulties included	NR	16 (55.2%)	9 (52.9%)	2 (50.0%)	5 (62.5%)
		Pain*	NR	12 (41.7%)	7 (41.2%)	1 (25.0%)	5 (62.5%)
		Limitation of mouth opening*	NR	5 (17.2%)	4 (23.5%)	1 (25.0%)	0 (0.0%)
		Presence of enamel hypoplasia	4 (13.7%)	7 (25.9%)	3 (17.6%)	3 (75.0%)	1 (12.5%)
		Gingival bleeding when brushing	3 (10.3%)	9 (31.3%)	7 (41.2%)	1 (25.0%)	1 (12.5%)
		Parental help with brushing	19 (66.7%)	26 (89.7%)	16 (94.1%)	4 (100.0%)	6 (75.0%)
Diet/function	Diet consistency*	Soft	NR	7 (24.1%)	5 (29.4%)	1 (25.0%)	1 (12.5%)
		Mixed	NR	22 (75.9%)	12 (70.6%)	3 (75.0%)	7 (87.5%)
	Sugar consumption	Once a day	7 (24.1%)	16 (55.2%)	11 (64.7%)	2 (50.0%)	3 (37.5%)
		Several times a day	10 (34.5%)	13 (44.8%)	6 (35.3%)	2 (50.0%)	5 (62.5%)
	Functional difficulties (y/n)*	To chew	NR	12 (41.4%)	7 (41.2%)	4 (100.0%)	1 (12.5%)
		To swallow	NR	8 (27.6%)	4 (23.5%)	3 (75.0%)	1 (12.5%)

DEB, dystrophic EB; JEB, junctional EB; NR, not reported; SEB, simplex EB.
*Items not evaluated in the control group because of non-relevance.

group, SEB and DEB patients < 12 years old had more severe symptoms than their over-12-years-old counterparts.

Periodontal examination

GI and "gingival bleeding when brushing" scores revealed gingival inflammation level and severity. EB participants showed higher mean GI and frequency of "gingival bleeding when brushing" than controls, regardless of age.[17] The mean GI and "gingival bleeding when brushing" frequency were higher for DEB than for SEB and JEB participants (1.8 ± 0.8; 47.8% vs 1.2 ± 0.7; 8.3%, and 1.1 ± 0.6; 40.0%); mean PI did not differ among groups (DEB, 1.7 ± 0.7; SEB, 1.6 ± 1.0; JEB, 1.80 ± 0.6). Participants < 12 years old showed similar results.

Dental examination

Sixty percent of JEB participants showed enamel hypoplasia, which was significantly higher than observed in DEB (12.0%), SEB (8.3%), and control participants (11.9%) (Table 2). Caries experience and enamel hypoplasia frequency did not differ significantly between EB participants and controls, regardless of age. Among all participants including controls, DEB participants had the lowest mean DMFT score (3.1±5.3). EB participants' and controls' DMFT scores did not differ (3.9±6.1 vs 5.03±5.5; $P=.100$), regardless of age (3.8±4.3 vs 5.1±4.3, $P=.100$ for patients <12 years old).

Discussion

This work on the global oral health condition of individuals with inherited EB highlighted that distribution of the lesion on mucosa or gingiva hinges on EB type while their severity hinges on age. Analysis with an age cutoff showed that for DEB and SEB patients, individuals under 12 years old were the ones most severely affected.

The size of the sample in this study is quite large for a rare condition and is one of the largest published among those that investigated the three major types of EB. The number and diversity of EB participants and the inclusion of a matched (by sex and age) control group adds value in comparison with previously published case series or cohort studies.[8,19,21,22] Furthermore, the present results were sustained by systematic examination according to validated scales for oral health (teeth, periodontium, mucosa) – key components and their daily oral maintenance habits records. Due to practical team and services organization, the control group including patients for regular treatment and oral check-up was only recruited at the Toulouse hospital, which could be considered a limitation of the study. There are no recent data on oral health patients in France, so it was decided to compare the EB population with one treated in the same conditions at the hospital. Given the authors' respective experiences and expertise as dental hospital professionals, it was considered representative of the oral health status of the population of all the authors' dental care centers. Furthermore, considering that EB patients came from all over France and Belgium, it would have been difficult to find matched patients in every town.

Most of the participants exhibited oral lesions, with a mean EBOS score of 3.3 (maximum 21.0), which is lower than the mean score reported by Fortuna et al[19] (12.9, maximum 23.8). This finding can be explained by the smaller size of the present sample (42 vs 92), a lower proportion of participants with DEB (60.0% vs 75.0%), and the regular (annual or semestrial) dental

follow-up of the participants. JEB and DEB individuals showed a different distribution of lesions and were the most severely affected.[11,13,18,19] Although the mucosal lesions' topographic distribution was the same regardless of age, the oral mucosal lesions' severity was higher for <12-year-old DEB and SEB patients. Age and EB type mainly contribute to lesion severity and distribution, respectively. This heterogeneity in lesion distribution and severity highlights the critical necessity to follow and document patients' oral health status.

Periodontal considerations have been mainly reported in people with Kindler EB subtype, displaying early and rapidly progressive periodontitis as a common feature.[23] In other EB types, plaque accumulation and gingival inflammation data were reported higher than in the present study,[8,9,13] which may have masked an intrinsic gingival inflammation. Indeed, the present finding that DEB participants showed substantial and constant gingival inflammation and high frequency of "gingival bleeding when brushing" could not be explained by clinical observation of oral hygiene (ie, the quantity of dental plaque).[17] In this situation, gingival inflammation cannot be associated with a lack of oral hygiene,[24] but rather reflects a specific feature of DEB.[17,25] The extent, severity, and progression of gingival lesions can be affected by systemic factors, such as impaired gingiva due to genetic mutation, which underlines changes in the organization of the periodontal tissues.[25] The present findings might be explained by the role of the mutated protein (collagen 7, for example, in DEB type) in oral mucosal physiology.[26] Because long-term gingival inflammation generally leads to periodontitis, management of the oral hygiene of these patients is mandatory to prevent periodontitis and tooth loss.

Enamel structural defects (ie, hypoplasia) have been described in EB patients and are related to EB genetic mutations that also affect ameloblastic differentiation.[8,27,28] However, the work of Kirkham et al[29] and Wright et al[7,12] concluded that the enamel of DEB patients was normal[12] and that only JEB patients display developmentally compromised enamel with mineral defects (more frequently in molars than incisors[29]), whereas SEB patients seemed less affected.[7] In the present work, significant differences were not observed in the prevalence of enamel hypoplasia between EB participants and controls. This finding might be explained by the increase in the enamel defect prevalence in the general population, especially molar incisor hypomineralization (affecting up to 40.0% of the population) and hypomineralized second primary molars (up to 7.0%),[30] and the low proportion of JEB individuals in our sample.

Only DEB patients showed ankyloglossia and microstomia, as previously reported.[8,24,25,28] These tissue retractions reduce access to the oral cavity and also explain the altered dietary

Table 3 Number, type, localization, and severity of oral lesions according to type of EB, for the total sample and for participants under 12 years

Patient characteristics		EB total (n = 42)	DEB (n = 25)	JEB (n = 5)	SEB (n = 12)	Total EB (n = 29)	DEB (n = 17)	JEB (n = 4)	SEB (n = 8)
		Total sample				**Children under 12 years of age**			
Microstomia		10 (23.8%)	10 (40.0%)	0 (0.0%)	0 (0.0%)	4 (13.8%)	4 (23.5%)	0 (0.0%)	0 (0.0%)
Ankyloglossia		12 (28.6%)	12 (48.0%)	0 (0.0%)	0 (0.0%)	6 (20.7%)	6 (35.3%)	0 (0.0%)	0 (0.0%)
Gingiva	Blistering	7 (16.7%)	4 (16.0%)	1 (20.0%)	2 (16.7%)	6 (20.7%)	3 (17.6%)	1 (25.0%)	2 (25.0%)
	Erythema	18 (42.9%)	16 (64.0%)	0 (0.0%)	2 (16.7%)	14 (48.3%)	12 (70.6%)	0 (0.0%)	2 (25.0%)
	Erosion/ulceration	7 (16.7%)	5 (20.0%)	0 (0.0%)	2 (16.7%)	6 (20.7%)	4 (23.5%)	0 (0.0%)	2 (25.0%)
	Atrophy	2 (4.8%)	2 (8.0%)	0 (0.0%)	0 (0.0%)	2 (6.9%)	2 (11.8%)	0 (0.0%)	0 (0.0%)
	No lesion	22 (52.4%)	9 (36.0%)	4 (80.0%)	9 (75.0%)	13 (44.8%)	5 (29.4%)	3 (75.0%)	5 (62.5%)
Lips	Blistering	10 (23.8%)	5 (20.0%)	2 (40.0%)	3 (25.0%)	8 (27.6%)	3 (17.6%)	2 (50.0%)	3 (37.5%)
	Erythema	5 (11.9%)	5 (20.0%)	0 (0.0%)	0 (0.0%)	5 (17.2%)	5 (29.4%)	0 (0.0%)	0 (0.0%)
	Erosion/ulceration	11 (26.2%)	10 (40.0%)	1 (20.0%)	0 (0.0%)	10 (34.5%)	9 (52.9%)	1 (25.0%)	0 (0.0%)
	Atrophy	1 (2.4%)	1 (4.0%)	0 (0.0%)	0 (0.0%)	1 (3.4%)	1 (5.9%)	0 (0.0%)	0 (0.0%)
	No lesion	26 (61.9%)	13 (52.0%)	3 (60.0%)	10 (83.3%)	16 (55.2%)	8 (47.1%)	2 (50.0%)	6 (75.0%)
Inner cheeks	Blistering	10 (23.8%)	9 (36.0%)	1 (20.0%)	0 (0.0%)	5 (17.2%)	4 (23.5%)	1 (25.0%)	0 (0.0%)
	Erythema	6 (14.3%)	6 (24.0%)	0 (0.0%)	0 (0.0%)	5 (17.2%)	5 (29.4%)	0 (0.0%)	0 (0.0%)
	Erosion/ulceration	15 (35.7%)	11 (44.0%)	0 (0.0%)	4 (33.3%)	15 (51.7%)	11 (64.7%)	0 (0.0%)	4 (50.0%)
	No lesion	26 (61.9%)	13 (52.0%)	4 (80.0%)	9 (75.0%)	17 (58.6%)	9 (52.9%)	3 (75.0%)	5 (62.5%)
Vesti-bules	Blistering	5 (11.9%)	3 (12.0%)	0 (0.0%)	2 (16.7%)	5 (17.2%)	3 (17.6%)	0 (0.0%)	2 (25.0%)
	Erythema	12 (28.6%)	11 (44.0%)	1 (20.0%)	0 (0.0%)	11 (37.9%)	10 (58.8%)	1 (25.0%)	0 (0.0%)
	Erosion/ulceration	5 (11.9%)	4 (16.0%)	1 (20.0%)	0 (0.0%)	4 (13.8%)	3 (17.6%)	1 (25.0%)	0 (0.0%)
	Atrophy	1 (2.4%)	1 (4.0%)	0 (0.0%)	0 (0.0%)	1 (3.4%)	1 (5.9%)	0 (0.0%)	0 (0.0%)
	No lesion	31 (73.8%)	17 (68.0%)	3 (60.0%)	11 (91.7%)	19 (65.5%)	10 (58.8%)	2 (50.0%)	7 (87.5%)
Palate	Blistering	8 (19.0%)	5 (20.0%)	1 (20.0%)	2 (16.7%)	7 (24.1%)	4 (23.5%)	1 (25.0%)	2 (25.0%)
	Erythema	8 (19.0%)	7 (28.0%)	1 (20.0%)	0 (0.0%)	8 (27.6%)	7 (41.2%)	1 (25.0%)	0 (0.0%)
	Erosion/ulceration	9 (21.4%)	7 (28.0%)	1 (20.0%)	1 (8.3%)	7 (24.1%)	5 (29.4%)	1 (25.0%)	1 (12.5%)
	Atrophy	1 (2.4%)	1 (4.0%)	0 (0.0%)	0 (0.0%)	1 (3.4%)	1 (5.9%)	0 (0.0%)	0 (0.0%)
	No lesion	27 (64.3%)	13 (52.0%)	4 (80.0%)	10 (83.3%)	16 (55.2%)	7 (41.2%)	3 (75.0%)	6 (75.0%)
Tongue	Blistering	9 (21.4%)	8 (32.0%)	0 (0.0%)	1 (8.3%)	3 (10.3%)	5 (29.4%)	0 (0.0%)	1 (12.5%)
	Erosion/ulceration	8 (19.0%)	6 (24.0%)	1 (20.0%)	1 (8.3%)	6 (53.3%)	6 (35.3%)	1 (25.0%)	1 (12.5%)
	Erythema	2 (4.8%)	2 (8.0%)	0 (0.0%)	0 (0.0%)	2 (6.9%)	2 (11.8%)	0 (0.0%)	0 (0.0%)
	Atrophy	1 (2.4%)	1 (2.4%)	0 (0.0%)	0 (0.0%)	1 (2.4%)	1 (2.4%)	0 (0.0%)	0 (0.0%)
	No lesion	27 (64.3%)	13 (52.0%)	4 (80.0%)	10 (83.3%)	17 (58.6%)	8 (47.1%)	3 (75.0%)	6 (75.0%)
Oral floor	Blistering	3 (7.1%)	2 (8.0%)	1 (20.0%)	0 (0.0%)	1 (3.4%)	0 (0.0%)	1 (25.0%)	0 (0.0%)
	Erythema	2 (4.8%)	2 (8.0%)	0 (0.0%)	0 (0.0%)	2 (6.9%)	2 (11.8%)	0 (0.0%)	0 (0.0%)
	Erosion/ulceration	2 (4.8%)	1 (4.0%)	1 (20.0%)	0 (0.0%)	2 (6.9%)	1 (5.9%)	1 (25.0%)	0 (0.0%)
	Atrophy	2 (4.8%)	2 (8.0%)	0 (0.0%)	0 (0.0%)	2 (6.9%)	2 (11.8%)	0 (0.0%)	0 (0.0%)
	No lesion	33 (78.6%)	18 (72.0%)	3 (60.0%)	12 (100.0%)	22 (75.9%)	12 (70.6%)	2 (50.0%)	8 (100.0%)
EBOS score	Mean ± SD	3.3 ± 3.0	4.4 ± 2.9	1.2 ± 3.1	1.4 ± 2.1	3.9 ± 3.1	4.5 ± 3.4	1.4 ± 1.3	2.1 ± 2.3
	Median	3.0	4.0	1.5	0.0	3.0	3.0	1.4	1.5
	Range distribution	0–21	0–10	0–8	0–6	0–10	0–10	1–8	0–6

DEB, dystrophic EB; EBOS, epidermolysis bullosa oropharyngeal severity; JEB, junctional EB; SEB, simplex EB.

habits because of chewing and swallowing difficulties.[5,12,14] Microstomia tends to worsen without interception if developed at a young age, so it requires attention and follow-up. Eventually, it will lead to severe difficulties in maintaining good oral hygiene and limitations in access to the posterior part of the oral cavity when dental treatment is needed. This situation will result in ethical reflections regarding the need for and timing of posterior teeth extractions before treatments become difficult. Although feeding through a gastrostomy is often implemented for individuals with severe microstomia, some still consume

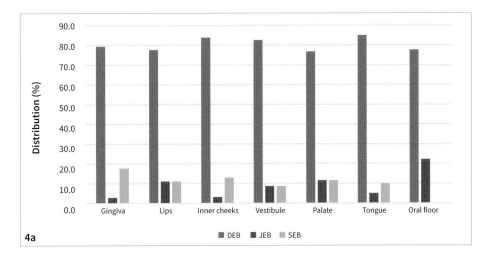

Figs 4a and 4b Topographical distribution of total oral lesions depending on the EB type, *(a)* for the all sample or *(b)* with a cut-off at 12 years old.

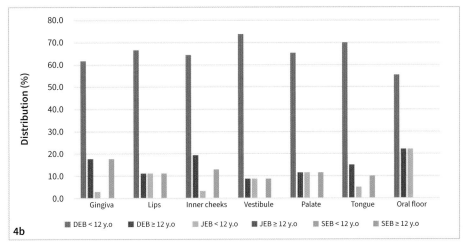

juices or other types of sugary food. In combination with poor oral hygiene, this consumption will increase the development of caries lesions. A protocol using exercises is currently being tested and shows encouraging results in interfering with the development and progression of microstomia.

The present study demonstrated no difference in sugar consumption frequency between EB and control groups, in accordance with Harris et al[13] but not with previous reports.[10] These seemingly conflicting results might be attributed to the increased attention given to children's sugar restriction in general. In line with Wright et al,[11] the present study confirms that caries development is not a specific sign of EB but rather a consequence of impaired oral health-related habits. The present participants had better oral health, dental care, and dietary habits, with better oral hygiene levels and lower caries experience, than reported in previous studies.[16,31] These results can be explained by the fact that these participants were included in

a multidisciplinary program with regular follow-up by a dental practitioner and dermatologist working collaboratively. Moreover, participants followed strict preventive recommendations,[31] including daily toothbrushing using a fluoride-containing toothpaste, fluoride applications every 6 months, and restriction of sugar intake. Despite frequent parental support with brushing (more frequent for EB groups), oral hygiene remains a point of attention requiring continuous education and motivation of patients and parents for brushing/cleaning techniques.

Some recommendations[31,32] are meant to help dental practitioners to care for these patients. Specific precautions are needed to be followed to treat those that suffer from the most sensitive mucosa and frequent oral lesions, such as lubricating the mouth or any dental instruments prior to treatment, and never using suction.

Investigating the oral health habits of patients raises an important element for professionals: the use of chlorhexidine mouthwash was widely advocated for gingivitis prevention in patients with EB due to its antiseptic properties.[31] However, two recent Cochrane meta-analyses concluded that there was insufficient evidence to prove that chlorhexidine (whatever its concentration) was efficient at reducing discrete to severe gingivitis,[33] and its role for caries prevention is very controversial.[34] Furthermore, side effects of long-term use of chlorhexidine, such as transient taste disturbance, extrinsic tooth staining, and calculus build up, are not negligible. Thus, systematic use of chlorhexidine mouthwashes is not recommended for EB or any patients. However, in case of extensive and severe mucosal lesion occurrence, chlorhexidine mouthwashes' anti-inflammatory property can help in reducing pain and inflammation, thus supporting tooth brushing[32] when used for a short period of time. ⊞

Conclusion

This large study highlights new appreciations regarding oral health involvement in people with EB, allowing improvements in patient care. Firstly, an EB type-dependent topographical distribution pattern of oral mucosal lesions was observed. Secondly, patients under 12 years old seem to exhibit more severe clinical signs than those over 12 years old, but long-term follow-up is needed to confirm this clinical trend. Thirdly, DEB participants displaying more severe lesions also showed stronger gingival reaction to dental plaque accumulation. Finally, oral health status seems to benefit from a close collaboration between the dermatologist and dental practitioner. General dental practitioners are qualified to treat these patients in the context of regular dental care, including prevention and oral health education. They can refer to a specialist when needed for heavier treatment, or for the most severely impaired patients, in particular in DEB type condition.

Acknowledgments

The authors thank Dr Sophie Caroline Campana for her help in collecting data, and Thibaut Canceill for the data analysis. The authors received no financial support for this research project, its authorship and/or publication. None of the authors have conflicts of interest to declare. The data supporting the findings of this study are available from the corresponding author upon reasonable request.

References

1. Silva LCP, Cruz RA, Abou-Id LR, Brini LNB, Moreira LS. Clinical evaluation of patients with epidermolysis bullosa: Review of the literature and case reports. Spec Care Dent 2004;24:22–27.

2. Tabolli S, Sampogna F, Di Pietro C, et al. Quality of life in patients with epidermolysis bullosa. Br J Dermatol 2009;161:869–877.

3. Rao R, Mellerio J, Bhogal BS, Groves R. Immunofluorescence antigen mapping for hereditary epidermolysis bullosa. Indian J Dermatol Venereol Leprol 2012;78:692–697.

4. Feijoo JF, Bugallo J, Limeres J, Peñarrocha D, Peñarrocha M, Diz P. Inherited epidermolysis bullosa: an update and suggested dental care considerations. J Am Dent Assoc 2011;142: 1017–1025.

5. Fortuna G, Lozada-Nur F, Pollio A, et al. Patterns of oral mucosa lesions in patients with epidermolysis bullosa: comparison and agreement between oral medicine and dermatology. J Oral Pathol Med 2013;42:733–740.

6. Wright JT, Johnson LB, Fine JD. Development defects of enamel in humans with hereditary epidermolysis bullosa. Arch Oral Biol 1993;38: 945–955.

7. Wright JT, Hall KI, Deaton TG, Fine J-D. Structural and compositional alteration of tooth enamel in hereditary epidermolysis bullosa. Connect Tissue Res 1996;34:271–279.

8. Wright JT, Fine JD, Johnson LB. Oral soft tissues in hereditary epidermolysis bullosa. Oral Surg Oral Med Oral Pathol 1991;71:440–446.

9. Wright JT, Fine JD, Johnson L. Hereditary epidermolysis bullosa: oral manifestations and dental management. Pediatr Dent 1993; 15: 242–248.

10. De Medeiros RA, Leal SC, Lia EN, et al. Higher dental caries prevalence and its association with dietary habits and physical limitation in epidermolysis bullosa patients: a case control study. J Contemp Dent Pract 2016;17: 211–216.

11. Wright JT, Fine JD, Johnson L. Dental caries risk in hereditary epidermolysis bullosa. Pediatr Dent 1994;16:427–432.

12. Kirkham J, Robinson C, Strafford SM, et al. The chemical composition of tooth enamel in recessive dystrophic epidermolysis bullosa: significance with respect to dental caries. J Dent Res 1996;75:1672–1678.

13. Harris JC, Bryan RA, Lucas VS, Roberts GJ. Dental disease and caries related microflora in children with dystrophic epidermolysis bullosa. Pediatr Dent 2001;23:438–443.

14. Louloudiadis AK, Louloudiadis KA. Case report: dystrophic epidermolysis bullosa: dental management and oral health promotion. Eur Arch Paediatr Dent 2009;10:42–45.

15. Stellingsma C, Dijkstra PU, Dijkstra J, Duipmans JC, Jonkman MF, Dekker R. Restrictions in oral functions caused by oral manifestations of epidermolysis bullosa. Eur J Dermatol 2011;21:405–409.

16. Scheidt L, Sanabe ME, Diniz MB. Oral manifestations and dental management of epidermolysis bullosa simplex. Int J Clin Pediatr Dent 2015;8:239–241.

17. Chiaverini C, Marty M, Dridi S-M, et al. Oral status in patients with inherited epidermolysis bullosa: A multicentric observational study. J Am Acad Dermatol 2022;87: 872–874.

18. World Health Organization. Oral Health Surveys: Basic Methods, 5th edition. Geneva: World Health Organization; 2013.

19. Fortuna G, Chainani-Wu N, Lozada-Nur F, et al. Epidermolysis Bullosa Oropharyngeal Severity (EBOS) score: A multicenter development and reliability assessment. J Am Acad Dermatol 2013;68:83–92.

20. Nelson SJ. Wheeler's Dental Anatomy, Physiology and Occlusion. First South Asia Edition. New Delhi: Reed Elsevier, 2015:394.

21. Serrano-Martínez MC, Bagán JV, Silvestre FJ, Viguer MT. Oral lesions in recessive dystrophic epidermolysis bullosa. Oral Dis 2003;9: 264–268.

22. Uitto J, Has C, Vahidnezhad H, Youssefian L, Bruckner-Tuderman L. Molecular pathology of the basement membrane zone in heritable blistering diseases. Matrix Biol 2017; 57–58:76–85.

23. Wiebe CB, Petricca G, Häkkinen L, Jiang G, Wu C, Larjava HS. Kindler syndrome and periodontal disease: review of the literature and a 12-year follow-up case. J Periodontol 2008;79:961–966.

24. Page RC, Schroeder HE. Pathogenesis of inflammatory periodontal disease. A summary of current work. Lab Investig J Tech Methods Pathol 1976;34:235–249.

25. Chapple ILC, Mealey BL, Van Dyke TE, et al. Periodontal health and gingival diseases and conditions on an intact and a reduced periodontium: Consensus report of workgroup 1 of the 2017 World Workshop on the Classification of Periodontal and Peri-Implant Diseases and Conditions. J Clin Periodontol 2018; 45(Suppl 20):S68–S77.

26. Abe M, Osawa T. The structure of the interstitial surfaces of the epithelial basement membranes of mouse oral mucosa, gingiva and tongue. Arch Oral Biol 1999; 44:587–594.

27. Pekiner FN, Yücelten D, Ozbayrak S, Sezen EC. Oral-clinical findings and management of epidermolysis bullosa. J Clin Pediatr Dent 2005;30:59–65.

28. Stavropoulos F, Abramowicz S. Management of the oral surgery patient diagnosed with epidermolysis bullosa: report of 3 cases and review of the literature. J Oral Maxillofac Surg 2008;66:554–559.

29. Kirkham J, Robinson C, Strafford SM, et al. The chemical composition of tooth enamel in junctional epidermolysis bullosa. Arch Oral Biol 2000;45:377–386.

30. Silva MJ, Scurrah KJ, Craig JM, Manton DJ, Kilpatrick N. Etiology of molar incisor hypomineralization: a systematic review. Community Dent Oral Epidemiol 2016;44:342–353.

31. Krämer SM, Serrano MC, Zillmann G, et al. Oral health care for patients with epidermolysis bullosa - best clinical practice guidelines: clinical guidelines for oral care in epidermolysis bullosa. Int J Paediatr Dent 2012;22:1–35.

32. Haute Autorité de Santé. Protocole National de Diagnostic et de Soins (PNDS) Épidermolyses bulleuses héréditaires. September 2021. https://www.has-sante.fr/jcms/c_2028188/fr/epidermolyses-bulleuses-hereditaires. Accessed 20 Sept 2022.

33. James P, Worthington HV, Parnell C, et al. Chlorhexidine mouthrinse as an adjunctive treatment for gingival health. Cochrane Database Syst Rev 2017;3:CD008676.

34. Walsh T, Oliveira-Neto JM, Moore D. Chlorhexidine treatment for the prevention of dental caries in children and adolescents. Cochrane Database Syst Rev 2015;4: CD008457.

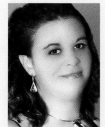

Clara Joseph

Clara Joseph   Associate Professor, Head, Department of Pediatric Dentistry, Centre Hospitalier Universitaire de Nice; Côte d'Azur University; Centre de Référence des Maladies Rares de la Peau et des Muqueuses d'Origine Génétique du Centre Hospitalier Universitaire de Nice; EA 7354, MICORALIS Laboratory, Nice, France. ORCID 0000-0002-1004-6163

Mathieu Marty   Associate Professor, Department of Pediatric Dentistry, Centre Hospitalier Universitaire de Toulouse, Paul Sabatier Toulouse III University, Competence Center of Oral Rare Diseases, Toulouse, France. ORCID 0000-0003-0579-341X

Sophie-Myriam Dridi   Full Professor, Department of Periodontology, Centre Hospitalier Universitaire de Nice, Côte d'Azur University, EA 7354, MICORALIS Laboratory, Nice, France. ORCID 0000-0001-6335-3370

Veroniek Verhaeghe   Staff Member, Department of Pediatric Dentistry and Special Care, University Hospitals Leuven, Leuven, Belgium

Isabelle Bailleul-Forestier   Full Professor, Department of Pediatric Dentistry, Centre Hospitalier Universitaire de Toulouse, Paul Sabatier Toulouse III University, Competence Center of Oral Rare Diseases, Toulouse, France. ORCID 0000-0002-9338-3017

Christine Chiaverini   Head of the Centre de Référence des Maladies Rares de la Peau et des Muqueuses d'Origine Génétique du Centre Hospitalier Universitaire de Nice; Department of Dermatology, Centre Hospitalier Universitaire de Nice, Côte d'Azur University, Nice, France. ORCID 0000-0002-6063-5409

Thomas Hubiche   Staff member, Centre de Référence des Maladies Rares de la Peau et des Muqueuses d'Origine Génétique du Centre Hospitalier Universitaire de Nice; Department of Dermatology, Centre Hospitalier Universitaire, Côte d'Azur University, Nice, France. ORCID 0000-0002-3247-7386

Juliette Mazereeuw-Hautier   Full Professor, Centre de Référence des Maladies Rares de la Peau et des Muqueuses d'Origine Génétique du Centre Hospitalier Universitaire de Toulouse, Department of Dermatology, Centre Hospitalier Universitaire de Toulouse, Toulouse, France. ORCID: 0000-0001-6259-9790

Olivier Deny   Staff member, Institut RESTORE, Paul Sabatier Toulouse III University, CNRS U-5070, EFS, ENVT, Inserm U1301; Department of Oral Biology, Institute of Oral Medicine and Science, Paul Sabatier Toulouse III University, Toulouse, France. ORCID: 0000-0002-7894-7240

Dominique Declerck   Full Professor, Department of Pediatric Dentistry and Special Care, University Hospitals Leuven, Leuven, Belgium. ORCID: 0000-0003-4637-0675

Philippe Kémoun   Full Professor, Oral Biology, Pediatric Dentistry, Institute of Oral Medicine and Science, Paul Sabatier Toulouse III University; Institut RESTORE, CNRS U-5070, EFS, ENVT, Inserm U1301, Toulouse III University; Competence Center of Oral Rare Diseases; Centre Hospitalier Universitaire de Toulouse, Toulouse, France. ORCID: 0000-0001-7373-2657

Correspondence: Dr Clara Joseph, Faculté de Chirurgie Dentaire, Université Côte d'Azur (UCA), Campus Saint Jean d'Angély, Bât SJA 2, 5 rue du 22ème BCA, 06357 Nice Cedex 4, France. Email: Clara.JOSEPH@univ-cotedazur.fr

First submission: 6 May 2022
Acceptance: 5 Aug 2022
Online publication: 11 Oct 2022

The relationship between periodontal and kidney disease: a critical review

Aditi Priyamvara, BDS, MHA/Amit K. Dey, MD/Abhiram Maddi, DDS, MS, PhD/Sorin Teich, DMD, MBA

Periodontal disease has been associated with various systemic diseases including kidney disease. However, a causal relationship is yet to be established. One possible association is that periodontitis may cause an increased inflammatory response in kidney disease patients which in turn destroys endothelial vasculature. This may contribute to development of risk factors of kidney disease such as diabetic neuropathy and cardiovascular events leading the progression and mortality in kidney disease patients. The role of periodontal inflammation driving kidney disease is still under investigation. This review article highlights the role of periodontal inflammation in the development and progression of kidney disease. It is crucial that dental practitioners and nephrologists understand the association between periodontal and kidney disease. Early periodontal screening and educating patients about the importance of good oral hygiene may play an important role in prevention of progression of kidney disease. *(Quintessence Int 2022;53: 178–187; doi: 10.3290/j.qi.b3320225)*

Key words: inflammation, kidney disease, periodontitis

Periodontal disease (PD) is associated with high health care burden and affects around 20% to 50% of the global population.[1] Moreover, this prevalence is much higher in the developing countries than in the developed countries and can account for much higher numbers. PD is interestingly associated with inflamed oral cavity as well as high systemic inflammation, and encompasses a variety of chronic inflammatory conditions including plaque-induced gingivitis and periodontitis (chronic periodontitis and aggressive periodontitis).[2] It results in progressive infection/inflammation followed by bone loss and consequent loss of teeth.[3] Thus PD can affect functionality and significantly affect the quality of life of patients.[4] PD is usually associated with Gram negative bacterial pathogens such as *Porphyromonas gingivalis*, *Tannerella forsythia*, *Campylobacter rectus*, *Fusobacterium nucleatum*, *Prevotella intermedia*, and *Aggregatibacter actinomycetemcomitans*,[5] and this microflora is found in a unique biofilm in the oral cavity called the dental plaque, giving rise to gingivitis or inflammation of the gums initially.[6,7] If untreated, this may further progress to the development of deeper periodontal pockets and loss of periodontal ligament. The bacteria then invade the bloodstream and migrate to various sites in the body leading to development of a persistent immune response in the form of a systemic chronic inflammatory state in the body, which may lead to initiation and/or progression of systemic diseases. Studies have discovered that PD has a number of systemic manifestations including cardiovascular disease (CVD), insulin resistance and diabetes, respiratory tract infections, and even cancer.[8,9] There is also an association of PD with obesity.[10] Furthermore, there is evidence that PD is also associated with kidney disease,[11] but this relationship has not been explored extensively. This article reviews the evidence showing the association between these two diseases states and the effect of PD on kidney disease.

CKD and PD

The overall prevalence of chronic kidney disease (CKD) in the United States as defined by the irreversible and progressive loss of kidney function was 14.8% in 2013 to 2016.[12] According to Kidney Disease: Improving Global Outcomes (KDIGO), it is classified based on severity of the condition into five stages (CKD Stage 1 to 5).[12] A diagnosis for CKD can be established by a glomerular filtration rate (GFR) of < 60 mL/min/1.73 m^2 or presence of markers of kidney damage, including albuminuria (albumin to creatinine ratio > 30 mg/g), hematuria, history of kidney transplantation, and structural abnormalities of electrolyte abnormalities due to tubular disorders for more than 3 months.[13,14] CKD eventually progresses to end stage kidney disease (ESKD), where the kidneys function at only 10% of their capacity. Some independent risk factors for kidney disease include diabetes and CVD.[15] This is interesting since PD has been linked with higher prevalence of diabetes and CVD and thus could in part lead to decline in kidney function through these pathways. Recent evidence also shows periodontitis as an independent risk factor for CKD,[16] and a causal relationship has been established between the incidence of CKD and PD.[11] Some studies state that there is an association between periodontitis and decline in kidney function;[17] however, this evidence is not consistent and can be explained by other common comorbidities. In addition, there is agreement that patients with kidney disease have higher prevalence of periodontitis than healthy individuals.[18] This is further supported by studies that showed that patients with diabetic nephropathy had deeper periodontal pockets as compared to healthy patients.[19]

Epidemiologic studies exploring the relation between periodontitis and kidney disease

Several studies have explored the relation between PD and kidney disease. Firstly, it is believed that there is a bidirectional relationship between PD and kidney disease.[20] Studies show that periodontitis can act as an important source of inflammation in both the CKD and ESKD population.[21,22] On the other hand, ESKD patients who are on renal replacement therapy (RRT) have an increased presence and degree of dental plaque, leading to gingival inflammation and increased severity of periodontitis.[23] Kidney disease can also induce a negative effect on oral tissues in form of delayed eruption of teeth, xerostomia, enamel hypoplasia, pulp chamber calcification, or altered pH of saliva.[23-25] Secondly, studies also depict that severe PD may be associated with a decline in kidney function or altered kidney function even when adjusted for confounders.[17,26-30] Interestingly, the relationship between PD and CKD has been shown to differentially modulate with age, sex, and race. A recent study showed that elderly males with severe periodontitis have a clinically significant incident decline in kidney function.[17] In addition, a second study quantified the decline in GFR and showed that patients above 65 years of age with PD showed an estimated GFR decline of ≥ 30% over a period of 2 to 3 years.[30]

There is also significant evidence to suggest that African Americans with severe periodontitis have up to four-fold higher chance of decrease in kidney function than those without periodontitis.[29] One more study demonstrated that in addition to an estimated GFR decline of ≥ 30% over a period of 2 to 3 years, there was an increase in all-cause and cardiovascular mortality in older patients with periodontitis in their study.[20]

In a recent study, the cross-sectional findings were extrapolated to how PD treatment would affect GFR, and showed that estimated GFR (eGFR) can be improved in CKD patients through periodontal specific therapy.[31] Finally, kidney disease patients with periodontitis have been associated with higher mortality rates. A 14-year follow up for the NHANES III data showed that CKD alone led to 1.5- to 1.7-fold increased risk for CV and all-cause mortality.[32] On sensitivity analyses of this study, periodontitis led to 1.4-fold increased risk for all-cause mortality and was not associated with cardiovascular mortality.[28] However, CKD patients with periodontitis were found to have a two-fold increased risk for both cardiovascular and all-cause mortality compared to CKD patients without periodontitis, suggesting that the presence of PD along with CKD independently as well as synergistically increased risk of mortality.[32]

Periodontal inflammation and kidney disease

Periodontal inflammation is initiated by oral bacteria and their virulence factors and leads to tissue destruction as a result of inflammatory cytokine production by host leukocytes.[33] Inflammation also plays an important role in the progression of kidney disease, and this has been shown time and time again. In addition, chronic inflammation in the form of elevated C-reactive protein (CRP) levels have been found to reduce renal function in CKD patients.[34] There is evidence that around 30% to 50% of patients who have CKD and ESKD have high levels of CRP and other inflammatory biomarkers such as interleukin (IL)-1, IL-6, and tumor necrosis factor (TNF)-α.[23]

In fact, a recent study showed that treating inflammation would lead to improvement in CKD status or degree over time. The present authors, as well as others, have shown before that PD is associated with higher systemic inflammation and is an ideal human model to study the role of inflammation in the progression of systemic disease.[5,35] Studies show that PD causes impairment in kidney disease patients through an inflammatory pathway, further proving the hypothesis that PD can have systemic manifestation somewhat mediated through increased inflammation.[35] This has been shown in the form of higher systemic inflammatory markers, such as elevated CRP levels in periodontitis, which in turn associates with endothelial dysfunction as well as contributes to mortality in kidney disease.[2,36] Prior studies have consistently demonstrated patients with periodontitis to have high levels of serum CRP in comparison to the general population.[37] In PD, the bacteria in the plaque biofilm disseminate into the bloodstream causing transient bacteremia, which leads to immune response in the form of chronic inflammation. Bacterial products trigger the production of inflammatory markers including IL-6 and TNF-α, which further stimulate hepatocytes to produce CRP. The bacteria invade and adhere to endothelial cells.[38-40] This leads to endothelial activation and the development of initial stages of atherosclerosis and atheroma formation.[41] This eventually destroys the endothelial vasculature which in turn is associated with worsening of CKD. Impairment of endothelial vasculature as seen in periodontitis leads to atherosclerotic complications seen in kidney disease.[36] Moreover, it is a known fact that CVD and atherosclerotic complications play a major role in mortality associated with kidney disease.[36,42]

Molecular mimicry of bacterial heat shock proteins contributing to renal atherogenesis

A proposed mechanism contributing to the association between PD and kidney disease suggests molecular mimicry.[43,44] It is postulated that periodontal bacteria are also responsible for producing a local immune response causing vascular inflammation and atherosclerosis by cross-reacting with self-antigens on the vascular endothelium. Similarities have been found between bacterial antigen and heat-shock protein (HSP), GroEL60, which is a protein of the HSP 60 family. An *Escherichia coli* GroEL60 homolog has been found in various bacteria,[45] including *P. gingivalis*, which is present in the plaque biofilm.[46] GroEL60 shares homology with human HSP60 and its antigens cross react with antibodies of human HSP60.[46] HSP60 is produced in response to endothelial damage and facilitates atherogenesis.[46] There is atheroma formation in renal arteries which contributes to a decrease in blood supply that causes ischemia, necrosis of glomeruli, and severe renal insufficiency.[47]

Association between risk factors for PD and kidney disease

Major risk factors for kidney disease include hypertension, diabetes, and smoking, which are also commonly seen in a patient with periodontitis. Understanding these risk factors when understanding the pathogenesis and relationship between PD and kidney disease is vital.

Hypertension

Studies show that patients with moderate to severe periodontitis have a higher susceptibility of developing hypertension and that there is an increased prevalence of periodontitis in patients who have hypertension.[48] Possible mechanisms include transient bacteremia through oral microflora, subsequent release of inflammatory biomarkers such as IL-1, IL-6, TNF-α, and CRP. This further leads to systemic inflammation and endothelial dysfunction, which can lead to increased susceptibility for hypertension. Asymmetric dimethylarginine (ADMA) is a biomarker of endothelial dysfunction and leads to impaired synthesis of nitric oxide synthase (NOS) which helps in the synthesis of nitric oxide (NO).[49] NO is a vasodilator and lowers blood pressure. It also plays a part in homeostasis and regulates platelet aggregation.[50] Decreased production of NO can thus lead to hypertension, CVD, and atherosclerotic complications. Sustained hypertension has been considered to be an important risk factor for organ damage leading to CVD and kidney disease,[51] especially in active PD.

Diabetes

It has been postulated that periodontitis is associated with higher incidence of CKD in part through higher insulin resistance and prevalent diabetes.[36,52] Diabetes is considered as one of the main risk factors for kidney disease. Type 2 diabetes mellitus patients with PD are more likely to have decreased kidney function and thus have a synergistic response. Many patients develop kidney dysfunction due to microvascular complications caused by hyperglycemia in PD. Diabetes shares a two-way relationship with periodontitis.[53] While studies state that risk of developing PD is greater if glycemic control is poor, there is also evidence that glycemic control is poor in periodontal inflammation. It is a known fact that long-term diabetes can lead to diabetic nephropathy.[54] Diabetic neuropathy and presence of persistent proteinuria, an important risk factor for progression of CKD to ESKD, occurs in 40% of type 1 and 2 diabetic patients.[55] A recent study showed that the incidence of proteinuria and ESKD in type 2 diabetes patients with periodontitis was higher compared with patients with no periodontitis depicting that presence or absence of periodontitis can predict the development of overt nephropathy.[28] Thus, glycemic control is important not only for PD but also for kidney disease, and especially important for CKD in PD patients.

Smoking

Smoking has been considered to be an independent risk factor for both PD[56] and kidney disease.[57] In periodontitis, it impairs inflammatory function, the functions of fibroblasts, and causes endothelial injury.[58] It has a similar endothelial dysfunction mechanism in kidneys where it activates fibroblasts and causes inflammatory and endothelial damage leading to fibrosis of the kidneys.[57] Nicotine in tobacco has vasoconstrictive characteristics that lead to an increase in blood pressure and a decreased GFR. Some adverse effects of smoking on kidneys include albuminuria, diabetic nephropathy in type 2 diabetes mellitus patients, cardiovascular complications, low creatinine values, and a decline in renal function.

Understanding the role of PD in different stages of kidney disease

KDIGO classifies kidney disease into five different stages based on GFR and albuminuria.[13] GFR categories G1 to G5:

- G1: Normal or high
  (≥ 90 mL/min/1.73 m^2)
- G2: Mildly decreased
  (60–89 mL/min/1.73 m^2)
- G3a: Mildly to moderately decreased
  (45–59 mL/min/1.73 m^2)
- G3b: Moderately to severely decreased
  (30–44 mL/min/1.73 m^2)
- G4: Severely decreased
  (15–29 mL/min/1.73 m^2)
- G5: Kidney failure
  (< 15 mL/min/1.73 m^2)

Persistent albuminuria categories A1 to A3:
- A1: Normal to mildly increased
  (< 30 mg/g; < 3 mg/mmol)
- A2: Moderately increased
  (30–300 mg/g; 3–30 mg/mmol)
- A3: Severely increased
  (> 300 mg/g; > 30 mg/mmol).[13]

Understanding the role of PD during the different stages of kidney disease might be helpful in adequately risk-stratifying these patients, and further helpful in targeted treatment of these patients.

PD and subclinical kidney disease

Acute kidney injury (AKI) refers to a sudden decrease in kidney function. It may be reversible; however, it may lead to the development of subacute or subclinical kidney disease. KDIGO clubs such disorders into the category of acute kidney disease (AKD) and disorders and defines them as kidney damage that is present for less than 3 months post AKI, GFR of < 60 mL/min/1.73 m^2 for less than 3 months, or GFR decrease of 35% or more or increase in serum creatinine by more than 50% for less than 3 months.[13,59] To date there is no evidence highlighting the potential association of PD and AKD, and further research is needed to understand this relationship.

PD and CKD

In addition to understanding the risk of developing CKD through PD it is also important to understand the effects of PD on renal function in a patient who already has baseline kidney disease. In a recent study severe PD had a direct association with severity of CKD (stage 4 and 5), with lower GFR values and a declined renal function, suggesting that there is a dose response relationship of CKD and PD.[60] This study was associational and thus could not establish a direct causal relationship. However, in a more recent study, it was found that a causal relationship exists between PD and CKD that is mediated through oxidative stress and inflammation.[61]

PD and ESKD

Higher incidence of ESKD has been found in individuals with severe periodontitis. In a study on type 2 diabetics, periodontitis has been shown to predict the development of overt nephropathy (macroalbuminuria ≥ 300 mg/g) and ESKD.[28] Common renal replacement therapies for survival of ESKD patients include hemodialysis (HD) and peritoneal dialysis. Inflammation plays an important role in periodontitis and CKD patients on hemodialysis (CKHD). Severe PD in these patients has been linked to increased left ventricular mass (LVM) and hypertension.[62] It has been found that kidney disease patients on HD who have advanced periodontitis have significantly high serum CRP levels and systemic inflammatory burden, which plays a role in atherosclerotic plaque formation in these patients.[55] This relationship between CVD and ESKD is important to understand since CVD is thought to be the leading cause of mortality in kidney disease patients.[63] However, some studies also postulate that there is not a significant relationship between high

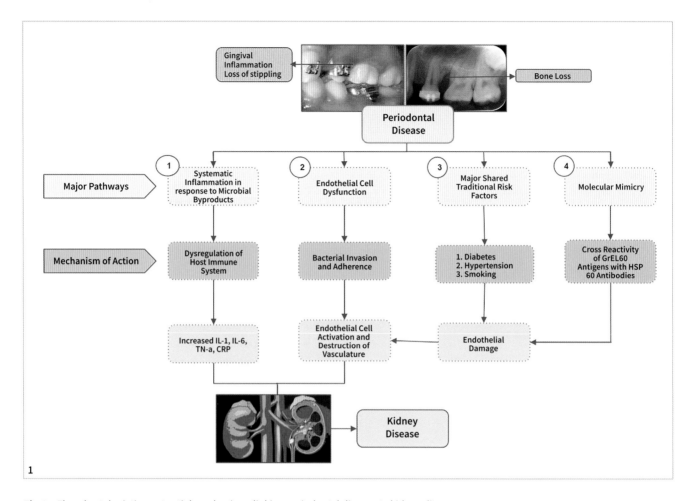

Fig 1 Flowchart depicting potential mechanisms linking periodontal disease to kidney disease.

serum CRP levels and severity of periodontitis in HD patients and thus this needs future research. Hypoalbuminemia is known as a predictor of mortality in HD patients since it affects the nutritional status in these patients. However, there is conflicting evidence suggesting HD patients with periodontitis may or may not have low serum albumin levels.

Limitations

Although there have been several hypotheses that have linked periodontitis to a decline in kidney function, there is limited/no consistent evidence that treating periodontitis actually slows the progression of CKD to ESKD or leads to improvement in kidney function. Indeed, PD is associated with an increase in inflammatory markers such as IL-1, IL-6, CRP, and TNF-a, and

periodontal therapy can help reduce these inflammatory markers and thus one would expect salutary effects for kidney disease. However, whether this systemic reduction of inflammation through nonsurgical periodontal therapy slows the decline in kidney function and thus progression of CKD remains debatable. To date, only one pilot randomized control trial (RCT), The Kidney and Periodontal Disease Study (KAPD), has been conducted to identify the impact of intensive periodontal therapy on slowing the progression of CKD in the United States.[64] In this 12-month trial, 51 eligible participants with CKD and periodontitis were provided with oral hygiene instructions at baseline and at 4, 8, and 12 months. Patients who were identified as requiring intensive periodontal therapy were provided full-mouth scaling and root planing, controlled release of antibiotics in deeper pockets, and extraction of hopeless teeth.[64] The trial was unblinded and did not have a true control group. It was less successful in measuring kidney disease biomarker variability and treatment adherence.[65]

Conclusions

Kidney disease exerts an overwhelming burden on health care and is a global health concern. There appears to be a positive correlation between kidney disease and PD through an inflammatory pathway. Even though the relationship is not clearly understood it would be reasonable to enhance efforts to diagnose and prevent periodontitis since epidemiologic evidence linking PD and kidney disease is irrefutable. In addition to treating the more commonly stated risk factors for kidney disease, periodontitis can potentially act as a novel, modifiable, and treatable risk factor. Periodontal screening should be included on assessment of kidney disease patients. Providers, especially nephrologists, should be encouraged to ask kidney disease patients about their last dental visit and whether they have a long-standing history of gum disease. A similar approach can be undertaken by dental practitioners who see CKD patients regularly. A more robust approach is needed to prevent PD through early screening and educating patients about oral hygiene during regular dental visits. Simple dental interventions such as scaling, root planning, and/ or even localized antibiotic therapy in deeper pockets when needed can help treat and maintain periodontal health in patients with PD. However, more investigation is needed to adequately risk stratify PD and CKD patients so that early and targeted treatment can be delivered along with effective monitoring of the disease.

Relevance to the general dental practitioner

The importance of the relationship between oral and systemic disease has been furthered by research in the fields of dentistry and medicine. There are several systemic conditions and drugs that have oral manifestations. Identically, managing the oral and dental needs of patients also is dependent on their systemic health conditions and their appropriate management. This applies to the management of PD and kidney disease for achieving oral and dental treatment outcomes and thus is relevant for the general dental practitioner to understand these relationships and apply them in their dental practice.

References

1. Nazir MA. Prevalence of periodontal disease, its association with systemic diseases and prevention. Int J Health Sci (Qassim) 2017;11:72–80.

2. Siribamrungwong M CP. Periodontitis: Tip of the iceberg in chronic kidney disease. World J Clin Urol 2014;3:295–303.

3. Zekeridou A, Mombelli A, Cancela J, Courvoisier D, Giannopoulou C. Systemic inflammatory burden and local inflammation in periodontitis: What is the link between inflammatory biomarkers in serum and gingival crevicular fluid? Clin Exp Dent Res 2019;5:128–135.

4. da Silva Araújo AC, Gusmão ES, Batista JE, Cimões R. Impact of periodontal disease on quality of life. Quintessence Int 2010;41: e111–e118.

5. Priyamvara A, Dey AK, Bandyopadhyay D, et al. Periodontal inflammation and the risk of cardiovascular disease. Curr Atheroscler Rep 2020;22:28.

6. Gunaratnam M, Smith GLF, Socransky SS, Smith CM, Haffajee AD. Enumeration of subgingival species on primary isolation plates using colony lifts. Oral Microbiol Immunol 1992;7:14–18.

7. Moore WEC, Moore LVH. The bacteria of periodontal diseases. Periodontology 2000 1994;5:66–77.

8. Bui FQ, Almeida-da-Silva CLC, Huynh B, et al. Association between periodontal pathogens and systemic disease. Biomed J 2019;42:27–35.

9. Maddi A, Scannapieco FA. Oral biofilms, oral and periodontal infections, and systemic disease. Am J Dent 2013;26:249–254.

10. Katz J, Bimstein E. Pediatric obesity and periodontal disease: a systematic review of the literature. Quintessence Int 2011;42: 595–599.

11. Deschamps-Lenhardt S, Martin-Cabezas R, Hannedouche T, Huck O. Association between periodontitis and chronic kidney disease: Systematic review and meta-analysis. Oral Dis 2019;25:385–402.

12. United States Renal Data System Volume 1: CKD in General Population. 2018. https://www.usrds.org/media/1723/v1_c01_genpop_18_usrds.pdf.

13. (KDIGO) KDiGO. 2012 Clinical Practice Guideline for the Evaluation and Management of Chronic Kidney Disease. Kidney Int Suppl (2011) 2013;3:1–150.

14. National Institute for Health and Care Excellence (NICE). Clinical Guideline [CG182]. Chronic kidney disease: early identification and management of chronic kidney disease in adults in primary and secondary care. London: NICE, 2014.

15. Luyckx VA, Tuttle KR, Garcia-Garcia G, et al. Reducing major risk factors for chronic kidney disease. Kidney Int Suppl (2011) 2017;7:71–87.

16. Lertpimonchai A, Rattanasiri S, Tamsailom S, et al. Periodontitis as the risk factor of chronic kidney disease: Mediation analysis. J Clin Periodontol 2019;46:631–639.

17. Grubbs V, Vittinghoff E, Taylor G, et al. The association of periodontal disease with kidney function decline: a longitudinal retrospective analysis of the MrOS dental study. Nephrol Dial Transplant 2016;31:466–472.

18. Miyata Y, Obata Y, Mochizuki Y, et al. Periodontal disease in patients receiving dialysis. Int J Mol Sci 2019;20:3805.

19.   Nylund K, Meurman JH, Heikkinen AM, Honkanen E, Vesterinen M, Ruokonen H. Oral health in predialysis patients with emphasis on periodontal disease. Quintessence Int 2015;46:899–907.

20.   Fisher MA, Taylor GW, West BT, McCarthy ET. Bidirectional relationship between chronic kidney and periodontal disease: a study using structural equation modeling. Kidney Int 2011;79:347–355.

21.   Kiany Yazdi F, Karimi N, Rasouli M, Roozbeh J. Effect of nonsurgical periodontal treatment on C-reactive protein levels in maintenance hemodialysis patients. Renal Failure 2013;35:711–717.

22.   Craig RG. Interactions between chronic renal disease and periodontal disease. Oral Dis 2008;14:1–7.

23.   Ismail G, Dumitriu HT, Dumitriu AS, Ismail FB. Periodontal disease: a covert source of inflammation in chronic kidney disease patients. Int J Nephrol 2013;2013:515796.

24.   Davidovich E, Davidovits M, Eidelman E, Schwarz Z, Bimstein E. Pathophysiology, therapy, and oral implications of renal failure in children and adolescents: an update. Pediatr Dent 2005;27:98–106.

25.   Proctor R, Kumar N, Stein A, Moles D, Porter S. Oral and dental aspects of chronic renal failure. J Dent Res 2005;84:199–208.

26.   Chang JF, Yeh JC, Chiu YL, Liou JC, Hsiung JR, Tung TH. Periodontal pocket depth, hyperglycemia, and progression of chronic kidney disease: a population-based longitudinal study. Am J Med 2017;130:61–69.e1.

27.   Iwasaki M, Taylor GW, Nesse W, Vissink A, Yoshihara A, Miyazaki H. Periodontal disease and decreased kidney function in Japanese elderly. Am J Kidney Dis 2012;59:202–209.

28.   Shultis WA, Weil EJ, Looker HC, et al. Effect of periodontitis on overt nephropathy and end-stage renal disease in type 2 diabetes. Diabetes Care 2007;30:306–311.

29.   Grubbs V, Vittinghoff E, Beck JD, et al. Association between periodontal disease and kidney function decline in African Americans: The Jackson heart study. J Periodontol 2015;86:1126–1132.

30.   Chen Y-T, Shih C-J, Ou S-M, et al. Periodontal disease and risks of kidney function decline and mortality in older people: a community-based cohort study. Am J Kidney Dis 2015;66:223–230.

31.   Chambrone L, Foz AM, Guglielmetti MR, et al. Periodontitis and chronic kidney disease: a systematic review of the association of diseases and the effect of periodontal treatment on estimated glomerular filtration rate. J Clin Periodontol 2013;40:443–456.

32.   Ricardo A, Athavale A, Chen J, et al. Periodontal disease, chronic kidney disease and mortality: results from the third National Health and Nutrition Examination Survey. BMC Nephrol 2015;16:97.

33.   Bascones A, Noronha S, Gómez M, Mota P, Moles MA, Dorrego MV. Tissue destruction in periodontitis: bacteria or cytokines fault? Quintessence Int 2005;36:299–306.

34.   Dungey M, Hull KL, Smith AC, Burton JO, Bishop NC. Inflammatory factors and exercise in chronic kidney disease. Int J Endocrinol 2013;2013:569831.

35.   Craig RG, Kotanko P, Kamer AR, Levin NW. Periodontal diseases: a modifiable source of systemic inflammation for the end-stage renal disease patient on haemodialysis therapy? Nephrology Dialysis Transplant 2006;22:312–315.

36.   Wahid A, Chaudhry S, Ehsan A, Butt S, Ali Khan A. Bidirectional relationship between chronic kidney disease & periodontal disease. Pak J Med Sci 2013;29:211–215.

37.   Bansal T, Pandey A, D D, Asthana AK. C-reactive protein (CRP) and its association with periodontal disease: a brief review. J Clin Diagn Res 2014;8:ZE21–ZE24.

38.   Amar S, Wu S-c, Madan M. "Is *Porphyromonas gingivalis* cell invasion required for atherogenesis? Pharmacotherapeutic implications". J Immunol 2009;182:1584–1592.

39.   Haffajee AD, Socransky SS. Microbial etiological agents of destructive periodontal diseases. Periodontol 2000 1994;5:78–111.

40.   Deshpande RG, Khan M, Genco CA. Invasion strategies of the oral pathogen *Porphyromonas gingivalis*: implications for cardiovascular disease. Invasion Metastasis 1998;18:57–69.

41.   Kurita-Ochiai T, Yamamoto M. Periodontal pathogens and atherosclerosis: implications of inflammation and oxidative modification of LDL. Biomed Res Int 2014;2014:595981.

42.   Gosmanova EO, Le N-A. Cardiovascular complications in CKD patients: role of oxidative stress. Cardiol Res Pract 2011;2011:156326.

43.   Ismail FB, Ismail G, Dumitriu AS, et al. Identification of subgingival periodontal pathogens and association with the severity of periodontitis in patients with chronic kidney diseases: a cross-sectional study. Biomed Res Int 2015;2015:370314.

44.   Kshirsagar AV, Offenbacher S, Moss KL, Barros SP, Beck JD. Antibodies to periodontal organisms are associated with decreased kidney function. Blood Purif 2007;25:125–132.

45.   Zügel U, Kaufmann SH. Role of heat shock proteins in protection from and pathogenesis of infectious diseases. Clin Microbiol Rev 1999;12:19–39.

46.   Seymour GJ, Ford PJ, Cullinan MP, Leishman S, West MJ, Yamazaki K. Infection or inflammation: the link between periodontal disease and systemic disease. Future Cardiol 2009;5:5–9.

47.   Caps MT, Zierler RE, Polissar NL, et al. Risk of atrophy in kidneys with atherosclerotic renal artery stenosis. Kidney Int 1998;53:735–742.

48.   Muñoz Aguilera E, Suvan J, Buti J, et al. Periodontitis is associated with hypertension: a systematic review and meta-analysis. Cardiovasc Res 2019;116:28–39.

49.   De Gennaro Colonna V, Bianchi M, Pascale V, et al. Asymmetric dimethylarginine (ADMA): an endogenous inhibitor of nitric oxide synthase and a novel cardiovascular risk molecule. Med Sci Monit 2009;15:Ra91–Ra101.

50.   Schini-Kerth VB. Vascular biosynthesis of nitric oxide: effect on hemostasis and fibrinolysis. Transfus Clin Biol 1999;6:355–363.

51.   Tedla FM, Brar A, Browne R, Brown C. Hypertension in chronic kidney disease: navigating the evidence. Int J Hypertens 2011;2011:132405.

52.   Kitamura M, Mochizuki Y, Miyata Y, et al. Pathological characteristics of periodontal disease in patients with chronic kidney disease and kidney transplantation. Int J Mol Sci 2019;20:3413.

53.   Preshaw PM, Alba AL, Herrera D, et al. Periodontitis and diabetes: a two-way relationship. Diabetologia 2012;55:21–31.

54.   Varghese RT, Jialal I. Diabetic Nephropathy. [Updated 28 Sep 2021]. In: StatPearls. Treasure Island (FL): StatPearls Publishing; 2022. https://www.ncbi.nlm.nih.gov/books/NBK534200/.

55.   Naruishi K, Oishi K, Inagaki Y, et al. Association between periodontal condition and kidney dysfunction in Japanese adults: A cross-sectional study. Clin Exp Dent Res 2016;2:200–207.

56.   Borojevic T. Smoking and periodontal disease. Materia socio-medica. 2012;24:274–276.

57.   Van Laecke S, Van Biesen W. Smoking and chronic kidney disease: seeing the signs through the smoke? Nephrol Dialysis Transplant 2017;32:403–405.

58.   Mozos I, Stoian D. Oral health and cardiovascular disorders. In: El-Esawi MA (ed). Understanding the Molecular Crosstalk in Biological Processes. London: IntechOpen, 2020.

59.   Mizuguchi KA, Huang CC, Shempp I, Wang J, Shekar P, Frendl G. Predicting kidney disease progression in patients with acute kidney injury after cardiac surgery. J Thorac Cardiovasc Surg 2018;155:2455–2463.e5.

60.   Schütz JdS, de Azambuja CB, Cunha GR, al. Association between severe periodontitis and chronic kidney disease severity in predialytic patients: A cross-sectional study. Oral Dis 2020;26:447–456.

61.   Sharma P, Fenton A, Dias IHK, et al. Oxidative stress links periodontal inflammation and renal function. J Clin Periodontol 2021; 48:357–367.

62.   Kolte RA, Kolte AP, Shah KK, Modak A, Sarda TS, Bodhare GH. Comparative evaluation of the left ventricular mass in patients with chronic kidney disease in periodontally healthy, chronic gingivitis, and chronic periodontitis patients. Int J Health Sci (Qassim) 2019;13:13–18.

63.   Kshirsagar AV, Craig RG, Moss KL, et al. Periodontal disease adversely affects the survival of patients with end-stage renal disease. Kidney Int 2009;75:746–751.

64.   Grubbs V, Garcia F, Jue BL, et al. The Kidney and Periodontal Disease (KAPD) study: A pilot randomized controlled trial testing the effect of non-surgical periodontal therapy on chronic kidney disease. Contemp Clin Trials 2017;53:143–150.

65.   Grubbs V, Garcia F, Vittinghoff E, et al. Nonsurgical periodontal therapy in CKD: findings of the Kidney and Periodontal Disease (KAPD) pilot randomized controlled trial. Kidney Med 2020;2:49–58.

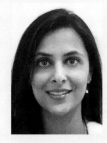

Aditi Priyamvara

Aditi Priyamvara   Student, University at Buffalo School of Dental Medicine, Buffalo, NY, USA

Amit K. Dey   Resident, Georgetown University Medical Center, Georgetown, DC, USA

Abhiram Maddi   Associate Professor, James B. Edwards College of Dental Medicine, Medical University of South Carolina, Charleston, SC, USA

Sorin Teich   Associate Dean/Professor, James B. Edwards College of Dental Medicine, Medical University of South Carolina, Charleston, SC, USA

Correspondence: Professor Sorin Teich, James B. Edwards College of Dental Medicine, Medical University of South Carolina, 29 Bee Street, DC 602, MSC 507, Charleston, SC 29425, USA. Email: teich@musc.edu

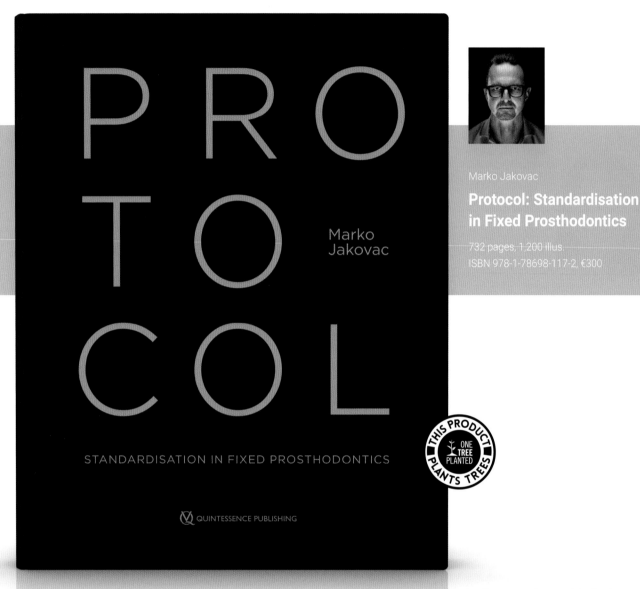

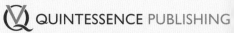

▦ RADIOLOGY/IMAGING

Radiographic analysis of the anterior mandible and its anatomical variations using cone-beam computed tomography

Felix Enderle, Dr med dent*/Florian D. Grill, Dr med Dr med dent*/

Niklas Rommel, Priv-Doz Dr med Dr med dent/Lucas M. Ritschl, Priv-Doz Dr med Dr med dent/

Andrea Grandoch, Dr med Dr med dent/Klaus-Dietrich Wolff, Prof Dr med Dr med dent/

Anton Sculean, Prof Dr med dent Dr hc MS/Herbert Deppe, Prof Dr med dent

Objective: The anterior loop, the mandibular incisive canal, and the lingual symphyseal foramen are important structures in the anterior mandible. The purpose of this study was to assess the prevalence of these structures using CBCT. **Method and materials:** A total of 170 projections were analyzed in different sectional planes. The study analyzed the prevalence and extension of the anterior loop and the prevalence of both the mandibular incisive canal and the lingual symphyseal foramen by using the GALAXIS software by Sirona. **Results:** In 98.2% (n = 167) a lingual symphyseal foramen was detected. An anterior loop was present in 31.2% (n = 53) with statistically significant higher detection rate in younger patients ($P = .001$). The median length was 1.26 mm (range 0.53–3.70 mm). No statistically significant differences regarding patient side or sex were found in either case. In 72.4% (n = 123) a mandibular incisive canal was detected. There was a statistically significant dependence of the mandibular incisive canal on patient sex ($P = .007$): female patients had a mandibular incisive canal significantly more often than male patients. Among male patients a significant difference of the mandibular incisive canal regarding the mandibular side ($P = .031$) was found; it was significantly less frequent on the right than on the left side. **Conclusion:** Anterior loop, mandibular incisive canal, and lingual symphyseal foramen are often present. Furthermore, the anatomical, neurovascular variability in the interforaminal area of the mandible emphasizes the importance of 3D imaging like CBCT in preoperative assessment, and confirms that a general safe zone should not solely be relied upon when performing surgery in this region. *(Quintessence Int 2022;53:874–882; doi: 10.3290/j.qi.b3315007)*

Key words: anterior loop, CBCT, interforaminal mandible, lingual foramen, mandibular incisive canal

---

The interforaminal area of the mandible, located between the left and right mental foramen (MF), is a popular surgical site. Here, implant placement is often possible without bone augmentation, even in edentulous mandibles.[1] Also, this region is an intraoral bone donor site in addition to the jaw angle and ascending branch of the mandible as well as the tuberosity region.[2] This popularity is because the interforaminal mandibular region is considered a safe surgical zone without significant sensory nerves or blood vessels, as is sometimes proposed in anatomical literature.[3,4] Despite this supposed safety there are reports of complications during or after surgery in the anterior mandible.

Both sensory disturbances[5-7] and severe bleedings[8,9] have occurred here after implantations. These complications happened because of damage to anatomically variable structures, which include the anterior loop (AL) of the mental canal, the mandibular incisive canal (MIC), and the lingual symphyseal foramen (LSF). The corresponding portion of the mental canal and nerve anterior to the MF which then loops back posterosuperiorly to exit the bone through the MF is defined as an AL. The mental nerve then innervates the lip and the chin.[4] The other branch of the now divided inferior alveolar nerve continues as the mandibular incisive nerve anteriorly in the mandible to supply the mandibular anter-

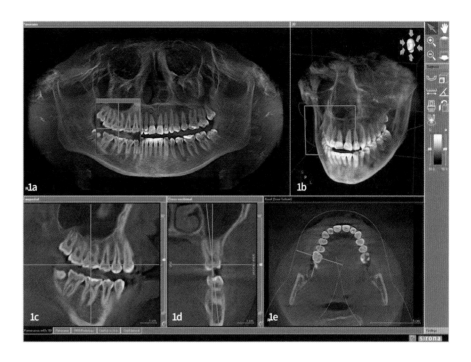

Fig 1 Overview page of the GALAXIS software. *(a)* Panoramic overview; *(b)* 3D view; *(c)* tangential plane; *(d)* cross-sectional plane; *(e)* axial plane (CBCT image from the archive of the Klinikum rechts der Isar).

ior teeth.[10] The LSF includes one or more foramina and its intramandibular canals in the midline of the lingual mandible. The prevalence and extension of these structures is a matter of controversy and there is a wide range of values in the literature. Thus, the values for the prevalence of the AL vary between 13.3%[11] and 100%.[12] To identify the presence of these structures, 3D imaging is necessary and CBCT seems suitable.[13] Therefore, the present study aimed to investigate and measure the interforaminal mandible using CBCT images from the authors' own collective to provide information on all three major structures (the AL, the MIC, and the LSF), in terms of prevalence and extension.

Method and materials

All procedures were conducted according to the principles expressed in the Declaration of Helsinki. Ethical approval for the retrospective study was granted by the Ethical Committee of the Technical University of Munich (Approval No. 611/19S). The data of this study were obtained retrospectively by analyzing a total of 170 CBCT scans, taken between 1 January 2015, and 31 December 2018, from patients of the Klinikum rechts der Isar of the Technical University of Munich, Clinic and Polyclinic for Oral and Maxillofacial Surgery. All CBCT images were taken using the GALILEOS Comfort CBCT unit (Sirona Dental Systems). The adjusted scan parameters were 85 kV and 7 mA. The exposure time was

adapted to the individual patient size and ranged from 3,000 to 5,000 ms. The voxel size was 0.3 × 0.3 × 0.3 mm, and the field of view was 15 × 15 × 15 cm³. Images that showed poor quality in the interforaminal area were excluded from this study. Reasons for poor image quality were operating errors, artifacts caused by inserted osteosynthesis material, or space-occupying lesions. Projections of patients who were under the age of majority at the time the image was taken were also excluded from the study. All CBCT images were analyzed in the Department of Oral and Maxillofacial Surgery of the Klinikum rechts der Isar of the Technical University of Munich. This analysis was performed using the GALILEOS Implant (version 1.9.2) of the GALAXIS 3D visualization software (Sirona Dental Systems). The CBCT images were analyzed in different sectional planes (tangential, cross-sectional, and axial). Figure 1 shows the structure of the software.

Anterior loop

To determine an AL, the most anterior point of the MF was marked in the axial view. Then the most anterior point of the mandibular canal was marked in both axial and tangential views. Two parallel lines were drawn in tangential plane using the length-measuring option of the software. The distance between these two lines was measured by drawing a perpendicular line between them and was considered as the length of the

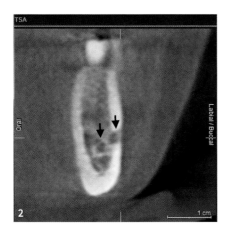

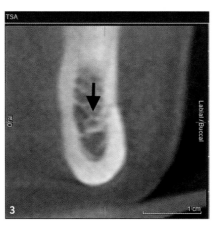

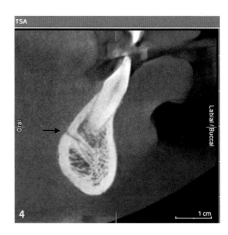

Fig 2 Two radiolucencies in the sense of an AL in the cross-sectional plane indicated by the two arrows (CBCT image from the archive of the Klinikum rechts der Isar).

Fig 3 MIC anterior to the MF indicated by the arrow in the cross-sectional plane (CBCT image from the archive of the Klinikum rechts der Isar).

Fig 4 LSF in the cross-sectional plane (CBCT image from the archive of the Klinikum rechts der Isar).

AL. The distance between the most anterior point of the MF and the most anterior point of the mandibular canal is defined as an AL if the mandibular canal extends further anteriorly than the MF. In the opposite case, there is no AL. Generally, if two radiolucencies were present in the cross-sectional view, an AL was assumed, as shown in Fig 2. In the case of one radiolucent structure anterior to the MF, this was seen as a MIC when the diameter was smaller than 3 mm.

Mandibular incisive canal

A possible MIC was examined directly at its origin. The decisive factor was whether a cortically limited radiolucency in the sense of a bony canal could be recognized anterior to the MF which could clearly be distinguished from an AL. The mentioned 3-mm diameter limit served as orientation. Figure 3 shows an MIC in region of the mandibular left first premolar (tooth 34) mesial of the MF.

Lingual symphyseal foramen

The lingual midline area was observed for LSF in all planes. Figure 4 shows an LSF in the cross-sectional plane.

Statistical analysis

Quantitative variables were presented descriptively using mean and standard deviation (SD), minimum and maximum, as well as quartiles, and were tested for normal distribution using the Kolmogorov–Smirnov test. Because of significant deviations from a normal distribution, the comparison of the sexes was made as two independent samples using the U-test. Age-dependency was investigated using a U-test, as well. Two dependent samples, as measurements on the left and right sides, were tested for differences using the Wilcoxon test for pair differences. Absolute and percentage frequencies were given for ordinally and nominally scaled variables. The chi-square test was used to test for statistical dependency. Alternatively, in cases of small patient numbers Fisher exact test was used. Two-sided testing was performed and the statistical significance level was set to $P < .05$. An alpha adjustment for multiple testing was not performed, so the results are exploratory and descriptive in nature. IBM SPSS Statistics (Version 26, SPSS, IBM) was used to perform the statistical analysis. Descriptive statistics were applied where appropriate. The McNemar test, chi-square test, and t test were performed to investigate statistically significant differences between patient side and sex. Again, the statistical significance level was set to $P < .05$.

Results

A total of 170 patients could be included in this study. Eighty patients (47.1%) were men, and 90 patients (52.9%) were women. The age of the study participants ranged from 18 to 76 years. The mean age was 36 (±16) years. The demographic patient data can be seen in Table 1.

Table 1 Demographic patient data (years)

Sex	N	Mean	SD	Minimum	Maximum	Interquartile range		
						25	50	75
Female	90	35.90	16.848	18	76	23.00	29.00	44.75
Male	80	35.21	14.757	18	75	24.00	32.00	41.75

Table 2 Mesial extension of the AL (mm)

Dimension	N	Mean	SD	Minimum	Maximum	Interquartile range		
						25	50	75
Extension AL	53	1.43	0.69	0.53	3.70	0.92	1.26	1.72

Anterior loop

An AL could be detected in 31.2% (n=53) of the patients. The remaining 68.8% did not show any AL. A statistical dependence on sex (Pearson chi-square test, $P=.755$) or body side (McNemar test, $P=.263$) was not found. The median anterior extension was 1.26 mm. The AL ranged from a minimum of 0.53 mm to a maximum of 3.70 mm. All numbers are shown in Table 2. Overall, no significant dependence on sex (U-test, $P=.313$) or mandibular side was found regarding AL extension (Wilcoxon test for pair differences, $P=.811$ for female and $P=.733$ for male patients). Concerning age-dependency, a statistical significance was detectable (U-test, $P=.001$) according to which an AL was visible more often in younger patients.

Mandibular incisive canal

A MIC was detected in 72.4% of the patients (n=123). The remaining 43 showed no MIC. Patient sex was found to be significant for the existence of an MIC (Pearson chi-square test, $P=.007$): female patients had a significantly higher incidence than male patients. Furthermore, the male patients showed an MIC significantly more frequently on the left than on the right side (McNemar test, $P=.031$). This was not detectable in female patients ($P>.999$). A statistical age-dependency could not be detected (U-test, $P=.252$).

Lingual symphyseal foramen

In the median plane one or more foramina could be detected in 98.2% of images. No sex dependence was detected (Pearson chi-square test, $P=.631$). A statistical age-dependency was not detected (U-test, $P=.181$).

Discussion

Materials, method, and study design

The CBCT images all originate from the database of the Department of Oral and Maxillofacial Surgery of the Klinikum rechts der Isar of the Technical University Munich. The images were randomly selected and were all acquired with the same standard parameters. However, the images were taken by different individuals, which may have resulted in differences in patient positioning and image quality. Also, the used CBCT unit uses a voxel size of 0.3 mm. More modern units can offer a voxel size of up to 0.08 mm[14] and may enable an even more accurate identification of the examined structures. Concerning the aforementioned dimensions, this may have only a minor impact. Further, the presented study was conducted retrospectively. Therefore, the included variables were not recorded specifically for this study and the CBCT scans were not performed by the same person, as mentioned above. Concerning the analysis of the CBCT, the same measures were applied for every scan analysis.

Anterior loop

The AL describes a curve of the mental canal, that bends anteriorly and back posteriorly before forming the MF.[15] This means that the mental nerve runs in this area more anteriorly than the position of the MF would suggest so that implantations in this area carry a high risk of iatrogenic nerve damage which can lead to a sensory disturbance in the area supplied by the mental nerve.[16] In the literature there is a wide range of values in studies using cadavers for assessment regarding the prevalence and extension of the AL, ranging from 13.3%[11] to 100%[12] prevalence and to as much as 11 mm anterior extension.[17]

In the present study, an AL was found in 31.2% of patients, with no significant dependence on sex (Pearson chi-square test, $P=.755$) or mandibular side (McNemar test, $P=.263$). The median anterior extension was 1.26 mm, with a maximum extension of 3.70 mm. Again, there was no significant dependence on sex (U-test, $P=.313$) or mandibular side (Wilcoxon test for pair differences, $P=.811$ for female and $P=.733$ for male patients).

In the above-mentioned comparative studies on cadavers in which an examination of the mental canal by probes was performed, very high numbers for both prevalence and extension of the AL are described, such as 100% and 6.95 mm[12] or 88% and 11 mm.[17] This could be due to an over-probing of the AL into a possible MIC since the presence of an MIC was not additionally analyzed. In comparison, cadaveric studies that used anatomical dissection for the identification of AL report much lower numbers for prevalence and extension. Mardinger et al[18] identified an AL in 28% of cases with an average length of 1.05 ± 0.47 mm. Kuzmanovic et al[15] detected an AL in 37% of cases with an average anterior extension of 1.2 ± 0.9 mm. These numbers are comparable to the results of the present study. However, significantly higher values have also been determined by anatomical preparation. Solar et al[19] identified an AL in 59.4% of patients and Uchida et al[13] in even 71% of cases.[11] In studies using panoramic radiography for the assessment the numbers are lower. Ngeow et al[20] detected an AL in 34.4% of cases and Kuzmanovic et al[15] in 27% of cases. However, Kuzmanovic et al[15] showed in a direct comparison of anatomical preparation and panoramic radiography that 2D radiography is not able to reliably identify the AL.

In contrast, Uchida et al[13] could prove that 3D imaging, such as CBCT, can reliably identify an AL. Nevertheless, there is high variation in the literature regarding prevalence and extent of the AL even among CBCT-based studies. Uchida et al[13] themselves identified an AL with an average extension of 2.7 ± 1.3 mm in 71% of cases. Sinha et al[21] reported only 9.7% prevalence, whereas

Yang et al[22] found an AL in 93.57% of cases. Other studies reported values for prevalence and extension like 25% and 1.63 mm (0.52 to 3.92 mm) in Raju et al,[23] or 53.13% and 1.07 ± 1.42 mm in Puri et al.[24] Kheir and Sheikhi[25] found an AL in 32.8% of cases with an anterior extension of 2.69 ± 1.56 mm on the right and 2.36 ± 1.16 mm on the left side. Do Nascimento et al[26] even found an AL in 41.6% of scans with 1.1 ± 0.8 mm anterior extension. A recent meta-analysis by Mishra et al[27] concluded a prevalence for the AL of 38% and an average anterior extension of 2.76 ± 1.15 mm. The authors also pointed out the high heterogeneity in the different studies regarding prevalence, length, and possible dependence on sex, age, or mandibular side in different populations.[27]

These differing results could be due to different definitions of the AL or divergent methodology in its determination. In the present study as well as in others, no dependence on side or sex was shown,[23-25] but such dependence was detected by do Nascimento et al.[26]

Further, the present statistical analysis revealed a significant age-dependency in the detection of the AL, with the AL being detectable more frequently in younger patients, while there was no positive correlation between age and length of the AL (Spearman correlation, $P=.37$). This, however, may not mean that in older patients it is not present. Concerning the visibility, similar findings were reported by Ngeow et al[20] in their investigation of radiography. Also, Velasco-Torres et al[28] found a reduced visibility and dimension with increasing age of the AL. As a possible explanation the authors mentioned the changing dimensions with increasing age of the MF and ongoing craniofacial growth.[28,29]

Overall, it can be concluded that the existing variability in the prevalence and extent of the AL, together with a possible MIC, requires an individual preoperative assessment and does not allow proposal of a general safety zone mesial of the MF as has been proposed in other studies.[15,18,30,31] Based on the present findings, a 3D imaging seems necessary when surgical interventions, such as interforaminal implantations, are planned. Despite the possibly reduced visibility with increasing age the existence of an AL still has to be considered.

Mandibular incisive canal

The inferior alveolar nerve splits into two branches. The mental nerve, together with the artery of the same name, leaves the mandible via the MF and provides the sensitive supply to the lip and chin.[4] The mandibular incisive nerve continues anteriorly for sensory supply of the mandibular anterior teeth.[10] Some authors reported its course in an intraosseous nerve plexus.[32-35] However, recent studies often identified a real cortically limited MIC in a large proportion of cases, in which the eponymous nerve runs anteriorly.[10,36,37] This is especially important since a study by Jacobs et al[38] has proven a neurovascular canal content by using high-resolution magnetic resonance imaging. The canal diameter is considered sufficiently large to cause significant trauma when injured.

In a case report by Romanos and Greenstein,[39] it is reported how, during implant bed drilling in region of the mandibular right canine region with a conspicuously large MIC present, the patient experienced severe pain when opening the canal roof under sufficient infiltration anesthesia. The occurrence of severe intraosseous bleeding from the burr hole also indicated the presence of a neurovascular structure. Implantation was not continued, and no permanent damage occurred.[39] Another case report describes the occurrence of a brisk, pulsatile arterial bleeding from the MIC after preparation and drilling of an implant osteotomy site in the left canine region. All local hemostatic measures were unsuccessful, which ultimately led to the patient's transport to the emergency department of a nearby hospital.[40] Kütük et al[41] obtained in a small collective computed tomography scans from 10 patients who reported postoperative neuropathic pain after implantation in the interforaminal mandible. They evaluated the relationship between dental implant and the MIC using a 3D software program and found that at least one implant perforated the MIC in all patients.[41] Jacobs et al[16] had similar experiences as they reported a case of severe chronic neuropathy and found the cause to be an implant that touched the roof the MIC.

In conclusion, direct trauma in the form of implantation into the canal may result in sensory disturbances or hemorrhage.[16,38-41] Furthermore, it was considered that placement of the implant into the MIC could result in an edema of the epineurium of the mandibular incisive nerve. This edema could then lead to retrograde damage of the main branch with sensory disturbances. In addition, there would be a risk of insufficient osseointegration due to the possible ingrowth of soft tissue from the canal interior.[42]

In the present study, an MIC was identified in 72.4% of cases (n = 127) and female patients were significantly more likely to have an MIC than male patients (Pearson chi-square test, $P=.007$), but only male participants were significantly more likely to have an MIC on the left mandibular side (McNemar test, $P=.031$).

Mraiwa et al[36] examined 50 cadavers and found an MIC in 96% of cases. The diameter at its origin was 1.8 ± 0.5 mm. The

canal tapered anteriorly and reached the mandibular midline in only 18% of cases.[36] Mardinger et al[43] even identified an MIC in all cadavers examined. In the same study the authors demonstrated the failure of panoramic radiography in detecting the MIC.

The unreliability of panoramic radiography is also confirmed in comparative radiographic studies. Pires et al[44] detected an MIC on only 11% of panoramic radiographs but on 83% of CT scans. De Brito et al[45] found an MIC on 24.4% of CT scans in comparison to 5.5% on the corresponding panoramic radiographs. Jacobs et al[37] detected an MIC on only 15% of panoramic radiographs, compared to 93% on CT scans.[46] Again, 3D images appear to provide a much more reliable determination. The CBCT-based studies by Panjnoush et al[47] (97.5%) and Puri et al[24] (93.75%) prove the high prevalence of the MIC and the reliable detectability by 3D imaging.

A sex- or patient-side-dependent distribution like in the present study could not be confirmed in any mentioned comparative study. Also, the present study shows a lower prevalence of the MIC. Reasons could be insufficient image quality to detect smaller canals or too small a case number. Also, different definitions or methods of assessment or differentiation from the AL may have played a role. Overall, the MIC must be noted as a constantly occurring structure, even if radiographic determination is not always possible.

In conclusion, it is worth considering to what extent and in what situations sensory disturbances occur, because it seems that the high prevalence of the MIC and the numbers of implantations in the anterior mandible does not correlate with the number of reports about sensory disturbances. This supposed discrepancy needs to be addressed to provide clear guidance for the clinician. However, the avoidance of iatrogenic damage should always be a top priority, especially in elective procedures such as implantation. Therefore, 3D imaging should be applied to identify a possible MIC and thus reliably prevent damage and consequent neurovascular complications.

Lingual symphyseal foramen

At least one LSF was found in 98.2% of patients. This high number is consistent with the results of other studies. As early as 1974, Sutton[48] demonstrated such a lingual foramen in 85% of the cadavers examined. In a study by von Arx et al,[49] a lingual foramen in the midline was present in 96.2% of cases, and Natsis et al[50] found at least one median lingual foramen in 97.9% of cases. Tagaya et al[51] even found an LSF in 100% of cases. In summary, it can be assumed that the LSF is a constantly present structure. Again, this is relevant because of its neurovascular content.[38] These lingual foramina are often further differentiated into cranial or caudal with respect to the mental spines. Furthermore, branches of the lingual artery, vein, and nerve were detected in the cranially located foramen, whereas vascular branches originating from the submental or sublingual artery and a branch of the mylohyoid nerve were detected in the caudal foramen. Here, the neurovascular structures appear to be large enough to sustain significant trauma when injured. Sensory disturbances or pain may result.[16,52,53]

In addition to sensitivity disturbances, there are many case reports describing the problem of life-threatening oral bleeding, which in most cases is due to perforation of the lingual cortex.[8,54-58] The floor of the mouth is supplied by a network of vessels from the lingual, sublingual, submental, and facial arteries. Hemorrhage occurring here can easily spread to the surrounding sublingual soft tissue, possibly causing life-threatening airway obstruction due to a hematoma of the floor of the mouth.[59] In addition to iatrogenic injury to the lingual cortical bone, injury to the neurovascular structures of the lingual foramina and their intraosseous canals, which remain to be further investigated, should also be avoided. One possibility would be to use shorter implants, whose survival rates were shown to have increased throughout recent years.[60] It has also been shown that reliable identification of the lingual foramina can be achieved by CBCT and thus damage and possible neurovascular consequences could be avoided.[7,36,38] ▦

Conclusion

The present study confirms the high anatomical variability of the anterior mandible. The dimensions of the AL can reach relevant values regarding surgical interventions. The MIC was found more frequently in female CBCTs, whereas in male patients it seems to be located more often on the left side. Due to the high neurovascular variability in the anterior mandible, appropriate preoperative 3D imaging like CBCT for individual assessment seems mandatory to avoid possible severe complications. Also, in elderly patients an AL has to be considered in surgical planning despite a possibly reduced visibility. ▦

Acknowledgments

This publication forms parts of the dental doctoral thesis of the first author (FE). The authors thank Mr Daniel Ross for language corrections. All authors declare that there are no financial or nonfinancial competing interests.

References

1. Soto-Penaloza D, Zaragozí-Alonso R, Penarrocha-Diago M, Penarrocha-Diago M. The all-on-four treatment concept: Systematic review. J Clin Exp Dent 2017;9:e474–e488.

2. Khoury F. Augmentative Verfahren in der Implantologie. Vol 1. Auflage. Berlin: Quintessence Publishing, 2009.

3. Agur AMR. Grant's Atlas of Anatomy. Vol 9. Baltimore: Williams and Wilkins, 1991.

4. Waschke J, Bröckers T, Paulsen F. Anatomie Das Lehrbuch. Munich: Elsevier, 2015.

5. Kohavi D, Bar-Ziv J. Atypical incisive nerve: clinical report. Implant Dent 1996;5:281–283.

6. Wismeijer D, van Waas MA, Vermeeren JI, Kalk W. Patients' perception of sensory disturbances of the mental nerve before and after implant surgery: a prospective study of 110 patients. Br J Oral Maxillofac Surg 1997;35: 254–259.

7. Liang X, Lambrichts I, Corpas L, et al. Neurovascular disturbance associated with implant placement in the anterior mandible and its surgical implications: literature review including report of a case. Chinese J Dent Res 2008;11:56.

8. Kalpidis CD, Setayesh RM. Hemorrhaging associated with endosseous implant placement in the anterior mandible: a review of the literature. J Periodontol 2004;75:631–645.

9. Longoni S, Sartori M, Braun M, et al. Lingual vascular canals of the mandible: the risk of bleeding complications during implant procedures. Implant Dent 2007;16:131–138.

10. De Andrade E, Otomo-Corgel J, Pucher J, Ranganath KA, St George N Jr. The intraosseous course of the mandibular incisive nerve in the mandibular symphysis. Int J Periodontics Restorative Dent 2001;21:591–597.

11. Benninger B, Miller D, Maharathi A, Carter W. Dental implant placement investigation: is the anterior loop of the mental nerve clinically relevant? J Oral Maxillofac Surg 2011;69:182–185.

12. Arzouman MJ, Otis L, Kipnis V, Levine D. Observations of the anterior loop of the inferior alveolar canal. Int J Oral Maxillofac Implants 1993;8:295–300.

13. Uchida Y, Noguchi N, Goto M, et al. Measurement of anterior loop length for the mandibular canal and diameter of the mandibular incisive canal to avoid nerve damage when installing endosseous implants in the interforaminal region: a second attempt introducing cone beam computed tomography. J Oral Maxillofac Surg 2009;67:744–750.

14. Dentsply. Orthophos S 3D. 2021; https://www.dentsplysirona.com/de-de/entdecken/bildgebende-systeme/panorama-roentgen/3d-roentgen/orthophos-s-3d.html. Accessed 13 April 2021.

15. Kuzmanovic DV, Payne AG, Kieser JA, Dias GJ. Anterior loop of the mental nerve: a morphological and radiographic study. Clin Oral Implants Res 2003;14:464–471.

16. Jacobs R, Quirynen M, Bornstein MM. Neurovascular disturbances after implant surgery. Periodontol 2000 2014;66:188–202.

17. Neiva RF, Gapski R, Wang HL. Morphometric analysis of implant-related anatomy in Caucasian skulls. J Periodontol 2004;75: 1061–1067.

18. Mardinger O, Chaushu G, Arensburg B, Taicher S, Kaffe I. Anterior loop of the mental canal: an anatomical-radiologic study. Implant Dent 2000;9:120–125.

19. Solar P, Ulm C, Frey G, Matejka M. A classification of the intraosseous paths of the mental nerve. Int J Oral Maxillofac Implants 1994;9:339–344.

20. Ngeow WC, Dionysius DD, Ishak H, Nambiar P. A radiographic study on the visualization of the anterior loop in dentate subjects of different age groups. J Oral Sci 2009;51:231–237.

21. Sinha S, Kandula S, Sangamesh N, Rout P, Mishra S, Bajoria A. Assessment of the anterior loop of the mandibular canal using cone-beam computed tomography in Eastern India: A record-based study. J Int Soc Preventive Community Dent 2019;9:290–295.

22. Yang XW, Zhang FF, Li YH, Wei B, Gong Y. Characteristics of intrabony nerve canals in mandibular interforaminal region by using cone-beam computed tomography and a recommendation of safe zone for implant and bone harvesting. Clin Implant Dent Relat Res 2017;19:530–538.

23. Raju N, Zhang W, Jadhav A, Ioannou A, Eswaran S, Weltman R. Cone-beam computed tomography analysis of the prevalence, length, and passage of the anterior loop of the mandibular canal. J Oral Implantol 2019;45:463–468.

24. Puri A, Verma P, Mahajan P, Bansal A, Kohli S, Faraz SA. CBCT evaluation of the vital mandibular interforaminal anatomical structures. Ann Maxillofac Surg 2020;10:149–157.

25. Kheir MK, Sheikhi M. Assessment of the anterior loop of mental nerve in an Iranian population using cone beam computed tomography scan. Dent Res J (Isfahan) 2017;14:418–422.

26. do Nascimento EH, Dos Anjos Pontual ML, Dos Anjos Pontual A, et al. Assessment of the anterior loop of the mandibular canal: A study using cone-beam computed tomography. Imaging Sci Dent 2016;46: 69–75.

27. Mishra SK, Nahar R, Gaddale R, Chowdhary R. Identification of anterior loop in different populations to avoid nerve injury during surgical procedures: a systematic review and meta-analysis. Oral Maxillofac Surg 2021;25:159–174.

28. Velasco-Torres M, Padial-Molina M, Avila-Ortiz G, García-Delgado R, Catena A, Galindo-Moreno P. Inferior alveolar nerve trajectory, mental foramen location and incidence of mental nerve anterior loop. Med Oral Patol Oral Cirug Bucal 2017; 22:e630–e635.

29. Daftary F, Mahallati R, Bahat O, Sullivan RM. Lifelong craniofacial growth and the implications for osseointegrated implants. Int J Oral Maxillofac Implants 2013;28:163–169.

30. Bavitz JB, Harn SD, Hansen CA, Lang M. An anatomical study of mental neurovascular bundle-implant relationships. Int J Oral Maxillofac Implants 1993;8:563–567.

31. Li X, Jin ZK, Zhao H, Yang K, Duan JM, Wang WJ. The prevalence, length and position of the anterior loop of the inferior alveolar nerve in Chinese, assessed by spiral computed tomography. Surg Radiol Anat 2013;35: 823–830.

32. Starkie C, Stewart D. The intra-mandibular course of the inferior dental nerve. J Anat 1931;65:319–323.

33. Denissen HW, Veldhuis HA, van Faassen F. Implant placement in the atrophic mandible: an anatomic study. J Prosthet Dent 1984;52: 260–263.

34. Haribhakti VV. The dentate adult human mandible: an anatomic basis for surgical decision making. Plast Reconstr Surg 1996;97: 536–541.

35. Polland KE, Munro S, Reford G, et al. The mandibular canal of the edentulous jaw. Clin Anat 2001;14:445–452.

36. Mraiwa N, Jacobs R, Moerman P, Lambrichts I, van Steenberghe D, Quirynen M. Presence and course of the incisive canal in the human mandibular interforaminal region: two-dimensional imaging versus anatomical observations. Surg Radiol Anat 2003;25: 416–423.

37. Jacobs R, Mraiwa N, Van Steenberghe D, Sanderink G, Quirynen M. Appearance of the mandibular incisive canal on panoramic radiographs. Surg Radiol Anat 2004;26: 329–333.

37. Jacobs R, Lambrichts I, Liang X, et al. Neurovascularization of the anterior jaw bones revisited using high-resolution magnetic resonance imaging. Oral Surg Oral Med Oral Pathol Oral Radiol Endod 2007;103: 683–693.

39. Romanos G, Greenstein G. The incisive canal. Considerations during implant placement: case report and literature review. Int J Oral Maxillofac Implants 2008;24: 740–745.

40. Lee CY, Yanagihara LC, Suzuki JB. Brisk, pulsatile bleeding from the anterior mandibular incisive canal during implant surgery: a case report and use of an active hemostatic matrix to terminate acute bleeding. Implant Dent 2012;21:368–373.

41. Kütük N, Demirbaş AE, Gönen ZB, et al. Anterior mandibular zone safe for implants. J Craniofac Surg 2013;24:e405–e408.

42. Rosenquist B. Is there an anterior loop of the inferior alveolar nerve? Int J Periodontics Restorative Dent 1996;16:40–45.

43. Mardinger O, Chaushu G, Arensburg B, Taicher S, Kaffe I. Anatomic and radiologic course of the mandibular incisive canal. Surg Radiol Anat 2000;22:157–161.

44. Pires CA, Bissada NF, Becker JJ, Kanawati A, Landers MA. Mandibular incisive canal: cone beam computed tomography. Clin Implant Dent Relat Res 2012;14:67–73.

45. de Brito A, Nejaim Y, Freitas D, Oliveira-Santos C. Panoramic radiographs underestimate extensions of the anterior loop and mandibular incisive canal. Imaging Sci Dent 2016;46:159–165.

46. Jacobs R, Mraiwa N, vanSteenberghe D, Gijbels F, Quirynen M. Appearance, location, course, and morphology of the mandibular incisive canal: an assessment on spiral CT scan. Dentomaxillofac Radiol 2002;31: 322–327.

47. Panjnoush M, Rabiee ZS, Kheirandish Y. Assessment of location and anatomical characteristics of mental foramen, anterior loop and mandibular incisive canal using cone beam computed tomography. J Dent (Tehran) 2016;13:126–132.

48. Sutton RN. The practical significance of mandibular accessory foramina. Aust Dent J 1974;19:167–173.

49. von Arx T, Matter D, Buser D, Bornstein MM. Evaluation of location and dimensions of lingual foramina using limited cone-beam computed tomography. J Oral Maxillofac Surg 2011;69:2777–2785.

50. Natsis K, Repousi E, Asouhidou I, Siskos C, Ioannidi A, Piagkou M. Foramina of the anterior mandible in dentate and edentulous mandibles. Folia Morphol (Warsz) 2016;75:204–210.

51. Tagaya A, Matsuda Y, Nakajima K, Seki K, Okano T. Assessment of the blood supply to the lingual surface of the mandible for reduction of bleeding during implant surgery. Clin Oral Implants Res 2009;20: 351–355.

52. Liang X, Jacobs R, Lambrichts I, et al. Microanatomical and histological assessment of the content of superior genial spinal foramen and its bony canal. Dentomaxillofac Radiol 2005;34:362–368.

53. Liang X, Jacobs R, Lambrichts I, Vandewalle G. Lingual foramina on the mandibular midline revisited: a macroanatomical study. Clin Anat 2007;20:246–251.

54. Laboda G. Life-threatening hemorrhage after placement of an endosseous implant: report of case. J Am Dent Assoc 1990;121: 599–600.

55. Mason ME, Gilbert Triplett R, Alfonso WF. Life-threatening hemorrhage from placement of a dental implant. J Oral Maxillofac Surg 1990;48:201–204.

56. Del Castillo-Pardo de Vera JL, López-Arcas Calleja JM, Burgueño-García M. Hematoma of the floor of the mouth and airway obstruction during mandibular dental implant placement: a case report. Oral Maxillofac Surg 2008;12:223–226.

57. Hwang HD, Kim JW, Kim YS, Kang DH, Kwon TG. Angiographic embolization for hemorrhage control after dental implantation. J Korean Assoc Oral Maxillofac Surg 2013; 39:27–30.

58. Sakka S, Krenkel C. Hemorrhage secondary to interforaminal implant surgery: anatomical considerations and report of a case. J Oral Implantol 2013;39:603–607.

59. Katsumi Y, Tanaka R, Hayashi T, Koga T, Takagi R, Ohshima H. Variation in arterial supply to the floor of the mouth and assessment of relative hemorrhage risk in implant surgery. Clin Oral Implants Res 2013;24: 434–440.

60. Karthikeyan I, Desai SR, Singh R. Short implants: A systematic review. J Indian Soc Periodontol 2012;16:302–312.

Felix Enderle* Dr med dent, Department of Oral and Maxillofacial Surgery, School of Medicine, Technische Universität München, Germany

Florian D. Grill* Dr med Dr med dent, Department of Oral and Maxillofacial Surgery, School of Medicine, Technische Universität München, Germany

Niklas Rommel Priv-Doz Dr med Dr med dent, Department of Oral and Maxillofacial Surgery, School of Medicine, Technische Universität München, Germany; and Medical Care Center for Oral and Maxillofacial Surgery, Memmingen, Germany

Lucas M. Ritschl Priv-Doz Dr med Dr med dent, Department of Oral and Maxillofacial Surgery, School of Medicine, Technische Universität München, Germany

Andrea Grandoch Dr med Dr med dent, Department of Oral and Maxillofacial Surgery, Universitätsklinik Köln, Germany

Klaus-Dietrich Wolff Prof Dr med Dr med dent, Department of Oral and Maxillofacial Surgery, School of Medicine, Technische Universität München, Germany

Anton Sculean Prof Dr med dent Dr hc mult, MS, Department of Periodontology, University of Bern, Switzerland

Herbert Deppe Prof Dr med dent, Department of Oral and Maxillofacial Surgery, School of Medicine, Technische Universität München, Germany

*Contributed equally and are shared first authors.

Correspondence: Dr Florian Dieter Grill, Technical University of Munich, School of Medicine, Klinikum rechts der Isar, Department of Oral and Maxillofacial Surgery, Ismaninger Str. 22, 81675 Munich, Germany. Email: florian.grill@tum.de

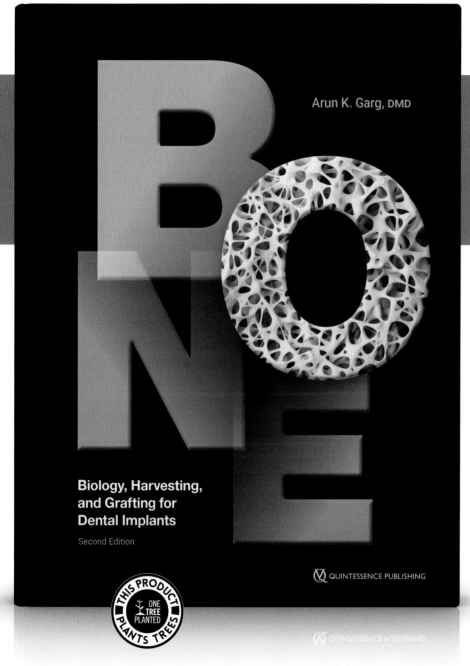

Arun K. Garg, DMD

Biology, Harvesting, and Grafting for Dental Implants

Second Edition

QUINTESSENCE PUBLISHING

Arun K. Garg

Bone

Biology, Harvesting, and Grafting for Dental Implants
2nd Edition 2024, 332 pages, 1,966 illus.
ISBN 978-1-64724-170-4
€158

Dental implant placement often requires bone grafting to ensure sufficient bony support for the implants being placed. Depending on the biologic conditions of the patient, including the level of bone atrophy and the status of the remaining teeth in the mouth, more adjunctive procedures like bone harvesting or sinus grafting may be required. This book covers it all, from the biology of bone and how dental implants work within that framework to the many procedures for harvesting bone and using it to augment sites for implant placement. The different types of bone grafts and membranes are discussed as well as procedures to preserve the alveolar ridge following tooth extraction. Dr Garg was a pioneer in dental bone grafting, and this new edition keeps him at the forefront of the field.

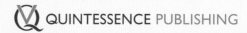

www.quint.link/bone   books@quintessenz.de   +49 (0)30 761 80 667   QUINTESSENCE PUBLISHING

Radiographic angle width as predictor of clinical outcomes following regenerative periodontal therapy with enamel matrix derivative: a retrospective cohort study with a mean follow-up of at least 10 years

Andrea Roccuzzo, DDS, MAS, PhDc*/Johanna Ettmayer, Med Dent*/Siro Pietro De Ry, Dr Med Dent, MAS/
Jean-Claude Imber, Dr Med Dent, MAS/Anton Sculean, Prof Dr Med Dent, MS, PhD, Dr hc mult/
Giovanni Edoardo Salvi, Prof Dr Med Dent

Objectives: To assess the association between the baseline radiographic defect angle and the long-term clinical outcomes following periodontal regenerative therapy with enamel matrix derivative (EMD). **Method and materials:** Baseline periapical radiographs obtained from a cohort of patients treated with periodontal regenerative therapy were digitized and the radiographic angle width between the root surface and the bony wall of the adjacent intraosseous defect was calculated and reported (in degrees). Changes in pocket probing depth (PD) and clinical attachment level (CAL) were assessed and reported (in mm). Clinical outcomes were evaluated at baseline (T0), 6 months following therapy (T1), and at the latest follow-up (T2). **Results:** Thirty-eight defects in 26 patients enrolled in supportive periodontal care for a mean period of 10.4 years (range 8.0 to 15.5 years) were available for analysis. The mean PD change between T0 and T2 was 2.33 ± 1.66 mm at teeth with a defect angle width <20 degrees and 0.86 ± 1.66 mm at teeth with a defect angle width >30 degrees ($P = .021$). When the baseline radiographic angle width was <20 degrees the probability of obtaining a CAL gain >3 mm was 1.5-times higher (95% CI 0.19 to 13.8) at T1 and 2.5-times higher (95% CI 0.40 to 15.6) at T2 compared with defects with a radiographic angle width >30 degrees. **Conclusion:** Within their limitations, these results indicate that pretherapeutic measurement of the radiographic defect angle width might provide relevant information on the short-/long-term clinical outcomes following regenerative periodontal therapy with EMD. (Quintessence Int 2023;54:384–392; doi: 10.3290/j.qi.b3824933)

Key words: enamel matrix derivative, intrabony defects, long-term results, periodontal regeneration, radiographic evaluation

Periodontitis is a multifactorial inflammatory chronic disease caused by bacterial biofilm resulting in progressive destruction of the tooth-supporting apparatus and ultimately leading to tooth loss.[1-5]

Despite the efficacy of the nonsurgical therapy (ie, scaling and root planing) in terms of clinical attachment level (CAL) gain and probing depth (PD) reduction, some patients' (ie, self-performed plaque control) tooth-related (ie, presence of multiple roots) and anatomical factors (ie, presence of intrabony defects) have been linked to persistent bleeding periodontal pockets and consequent increased risk for tooth loss.[6-9]

Consequently, surgical interventions have been adopted with the aim to decontaminate root surface and whenever possible regenerate lost periodontal tissues by means of bioactive agents such as enamel matrix derivative (EMD).[10-14] In this respect, as reported by Falk,[15] in a large retrospective clinical study on guided tissue regeneration procedures, the radiographic intrabony defect width was strictly correlated to a CAL gain of at least 3 mm. Later on, similar results have been published by Tsitoura et al[16] after periodontal regenerative procedures with EMD. However, although the existing evidence suggests a positive correlation between the defect angle and the

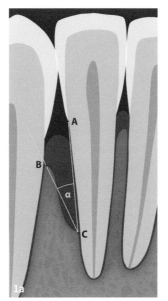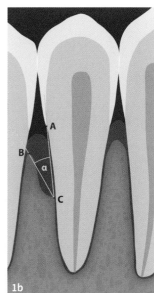

Figs 1a and 1b Linear radiographic reference points and lines used to measure the width of the intrabony defect angle (alpha) at defect site. *(a)* Incisors. *(b)* Premolars.

clinical outcome after regenerative periodontal therapy in the short-term (ie, 12 months follow-up), no studies reported the potential impact of the intrabony radiographic angle width in the long-term (ie, > 8 years).[16]

Hence, the aim of the present study was to investigate the correlation between the radiographic angle width of the intrabony defect and both the short- and long-term clinical outcomes of such periodontal defects treated with EMD in patients enrolled in a supportive periodontal care (SPC) program up to 15 years in the Department of Periodontology of the University of Bern, Switzerland.

Method and materials

The study protocol was submitted to and approved by the Ethics Committee of the Canton of Bern (KEK), Switzerland (Nr. 2018-01877). The investigation was conducted according to the revised principles of the Helsinki Declaration (2013) and signed informed consent was obtained from each patient before study initiation.

Study design

For the present single-center retrospective study, conventional periapical radiographs were used to measure the width of the intrabony defect angle and to correlate it with the change in clinical outcomes following regenerative periodontal therapy by means of EMD. Over the entire follow-up period up to 15 years, patients were enrolled in a university-based SPC program. Clin-

ical outcomes were evaluated at three different time points (ie, T0, T1, T2) as previously reported by De Ry et al:[17]

- T0: 6 months following nonsurgical periodontal therapy and before periodontal surgery
- T1: 6-month follow-up examination
- T2: latest follow-up examination performed between January 2019 and December 2020.

Clinical measurements

The following clinical parameters were assessed at three different time points (ie, T0, T1, T2), at six sites per tooth by means of a XP23/UNC 15 probe (Hu-Friedy):

- CAL: distance in millimeters from the cementoenamel junction (CEJ) to the bottom of the pocket
- PD: distance in millimeters from the gingival margin to the bottom of the pocket
- gingival recession (GR): distance in millimeters from the gingival margin to the CEJ
- presence or absence of dental plaque (Plaque Index, PI)[18]
- presence or absence of bleeding on probing (BoP).[19]

In addition, for each patient the following full-mouth periodontal variables were recorded:

- full-mouth plaque score (FMPS): percentage of tooth sites revealing the presence of dental biofilm[18]
- full-mouth bleeding score (FMBS): percentage of tooth sites revealing the presence of bleeding on probing.[19]

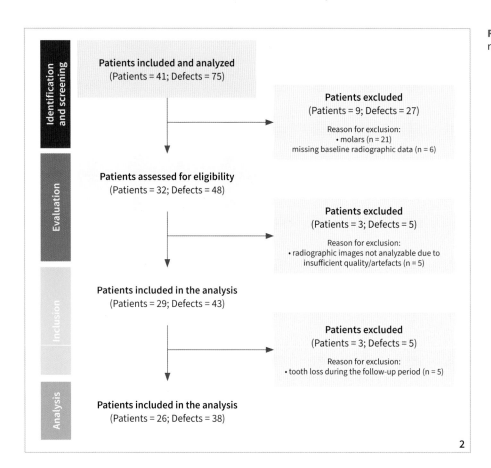

Fig 2 Flowchart of the identified, re-evaluated and analyzed patients.

Radiographic assessment

Nonindividualized 2D analog periapical radiographs (Kodak Ultraspeed DF 58, Eastman Kodak Company) were taken with the long cone paralleling technique using Rinn holders.[20] Baseline radiographs collected from patients' dental charts were scanned and digitized using Microtek TMA 1600 and Microtek ScanPotter (settings on Mac OS X: 1600 dpi, Diafilm, format .tif). Subsequently, each radiographic image was anonymously stored in a dedicated personal computer and evaluated by means of the software ImageJ (National Institutes of Health). All radiographic measurements were assessed in duplicate by two experienced examiners (JE, J-CI) not involved in any part of the treatment and follow-up examinations.

Radiographic assessment of the baseline defect angle width

The following anatomical references points of the intrabony defect were identified on the scanned images based on meth-

odology validated by Tsitoura et al[16] following the criteria proposed by Björn et al[21] and Schei et al:[22]

- A: The CEJ of the tooth involved in the intrabony defect.
- B: The most coronal position of the alveolar bone crest of the intrabony defect when it touches the root surface of the adjacent tooth before treatment (the top of the crest).
- C: The most apical extension of the intrabony destruction where the periodontal ligament space still retained its normal width before treatment (the bottom of the defect). If restorations were present, the apical margin of the restoration was used to replace the CEJ as a fixed reference point. The radiographic defect angle (alpha) was then defined by the two lines that represent the root surface of the involved tooth and the bone defect surface, as described by Steffensen and Webert[23] and Tonetti and colleagues.[24,25] Details of the linear measurements are graphically described in Fig 1a (incisors/canines) and Fig 1b (premolars).

Data were reported in accordance with the STROBE checklist.[26]

Table 1 Baseline patient, teeth, and defect characteristics

Characteristic		n (%)	Average (mean ± SD)	Range
Patients, n (%)		29 (100.0)	NA	
N teeth, n (%)		43 (100.0)	NA	
Age, y		NA	50.6±9.0	33.0 – 65.0
Smoking status	Nonsmoker	11 (37.9)	NA	
	Smoker	11 (37.9)		
	Former smoker	7 (24.1)		
Full-mouth no. of teeth		29 (100.0)	24.6±3.7	16.0 – 32.0
No. of teeth with PD>5mm		29 (100.0)	6.0±3.2	1.0 – 13.0
Radiographic angle width intervals	<20 degrees	11 (25.6)	NA	
	20–30 degrees	20 (46.5)		
	>30 degrees	12 (27.9)		

NA, not applicable.

Table 2 (A) Full mouth plaque score (FMPS) and full mouth bleeding score (FMBS) at baseline, at reevaluation after periodontal regeneration, and at latest follow-up (means±SD) (n=26 patients who completed follow-up). 95% CI and *P* values corrected by Bonferroni from the ANOVA of repeated measurements model. (B) Mean clinical parameters and frequency distribution of the treated teeth which reached the latest follow-up examination (means±SD) (n=38). 95%CI and *P* values corrected by Bonferroni from the GEE model

	Measurement	T0	T1	T2	Mean difference (95% CI), *P* value		
					T0 vs T1	T1 vs T2	T0 vs T2
A	FMPS (%)	19.00±9.02 (15.40–22.60)	13.90±6.22 (11.40–16.40)	27.00±10.50 (22.80–31.30)	5.12±7.32 (1.43–8.80), P=.005**	−13.20±11.30 (−18.80−−7.47), P<.001***	−8.04±11.70 (−13.9−−2.14), P=.005**
	FMBS (%)	22.60±10.10 (18.50–26.70)	10.30±5.99 (7.93–12.80)	9.85±7.58 (6.79–12.90)	12.30±11.90 (6.29–18.20), P<.001***	0.50±9.67 (−4.37–5.37), P=1.000	12.80±12.40 (6.55–19.0), P<.001***
B	Mean deepest PD (mm)	6.68±1.45 (6.23–7.14)	3.95±1.25 (3.58–4.31)	3.87±1.23 (3.50–4.24)	2.74±1.45 (2.21–3.26), P<.001***	0.08±1.75 (−0.45–0.61), P=.771	2.82±1.77 (2.25–3.38), P<.001***
	Mean deepest CAL (mm)	8.13±2.03 (7.54–8.73)	6.47±1.96 (5.85–7.09)	5.95±1.75 (5.42–6.47)	1.66±1.48 (1.18–2.14), P<.001***	0.53±1.89 (−0.07–1.12), P=.083	2.18±1.96 (1.59–2.78), P<.001***

*P<.05.
**P<.01.
***P<.001.

Statistical analysis

All statistical analyses were performed using IBM SPSS Statistics for Windows, version 26.0.0.0 (IBM). In the calculations the deepest PD measure at T0 (ie, baseline) per tooth was considered. The same site was measured at the follow-up time points (ie, T1 and T2). Descriptive statistics were expressed using means with standard deviation (SD) and ranges for continuous variables and relative frequencies (%) for categorical variables. Additionally, 95% confidence intervals (CIs) were calculated for mean differences of parameters between time-points. Linear models of repeated measurements using generalized estima-

tion equations (GEE) were performed to analyze changes over time of the clinical outcomes, according to the radiographic angle, due to the within-subjects dependence of observations. *P* values were corrected by Bonferroni in multiple pairwise comparisons. Smoking status and FMPS (%) at T0 were also considered as independent variables in similar models. A CAL gain >3mm was the considered the outcome in a binary logistic regression model depending on the measurement of angle, as well estimated using GEE approach. Odds ratio (OR) and 95% CIs were calculated. ANOVA for repeated measurements was conducted to analyze changes in FMPS and FMPS over time. Inter-examiner reliability for radiographic angle was estimated

Table 3 (A) Mean PD±SD (six sites and in deepest site) and mean PPD differences±SE between angle groups of the treated teeth which reached the latest follow-up. (B) Mean CAL±SD (six sites and in deepest site) and mean CAL differences±SE between angle groups of the treated teeth which reached the latest follow-up. 95%CI and P values corrected by Bonferroni from the GEE model

Measurement			< 20 degrees	20–30 degrees	> 30 degrees	Mean difference ± SE (95% CI), P value		
						< 20 degrees vs 20–30 degrees	20–30 degrees vs > 30 degrees	< 20 degrees vs > 30 degrees
A	Mean PD (mm)	T1–T0	−1.78±1.01 (−2.34 – −1.21), P<.001***	−0.78±0.61 (−1.12 – −0.45), P<.001***	−1.01±0.63 (−1.33 – −0.70), P<.001***	−0.99±0.34 (−1.67 – −0.32), P=.012*	0.23±0.24 (−0.24 – 0.69), P=1.000	−0.76±0.34 (−1.45 – −0.08), P=.085
		T2–T1	−0.56±1.11 (−1.18 – 0.06), P=.079	−0.60±0.86 (−0.99 – −0.21), P=.003**	0.15±0.76 (−0.22 – 0.53), P=.427	0.04±0.38 (−0.70 – 0.79), P=1.000	−0.75±0.24 (−1.23 – 0.27), P=.006**	−0.71±0.38 (−1.45 – 0.04), P=.187
		T2–T0	−2.33±1.66 (−3.24 – −1.43), P<.001***	−1.38±0.73 (−1.73 – −1.03), P<.001***	−0.86±0.88 (−1.31 – −0.42), P<.001***	−0.95±0.51 (−1.95 – 0.05), P=.184	−0.52±0.27 (−1.05 – 0.01), P=.162	−1.47±0.54 (−2.54 – −0.40), P=.021*
	PD (mm) in deepest site	T1–T0	−3.78±1.56 (−4.83 – −2.73), P<.001***	−2.18±1.19 (−2.69 – −1.66), P<.001***	−2.75±1.36 (−3.47 – −2.03), P<.001***	−1.60±0.61 (−2.80 – −0.40), P=.027*	0.57±0.45 (−0.32 – 1.47), P=.622	−1.03±0.69 (−2.37 – 0.32), P=.403
		T2–T1	−0.22±1.92 (−1.32 – 0.88), P=.693	−0.71±1.61 (−1.31 – −0.10), P=.022*	0.92±1.44 (0.20 – 1.63), P=.012*	0.48±0.66 (−0.80 – 1.77), P=1.000	−1.62±0.48 (−2.57 – −0.68), P=.002**	−1.13±0.69 (−2.49 – 0.21), P=.295
		T2–T0	−4.00±2.12 (−5.19 – −2.81), P<.001***	−2.88±1.32 (−3.44 – −2.32), P<.001***	−1.83±1.59 (−2.72 – −0.95), P<.001***	−1.12±0.69 (−2.47 – 0.24), P=.316	−1.05±0.57 (−2.17 – 0.07), P=.200	−2.17±0.82 (−3.77 – −0.56), P=.024*
B	Mean CAL (mm)	T1–T0	−0.81±1.04 (−1.38 – −0.25), P=.005**	−0.32±0.63 (−0.68 – 0.03), P=.075	−0.26±0.74 (−0.63 – 0.10), P=.159	−0.49±0.35 (−1.17 – 0.19), P=.477	−0.06±0.25 (−0.56 – 0.44), P=1.000	−0.56±0.36 (−1.25 – 0.15), P=.373
		T2–T1	−1.22±1.83 (−2.17 – −0.28), P=.011*	−0.54±1.13 (−1.12 – 0.04), P=.069	−0.33±0.88 (−0.77 – 0.11), P=.136	−0.68±0.58 (−1.81 – 0.45), P=.710	−0.21±0.34 (−0.87 – 0.46), P=1.000	−0.89±0.55 (−1.96 – 0.18), P=.312
		T2–T0	−2.04±1.94 (−3.06 – −1.01), P<.001***	−0.86±1.15 (−1.51 – −0.22), P=.009**	−0.60±0.94 (−1.06 – −0.14), P=.011*	−1.17±0.63 (−2.41 – 0.06), P=.189	−0.27±0.38 (−1.02 – 0.49), P=1.000	−1.44±0.59 (−2.60 – −0.28), P=.046*
	CAL (mm) in deepest site	T1–T0	−2.67±1.32 (−3.48 – −1.86), P<.001***	−1.29±1.26 (−1.82 – −0.77), P<.001***	−1.42±1.62 (−2.27 – −0.57), P=.001**	−1.37±0.50 (−2.36 – −0.39), P=.019*	0.12±0.51 (−0.88 – 1.13), P=1.000	−1.25±0.62 (−2.47 – −0.03), P=.136
		T2–T1	−0.56±2.46 (−1.94 – 0.83), P=.431	−1.12±1.73 (−1.79 – −0.44), P=.001**	0.33±1.37 (−0.40 – 1.06), P=.371	0.56±0.81 (−1.02 – 2.14), P=1.000	−1.45±0.53 (−2.49 – −0.41), P=.019*	−0.89±0.82 (−2.50 – 0.73), P=.843
		T2–T0	−3.22±2.17 (−4.38 – −2.07), P<.001***	−2.41±1.42 (−3.04 – −1.78), P<.001***	−1.08±2.07 (−2.27 – 0.10), P=.073	−0.81±0.69 (−2.16 – 0.54), P=.716	−1.33±0.76 (−2.83 – 0.17), P=.716	−2.14±0.86 (−3.83 – −0.45), P=.040*

*P<.05.
**P<.01.
***P<.001.
SE, standard error.

using paired t test for mean differences, Dahlberg d, and intraclass correlation coefficient (ICC). All tests were two-tailed, and P values <.05 were defined as statistically significant.

Results

Subject accountability and missing data

From the identified and screened sample of 41 patients with 75 defects 32 patients (48 defects) were assessed for eligibility. In nine patients, 21 defects at molar sites and six defects with missing baseline radiographic data were excluded prior to evaluation.

In addition, three patients (five defects) had to be excluded since the assessment of the preoperative defect angle width was not possible due to radiographic artefacts.

Following the additional exclusion of three patients (five defects) suffering from tooth loss after regenerative therapy, 26 patients with 38 defects were followed for a mean observation period of 10.4 years (range 8.0 to 15.5 years). The study flowchart is illustrated in Fig 2.

Baseline subject characteristics

Details of patients' baseline characteristics are displayed in Table 1. There were 15 female and 14 male patients with a mean age of 50.6 ± 9.0 years. Eleven patients (37.9%) who underwent surgical intervention with application of EMD were smokers.

FMPS and FMBS

Mean FMPS and FMBS recorded at the three different time-points are listed in Table 2. The mean FMPS at T0 was 19.0% ± 9.02% (range 15.4% to 22.6%), and at T1 and T2 it was 13.9% ± 6.22% (range 11.4% to 16.4%) and 27.0 ± 10.5 (range 22.8 to 31.3), respectively (P < .001). With respect to the mean FMBS, a statistically significant reduction was observed from T0 (22.6% ± 10.1%, range 18.5% to 26.7%) to T1 (10.3% ± 5.99%, range 7.9% to 12.8%) and T2 (9.85% ± 7.58%, range 6.79% to 12.9%), respectively (P < .001).

Baseline defect characteristics

All intrabony defects were self-contained with a two- to three-wall intraosseous component at baseline and the mean PD value was 6.68 ± 1.45 mm (range 6.23 to 7.14 mm), as shown in Table 2. At follow-up T1, a statistically significant decrease in PD of 2.74 ± 1.45 mm was detected compared to T0 (from 6.68 ± 1.45 mm to 3.95 ± 1.25 mm) (P < .001). The mean PD was still statistically significantly reduced at the latest follow-up T2, compared to baseline (P < .001), but did not statistically significantly change between T1 and T2 (PD change 0.08 ± 1.75 mm; P = .771).

The mean CAL at baseline was 8.13 ± 2.03 mm (range 7.54 to 8.73 mm). Both at T1 (1.66 ± 1.48 mm) and T2 (2.18 ± 1.96 mm) the mean CAL change revealed statistically significant improvements compared with T0 (P < .001). There was no statistically significant difference in mean CAL change between T1 and T2 (0.53 ± 1.89 mm; P = .083). All clinical parameters are reported in Table 2.

Inter-examiner reliability

The calculated inter-examiner agreement between the two examiners who performed the radiographic analysis with Dahlberg d test was in the range of 0.09 to 0.14 mm and the ICC was calculated at 0.904 (P = .872; 95% CI 0.830 to 0.947), suggesting a low random error (ie, 0.95 to 0.98) thus providing a very high level of reproducibility of the performed measurements.

Table 4 CAL gain > 3 mm at T2 by angle group: OR from simple binary logistic regression analysis (95% CI and P value of Wald test) for probability of gain > 3 mm from GEE model

	OR	95% CI	P value
Angle group			.330
> 30 degrees	1		
20–30 degrees	0.67	0.09 – 4.81	.687
< 20 degrees	2.50	0.40 – 15.60	.327

*P < .05.
**P < .01.
***P < .001.
A CAL gain of > 3 mm was considered as dependent variable.

Correlation of clinical outcomes at T1 and T2 with the radiographic defect angle width

The clinical improvements obtained following regenerative surgery with EMD regarding PD reduction and mean CAL gain are listed in Table 3. Three intervals for the angle were considered based on its distribution in quartiles (ie, 1st quartile, < 20 degrees; 2nd quartile, 20 to 30 degrees; 3rd quartile, > 30 degrees). Angle widths < 20 degrees were defined as "narrow," "intermediate" between 20 and 29 degrees, and angles > 30 degrees were defined as "wide." The mean PD change between T0 and T2 was 2.33 ± 1.66 mm at teeth with a defect angle width < 20 degrees, and 0.86 ± 0.88 mm at teeth with a defect angle width > 30 degrees, involving significant differences (P = .021).

From T0 to T2, a statistically significant decrease in PD of 4.00 + 2.12 mm was observed at the deepest site of teeth with a defect angle width < 20 degrees (P = .024). A statistically significantly higher gain in CAL was observed from T0 to T2 at teeth with a defect angle width < 20 degrees (2.04 ± 1.94 mm) compared with that of teeth with a defect angle width > 30 degrees (0.60 ± 0.94 mm) (P = .046).

From T0 to T2 a statistically significant gain in CAL of 3.22 + 2.17 mm was observed at the deepest site of teeth with a defect angle width < 20 degrees (P = .040).

The probability of CAL gain > 3 mm was 2.5-times higher (95% CI 0.4 to 15.60) (P = .327) when the radiographic defect angle width was < 20 degrees compared with that of teeth with a radiographic angle width > 30 degrees (Table 4).

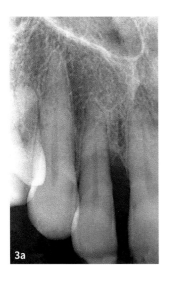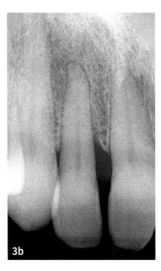

Figs 3a and 3b Preoperative radiograph prior to regenerative surgery with EMD depicting a deep intrabony defect located at a maxillary right lateral incisor (tooth 12). At 10 years following regenerative surgery with EMD, complete fill of the intrabony defect has occurred.

Discussion

This study investigated the potential association between the radiographic angle width of intrabony defects and the long-term clinical outcomes after regenerative periodontal therapy with application of EMD. The results revealed stable clinical outcomes and that defects with a "narrow" angle width < 20 degrees had a 2.5-times greater chance to reach a CAL gain of > 3 mm compared with defects with a "wide" angle > 30 degrees after a mean follow-up period of 10 years.

Despite the body of evidence on the use of EMD to successfully treat periodontal intrabony defects both in the short and long term, only a few studies have specifically addressed the potential effect of this variable in the long term.[27-35] In the present study, three different ranges were defined following a methodology proposed by Tsitoura et al.[16] Despite a general improvement of the clinical parameters both at T1 and T2, a statistically significant difference was found with respect to the mean clinical outcomes (Fig 3). These results are in accordance with previous findings reporting better clinical outcomes in terms of PD reduction and CAL gain after periodontal surgery with EMD due to the higher self-regenerative potential of contained defects compared to the not-contained ones.[16,36,37] When focusing on the magnitude of the clinical improvements of the present data, these are in accordance with previous studies that have shown better clinical results of the regenerative procedures versus access flap interventions.[31,36,37]

The present study has several limitations. Firstly, the retrospective study design and the limited sample size affected the obtained outcomes. A post hoc power calculation using the same radiographic angle groups yielded a sample size of n = 222

defects necessary to reach statistical significance to detect a CAL gain > 3 mm with an OR = 2.5 when comparing defects with an angle width < 20 degrees to those with > 30 degrees. Consequently, the obtained data must be interpreted with caution and do not allow any generalizability to a population-based setting and preclude from external validity. Moreover, one aspect that has to be underlined is that the performed analysis was limited to single-rooted teeth. The rationale behind this choice was based on the assumption that anatomical characteristics related to tooth morphology (ie, single vs multi-rooted tooth and presence of furcation involvement) have a major impact on the 2D radiographic assessment of the periodontal defects and therefore were excluded from the analysis.[38]

Out of the 48 radiographic images originally evaluated, five (10.4%) could not be analyzed due to technical issues. These findings are in agreement with a previous study which revealed that preoperatively routinely used 2D radiographic images do provide clinicians sufficient information to visualize the radiographic angle of the defect.[16]

2D radiographic interpretation of periodontal intrabony defects might be challenging indeed since several technical (ie, time of exposition and contrast) and geometric (ie, x-ray angulation and tooth-film distance) features might preclude from the correct assessment of the intrabony defect.[39] Moreover, it has to be underlined that detection of a periodontal intrabony defect located on the buccal or lingual tooth surface is almost impossible due to the presence of anatomical masking structures.[40] In the present study, in order to increase the reliability of the performed measurements, all images were evaluated in duplicate by two experienced periodontists blinded to the treatment provided, resulting in a good level of inter-examiner agreement.

It has been vastly assessed that smoking status and plaque control do have a great impact both on the short- and long-term clinical outcomes of regenerative procedures with EMD.[41-43] In the present study, low FMPS values were reported through the observation period as result of a strict SPC program. With respect to smoking status, it must be underlined that it was assessed only once before surgery and that changes in smoking habits over the study period cannot be excluded.

Nevertheless, when adjusting the obtained results for these two important confounding factors, no statistically significant differences were detected among the three different defect angle widths consequently providing a good level of comparability. ▦

Conclusion

In conclusion, within their limitations, the present results indicate that baseline radiographic angle width of intrabony de-

fects treated with periodontal regeneration was significantly associated with a CAL gain > 3 mm both in the short and in the long term. In particular, intrabony defects with a "narrow" angle width (ie, < 20 degrees) experienced greater improvements in terms of CAL gain and PD reduction compared with those with a "wide" angle width (ie, > 30 degrees). The use of this preoperative tool might be used to estimate the short- and long-term clinical outcomes following regenerative periodontal therapy.

Disclosure

The authors declare not to have any potential conflict of interest. The present study was funded by the author's own institutions. AR and JE are the recipients of a 3-year scholarship from the Clinical Research Foundation (CFR) for the Promotion of Oral Health, Brienz, Switzerland. AR is the recipient of a 1-year scholarship from the International Team of Implantology (ITI).

References

1. Papapanou PN, Sanz M, Buduneli N, et al. Periodontitis: Consensus report of workgroup 2 of the 2017 World Workshop on the Classification of Periodontal and Peri-Implant Diseases and Conditions. J Clin Periodontol 2018;45:162–170.

2. Jakubovics NS, Goodman SD, Mashburn-Warren L, Stafford GP, Cieplik F. The dental plaque biofilm matrix. Periodontol 2000 2021;86:32–56.

3. Joseph S, Curtis MA. Microbial transitions from health to disease. Periodontol 2000 2021;86:201–209.

4. Darveau RP, Curtis MA. Oral biofilms revisited: A novel host tissue of bacteriological origin. Periodontol 2000 2021;86:8–13.

5. Wade WG. Resilience of the oral microbiome. Periodontol 2000 2021;86:113–122.

6. Badersten A, Nilveus R, Egelberg J. Effect of nonsurgical periodontal therapy. II. Severely advanced periodontitis. J Clin Periodontol 1984;11:63–76.

7. Lang NP, Salvi GE, Sculean A. Nonsurgical therapy for teeth and implants-When and why? Periodontol 2000 2019;79:15–21.

8. Lindhe J, Nyman S. Long-term maintenance of patients treated for advanced periodontal disease. J Clin Periodontol 1984; 11:504–514.

9. Papapanou PN, Wennström JL. The angular bony defect as indicator of further alveolar bone loss. J Clin Periodontol 1991;18:317–322.

10. Sanz M, Herrera D, Kebschull M, et al. Treatment of stage I-III periodontitis-The EFP S3 level clinical practice guideline. J Clin Periodontol 2020;47(Suppl 22):4–60.

11. Roccuzzo A, Imber JC, Stähli A, Kloukos D, Salvi GE, Sculean A. Enamel matrix derivative as adjunctive to non-surgical periodontal therapy: a systematic review and meta-analysis of randomized controlled trials. Clin Oral Investig 2022;26:4263–4280.

12. Lindskog S, Hammarström L. Evidence in favor of an anti-invasion factor in cementum or periodontal membrane of human teeth. Scand J Dent Res 1980;88:161–163.

13. Slavkin HC, Bessem C, Fincham AG, et al. Human and mouse cementum proteins immunologically related to enamel proteins. Biochim Biophys Acta 1989;991:12–18.

14. De Ry S, Pagnamenta M, Ramseier C, Roccuzzo A, Salvi G, Sculean A. Five-year results following regenerative periodontal surgery with an enamel matrix derivative in patients with different smoking status. Quintessence Int 2022;53:832–838.

15. Falk H, Laurell L, Ravald N, Teiwik A, Persson R. Guided tissue regeneration therapy of 203 consecutively treated intrabony defects using a bioabsorbable matrix barrier. Clinical and radiographic findings. J Periodontol 1997;68:571–581.

16. Tsitoura E, Tucker R, Suvan J, Laurell L, Cortellini P, Tonetti M. Baseline radiographic defect angle of the intrabony defect as a prognostic indicator in regenerative periodontal surgery with enamel matrix derivative. J Clin Periodontol 2004;31:643–647.

17. De Ry SP, Roccuzzo A, Lang NP, Sculean A, Salvi GE. Long-term clinical outcomes of periodontal regeneration with enamel matrix derivative: A retrospective cohort study with a mean follow-up of 10 years. J Periodontol 2022;93:548–559.

18. O'Leary TJ, Drake RB, Naylor JE. The plaque control record. J Periodontol 1972; 43:38.

19. Lang NP, Joss A, Orsanic T, Gusberti FA, Siegrist BE. Bleeding on probing. A predictor for the progression of periodontal disease? J Clin Periodontol 1986;13:590–596.

20. Updegrave WJ. The paralleling extension-cone technique in intraoral dental radiography. Oral Surg Oral Med Oral Pathol 1951;4:1250–1261.

21. Björn H, Halling A, Thyberg H. Radiographic assessment of marginal bone loss. Odontol Revy 1969;20:165–179.

22. Schei O, Waerhaug J, Lovdal A, Arno A. Alveolar bone loss as related to oral hygiene and age. J Periodontol 1959;30:716.

23. Steffensen B, Webert HP. Relationship between the radiographic periodontal defect angle and healing after treatment. J Periodontol 1989;60:248–254.

24. Tonetti MS, Pini Prato G, Williams RC, Cortellini P. Periodontal regeneration of human infrabony defects. III. Diagnostic strategies to detect bone gain. J Periodontol 1993;64:269–277.

25. Tonetti MS, Pini-Prato G, Cortellini P. Periodontal regeneration of human intrabony defects. IV. Determinants of healing response. J Periodontol 1993;64:934–940.

26. von Elm E, Altman DG, Egger M, Pocock SJ, Gøtzsche PC, Vandenbroucke JP. The Strengthening the Reporting of Observational Studies in Epidemiology (STROBE) statement: guidelines for reporting observational studies. Lancet 2007;370:1453–1457.

27. Sculean A, Kiss A, Miliauskaite A, Schwarz F, Arweiler NB, Hannig M. Ten-year results following treatment of intra-bony defects with enamel matrix proteins and guided tissue regeneration. J Clin Periodontol 2008;35:817–824.

28. Sculean A, Schwarz F, Chiantella GC, Arweiler NB, Becker J. Nine-year results following treatment of intrabony periodontal defects with an enamel matrix derivative: report of 26 cases. Int J Periodontics Restorative Dent 2007;27:221–229.

29. Silvestri M, Rasperini G, Milani S. 120 infrabony defects treated with regenerative therapy: long-term results. J Periodontol 2011;82:668–675.

30. Roccuzzo M, Marchese S, Dalmasso P, Roccuzzo A. Periodontal regeneration and orthodontic treatment of severely periodontally compromised teeth: 10-year results of a prospective study. Int J Periodontics Restorative Dent 2018;38:801–809.

31. Sculean A, Windisch P, Chiantella GC, Donos N, Brecx M, Reich E. Treatment of intrabony defects with enamel matrix proteins and guided tissue regeneration. A prospective controlled clinical study. J Clin Periodontol 2001;28:397–403.

32. Wachtel H, Schenk G, Böhm S, Weng D, Zuhr O, Hürzeler MB. Microsurgical access flap and enamel matrix derivative for the treatment of periodontal intrabony defects: a controlled clinical study. J Clin Periodontol 2003;30:496–504.

33. Sculean A, Donos N, Schwarz F, Becker J, Brecx M, Arweiler NB. Five-year results following treatment of intrabony defects with enamel matrix proteins and guided tissue regeneration. J Clin Periodontol 2004;31:545–549.

34. Pietruska M, Pietruski J, Nagy K, Brecx M, Arweiler NB, Sculean A. Four-year results following treatment of intrabony periodontal defects with an enamel matrix derivative alone or combined with a biphasic calcium phosphate. Clin Oral Investig 2012;16:1191–1197.

35. Sculean A, Pietruska M, Arweiler NB, Auschill TM, Nemcovsky C. Four-year results of a prospective-controlled clinical study evaluating healing of intra-bony defects following treatment with an enamel matrix protein derivative alone or combined with a bioactive glass. J Clin Periodontol 2007;34:507–513.

36. Sanz M, Tonetti MS, Zabalegui I, et al. Treatment of intrabony defects with enamel matrix proteins or barrier membranes: results from a multicenter practice-based clinical trial. J Periodontol 2004;75:726–733.

37. Tonetti MS, Lang NP, Cortellini P, et al. Enamel matrix proteins in the regenerative therapy of deep intrabony defects. J Clin Periodontol 2002;29:317–325.

38. Rams TE, Listgarten MA, Slots J. Radiographic alveolar bone morphology and progressive periodontitis. J Periodontol 2018;89:424–430.

39. Lang NP, Hill RW. Radiographs in periodontics. J Clin Periodontol 1977;4:16–28.

40. Rams TE, Listgarten MA, Slots J. Utility of radiographic crestal lamina dura for predicting periodontitis disease-activity. J Clin Periodontol 1994;21:571–576.

41. Heijl L, Heden G, Svärdström G, Ostgren A. Enamel matrix derivative (EMDOGAIN®) in the treatment of intrabony periodontal defects. J Clin Periodontol 1997;24:705–714.

42. Heden G, Wennström JL. Five-year follow-up of regenerative periodontal therapy with enamel matrix derivative at sites with angular bone defects. J Periodontol 2006;77:295–301.

43. Cortellini P, Pini-Prato G, Tonetti M. Periodontal regeneration of human infrabony defects (V). Effect of oral hygiene on long-term stability. J Clin Periodontol 1994;21:606–610.

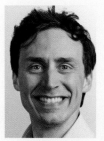

Andrea Roccuzzo

Andrea Roccuzzo* Staff member, Department of Periodontology, School of Dental Medicine, University of Bern, Bern, Switzerland

Johanna Ettmayer* Postgraduate Student, Department of Periodontology, School of Dental Medicine, University of Bern, Bern, Switzerland

Siro Pietro De Ry Postgraduate Student, Department of Periodontology, School of Dental Medicine, University of Bern, Bern, Switzerland

Jean-Claude Imber Staff member, Department of Periodontology, School of Dental Medicine, University of Bern, Bern, Switzerland

Anton Sculean Professor and Chairman, Department of Periodontology, School of Dental Medicine, University of Bern, Bern, Switzerland

Giovanni Edoardo Salvi Associate Professor, Department of Periodontology, School of Dental Medicine, University of Bern, Bern, Switzerland

*AR and JE contributed equally to the manuscript and share first author position.

Correspondence: Prof Anton Sculean, Department of Periodontology, School of Dental Medicine, University of Bern, Freiburgstrasse 7, 3010 Bern, Switzerland. Email: anton.sculean@unibe.ch

First submission: 1 Jan 2023
Acceptance: 2 Jan 2023
Online publication: 20 Jan 2023

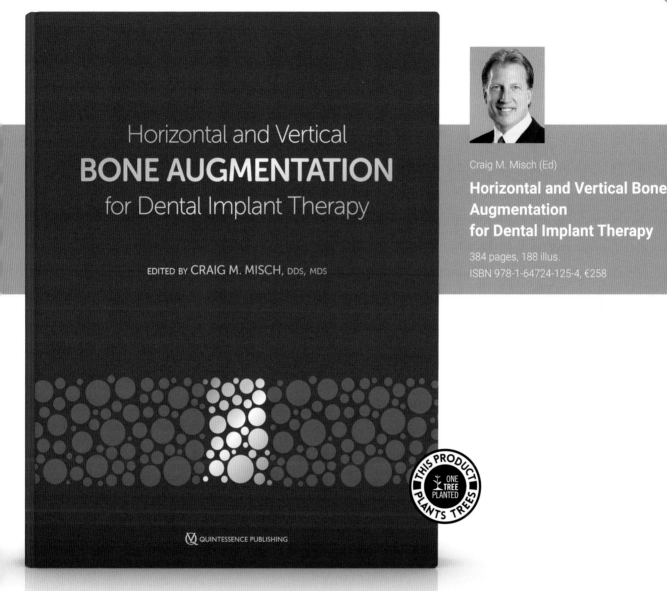

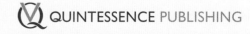

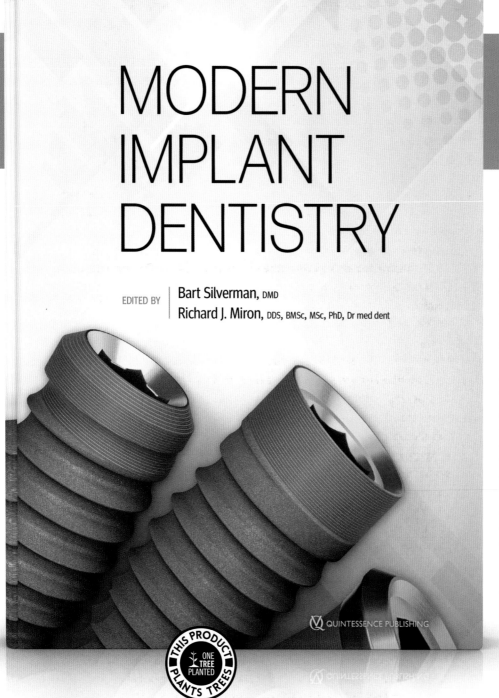

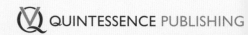